# Nano Biosensors for Non-Invasive Diagnosis of Cancer

Online at: https://doi.org/10.1088/978-0-7503-6234-4

IPEM–IOP Series in Physics and Engineering in Medicine and Biology

## Editorial Advisory Board Members

## About the Series

The series in Physics and Engineering in Medicine and Biology will allow the Institute of Physics and Engineering in Medicine (IPEM) to enhance its mission to 'advance physics and engineering applied to medicine and biology for the public good'.

It is focused on key areas including, but not limited to:
- clinical engineering
- diagnostic radiology
- informatics and computing
- magnetic resonance imaging
- nuclear medicine
- physiological measurement
- radiation protection
- radiotherapy
- rehabilitation engineering
- ultrasound and non-ionising radiation.

A number of IPEM–IOP titles are being published as part of the EUTEMPE Network Series for Medical Physics Experts.

A full list of titles published in this series can be found here: https://iopscience.iop.org/bookListInfo/physics-engineering-medicine-biology-series.

# Nano Biosensors for Non-Invasive Diagnosis of Cancer

**Edited by**
**Nidhi Puranik**
*Department of Life Science, Yeungnam University, Gyeongsan 38541, South Korea*

**Shiv Kumar Yadav**
*Department of Botany, Government Lal Bahadur Shastri PG College, Sironj,
Vidisha 464228, Madhya Pradesh, India*

**IOP** Publishing, Bristol, UK

ISBN    978-0-7503-6234-4 (ebook)
ISBN    978-0-7503-6232-0 (print)
ISBN    978-0-7503-6235-1 (myPrint)
ISBN    978-0-7503-6233-7 (mobi)

DOI    10.1088/978-0-7503-6234-4

Version: 20241201

IOP ebooks

British Library Cataloguing-in-Publication Data: A catalogue record for this book is available from the British Library.

Published by IOP Publishing, wholly owned by The Institute of Physics, London

IOP Publishing, No.2 The Distillery, Glassfields, Avon Street, Bristol, BS2 0GR, UK

US Office: IOP Publishing, Inc., 190 North Independence Mall West, Suite 601, Philadelphia, PA 19106, USA

*Dedicated to the Almighty, who gave us the strength to complete this work.*

# Contents

## 3  Invasive and non-invasive techniques and their challenges    3-1
## in the early detection of cancer

*Rashmi Gupta, Bimal Prasad Jit, Alisha Behara, Rohit Kumar Singh*
*and Ashok Sharma*

# Preface

Early identification of cancer raises the chances of recovery and survival dramatically. Liquid biopsy, which is based on the examination of body fluids, has received a lot of attention in the quest for cancer biomarkers. Thanks to recent advances in analytical techniques, it has gradually become possible to diagnose breast cancer early through the biomarker analysis of blood, nipple aspirate fluid, perspiration, urine, tears, and breath.

In recent years, very sensitive and robust innovative cancer diagnosis methods have been created for clinical use, and they may offer an alternative cancer diagnosis strategy. This book includes the most up-to-date point-of-care cancer detection technologies and processes, which are based on biomedical sensors, microfluidics, and integrated systems engineering. It also includes current advancements and diagnostic tests that can be conducted outside of the laboratory in remote areas. Electrochemical sensors, paper-based microfluidics, and other kit-based diagnostic techniques are just a few of the technologies that can be tweaked to bring cancer detection and diagnosis to more remote parts of the globe.

The book compiles detailed literature on various novel applications of nanobiosensors in cancer diagnosis, mainly focusing on noninvasive biomarker detection, the use of nanoparticles, and biosensors applications. It provides room for researchers to further explore nanobiosensors and their broad range of applications in detection and diagnosis. There are many books available on nanosensors and cancer diagnosis, but to date, there is no book that brings together the literature on the broad-spectrum applications of noninvasive nanobiosensors and, therefore, this book is one of a kind. The book will help in bridging the gap of knowledge in the biotechnology, nanotechnology, and nanobiotechnology domains, and targets a variety of readers from different domains. It will help various experts to explore appropriate information on applications of the noninvasive detection of diagnosis of cancer. The book aims to combine, promote, and increase the potential of nanobiosensors in the detection and diagnosis fields.

# Acknowledgements

All contributors to the respective chapters in this book are gratefully acknowledged by the editors. Their honest efforts, hard work, and analytical approach have been appreciated and recognized. Dr Nidhi Puranik is grateful to Yeungnam University, Gyeongsan, South Korea, and Professor Shiv Kumar Yadav is grateful to the Government Lal Bahadur Shastri PG College, Sironj, Vidisha, Madhya Pradesh, India for providing infrastructure facilities and all relevant assistance.

# Editor biographies

## Nidhi Puranik

Dr Nidhi Puranik is a Research Assistant Professor in the Department of Life Science at Yeungnam University in Gyeongsan, South Korea. She studied for her PhD at the Defence Research and Development Establishment (DRDO) (a research center) and her degree was awarded by Bharathair University, Coimbatore, Tamil Nadu, India. She has more than ten years of research and teaching experience in the field of disease therapeutics and diagnostics. Her current research is focused on the screening and development of plant-based drugs for various diseases. She has been awarded the prestigious GATE, CSIR-NET, ICAR-NET, DRDO Junior Research Fellowship, MPCST Young Scientist Award, MPCST Young Scientist Training Fellowship (national), and Young Investigator Award (international). She has worked in various prestigious institutes in India, including ICMR-NIREH (Bhopal), ICAR-IISR (Indore), Jiwaji University (Gwalior), and Barkatullah University (Bhopal). She has published over 40 research articles with high citation scores one edited book with IOP, and hold one Indian patent. The overall relevance and importance of her research work to human clinician medicine in the treatment and diagnosis of diseases cannot be underestimated.

## Shiv Kumar Yadav

Professor Shiv Kumar Yadav is currently working as an Assistant Professor at Government Lal Bahadur Shastri PG College, Sironj, Vidisha, Madhya Pradesh, India. He has more than seven years of R&D experience. He has published more than ten articles in SCI journals. He received his MSc degree in Biotechnology from Jiwaji University, Madhya Pradesh, India, in 2010 and has submitted a PhD in Biological Sciences at Bharathiar University, Coimbatore, Tamil Nadu. He received an ICMR-JRF fellowship for his PhD. He has qualified for various national exams in the life sciences, such as CSIR-NET-JRF, ICMR-JRF, UGC-NET, GATE, ASRB NET, and South Asian University PhD entrance exam. He has worked in reputed research and academic institutes such as DRDO-DRDE (Gwalior), Jiwaji University (Gwalior), and Barkatullah University (Bhopal). He is currently working on immunological diagnosis, computational biology, and cancer.

# List of contributors

**Pavitra Banan**
GN Khalsa College, University of Mumbai, India

**Sharmistha Banerjee**
Chhattisgarh Swami Vivekanand Technical University, Bhilai, India

**Alisha Behara**
Department of Biochemistry, AIIMS, New Delhi, India

**Divya Bisht**
Biochemistry Discipline, School of Sciences, Indira Gandhi National Open University, New Delhi 110068, India

**Gresh Chander**
ICMR-CAR School of Biotechnology, Shri Mata Vaishno Devi University, Katra, J&K 182320, India

**Priya Chauhan**
Department of Basic Science and Humanities (Chemistry), Maharana Pratap Group of Institution, Kanpur 209217, India

**N Ganesh**
Department of Research and Clinical Genetics, Jawaharlal Nehru Cancer Hospital and Research Centre, Idgah Hills, Bhopal, India

**Rashmi Gupta**
Department of Biochemistry, AIIMS, New Delhi, India

**Rohit Gupta**
CSIR-Institute of Genomics and Integrative Biology, New Delhi 110025, India

**Bimal Prashad Jit**
Department of Biochemistry, AIIMS, New Delhi, India

**Khushboo Joshi**
Amity Institute of Biotechnology, Amity University Madhya Pradesh, INDIA

**Abhinav Kant**
Department of Oncopathology, Molecular Pathology Laboratory, Mahamana Pandit Madan Mohan Malviya Cancer Centre, Varanasi 221005, India

**Shuchi Kaushik**
State Forensic Science Laboratory, Madhya Pradesh, India

**Pankaj Keshari**
School of Life Sciences, Jawaharlal Nehru University, New Delhi 110067, India

**Ajay Kumar**
Special Centre for Molecular Medicine, Jawaharlal Nehru University, New Delhi 110067, India

**Rahul Kumar**
Department of Zoology, Sheodeni Sao College (Magadh University), Kaler 824127, India
School of Life Sciences, Jawaharlal Nehru University, New Delhi 110067, India

**Santosh Kumar**
Department of Biochemistry, AIIMS, New Delhi, India

**Priya Kumari**
School of Bioscience, IIT Kharagpur 721302, West Bengal, India
Department of Chemistry, Dayalbagh Educational Institute, Agra 282005, India

**Raghvendra Kumar Mishra**
Amity Institute of Biotechnology, Amity University Madhya Pradesh, India

**Annu Pandey**
KTH Royal Institute, School of Chemical Science and Engineering, Teknikringen 56-58, 10044 Stockholm, Sweden

**Vikas Pitre**
Department of Zoology, Government PG College, Guna, Madhya Pradesh, India

**Deena Prakash**
Biochemistry Discipline, School of Sciences, Indira Gandhi National Open University, New Delhi 110068, India

**Nidhi Puranik**
Department of Life Science, Yeungnam University, Gyeongsan 38541, South Korea

**Gayatri Rai**
Department of Zoology, Government PG College, Guna, Madhya Pradesh, India

**Alibha Rawat**
Department of Research and Clinical Genetics, Jawaharlal Nehru Cancer Hospital and Research Centre, Idgah Hills, Bhopal, India

**Bharti Sahu**
Department of Pharmacy, Ram Krishna Dharmarth Foundation University, Bhopal 462033, India

**Manish S Sengar**
Department of Physics, IIT Delhi 110016, India
School of Medical Science and Technology (SMST), IIT Kharagpur 721302, West Bengal, India
Department of Chemistry, Dayalbagh Educational Institute, Agra 282005, India

**Neha Sengar**
Department of Chemistry, Delhi University, Delhi 110007, India

**Anushri Sharma**
Department of Biochemistry and Genetics, Barkatullah University, Bhopal 462026, India

**Arun Sharma**
Department of Chemistry, School of Basic and Applied Sciences, Career Point University, Kota, Rajasthan 325001, India

**Ashok Sharma**
Department of Biochemistry, AIIMS, New Delhi, India

**Neha Sharma**
Amity Institute of Biotechnology, Amity University, Madhya Pradesh, India

**Swati Sharma**
School of Studies in Environmental Chemistry, Jiwaji University, Gwalior 474011, India

**Kavita Shukla**
Hitkarini College of Pharmacy, Jabalpur 482001, India

**Rohit Kumar Singh**
Agricultural Research Organization, Volcani Institute, Israel

**Surabhi Singh**
Department of Chemistry, School of Basic and Applied Sciences, Career Point University, Kota, Rajasthan 325001, India

**Minseok Song**
Department of Life Science, Yeungnam University, Gyeongsan 38541, South Korea

**Amit Kumar Sonkar**
Department of Biochemistry, All India Institute of Medical Sciences, Guwahati, India

**Priyanka Sonkar**
Department of Biosciences, Bharathiar University, Coimbatore, India

**Megha Srivastava**
Department of Zoology, Government PG College, Guna, Madhya Pradesh, India

**Karishma Thakur**
Department of Basic Science and Humanities, Maharana Pratap Group of Institution, Kanpur 209217, India

**Shiv Kumar Yadav**
Department of Botany, Government Lal Bahadur Shastri PG College, Sironj, Madhya Pradesh 464228, India

**Subhash Chandra Yadav**
Department of Anatomy, Nanotechnology Lab, Electron Microscopy Facility, All India Institute of Medical Sciences, New Delhi 110029, India

# Chapter 1

## Cancer: an overview of its development, progression, detection and diagnosis

**Nidhi Puranik and Minseok Song**

Cancer is a global health concern that causes millions of deaths each year. Even though several treatments are available, the death rate is still quite high. Furthermore, even though a variety of techniques are employed in clinical settings for the detection and treatment of cancer, many cancers have poor survival rates and do not respond to therapy. Tissue biopsy is regarded as the gold standard among the pathological investigations used to diagnose tumors. However, there are a lot of drawbacks to tumor diagnosis based on tissue biopsy. In contrast, using liquid biopsy, cancer can be examined and tracked in different body fluids including blood and urine through the presence of specific cancer markers that could be exosomes, tumor-relevant proteins, circulating tumor cells (CTCs), cell-free nucleic acids, and other metabolites. The small amounts of these biomarkers prevents them from being widely used in clinical practice. However, nanosensors have improved biomarkers' specificity and sensitivity in cancer detection. This chapter is an overview of cancer pathogenesis, progression, and detection methods, and the role of nanomaterials in diagnosis is covered in brief.

## 1.1 Introduction

Cancer is a serious global public health issue and, for example, is the second largest cause of mortality in the USA. Delayed diagnosis and treatment leads to advanced-stage diagnosis and increased mortality rates (Siegel *et al* 2023). More than 277 distinct forms of cancer disease are referred to as cancer in the broadest sense. Researchers have distinguished between various cancer phases and have suggested that several gene alterations contribute to the etiology of cancer. Anomalous cell proliferation results from these gene alterations. Cell growth is significantly accelerated by genetic abnormalities brought on by hereditary factors (Hassanpour and Dehghani 2017).

doi:10.1088/978-0-7503-6234-4ch1

1-1

**Table 1.1.** Common cancers and their main sites of metastasis.

| Cancer type | Main sites of metastasis |
| --- | --- |
| Lung | Adrenal gland, bone, brain, liver and other organs |
| Melanoma | Bone, brain, liver, lung, skin, muscle |
| Ovary | Liver, lung, peritoneum |
| Pancrease | Liver, lung, peritoneum |
| Prostate | Adrenal gland, bone, liver, lung |
| Rectal | Liver, lung, peritoneum |
| Stomach | Liver, lung, peritoneum |
| Thyroid | Bone, liver, lung |
| Uterus | Bone, brain, liver, lung, peritoneum, vagina |

Tumors classified as benign remain in their original location without spreading to other distant or localized areas of the body. Benign tumors typically have defined edges and develop slowly. They typically present no problems, however, if they become large they may compress neighboring structures, resulting in pain or other health issues. Cells in malignant tumors proliferate uncontrollably and may disperse locally or throughout the body via either the lymphatic or circulatory systems; this spread of tumor cells is known as metastasis (Fares *et al* 2020). Although it can happen anywhere in the body, the liver, lungs, brain, and bones are the most typical places for metastasis to develop. Because malignant tumors spread quickly, treatment is necessary to stop them from spreading. Major type of cancers and their metastasis sites are mentioned in table 1.1. The most common treatment is surgery with the possibility of chemotherapy or radiation (Patel 2020). Over 90% of cancer-related deaths are caused by metastatic illness, which is also frequently linked to high patient mortality since it is challenging to treat surgically or with traditional chemotherapy and radiation therapy (Rankin and Giaccia 2016).

## 1.2 The hallmarks of cancer

According to theory, the hallmarks of cancer are a collection of functional abilities that human cells pick up along the route from normalcy to neoplastic development states, as shown in figure 1.1. These abilities are particularly important for the cells' capacity to develop malignant tumors. The eight hallmarks that are currently recognized include the abilities to maintain proliferative signaling, avoid immune destruction, resist cell death, enable replicative immortality, induce/access vasculature, activate invasion and metastasis, and reprogram cellular metabolism. Deregulating cellular metabolism and preventing immune destruction were described as 'emerging hallmarks' in the most current iteration of this theory (Hanahan 2022).

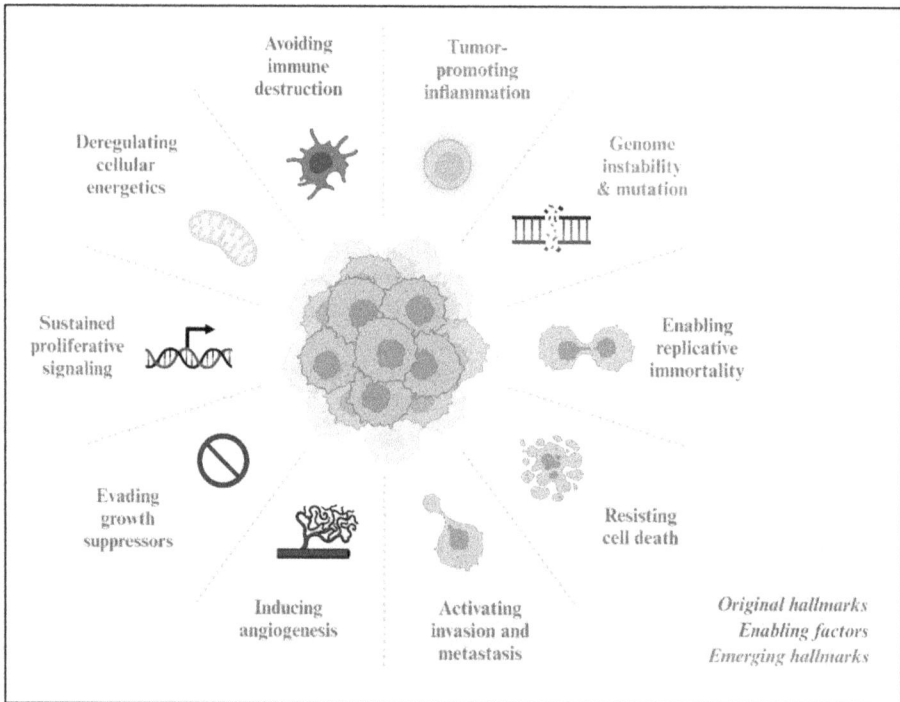

**Figure 1.1.** The hallmarks of cancer. (Created with biorender.com.)

## 1.3 The tumor microenvironment

A tumor is a diverse combination of extracellular matrix (ECM), secreted factors, and resident and invading host cells, rather than just a collection of cancer cells. To promote tumor development and progression, tumor cells induce notable changes in the host tissues' chemistry, physiology, and molecular makeup. A developing tumor microenvironment (TME) is a dynamic, multifaceted system. The tumor micro-environment makeup varies depending on the type of tumor, but common elements include blood vessels, stromal cells, immune cells, and ECM, as shown in figure 1.2. According to Anderson and Simon (2020), the 'tumor microenvironment is not just a silent bystander, but rather an active promoter of cancer progression'. The cellular environment that tumors or cancer stem cells reside in is referred to as the TME. Tumor stem cells possess the capacity to proliferate and initiate new tumor growth. In the past, research has identified distinct cancer stem cells in patient samples from malignancies of the breast, blood, colon, lung, and brain. The TME is made up of various cellular components. The first is endothelial cells, which are essential for both the growth of tumors and the defense of tumor cells from the immune system. Typically, tumor angiogenic vessels originate from endothelial progenitor cells or grow outward from pre-existing vessels. These cells provide nutritional support for the growth and development of tumors in this way. Immune cells, including lymphocytes, macrophages, and granulocytes, make up the second main component.

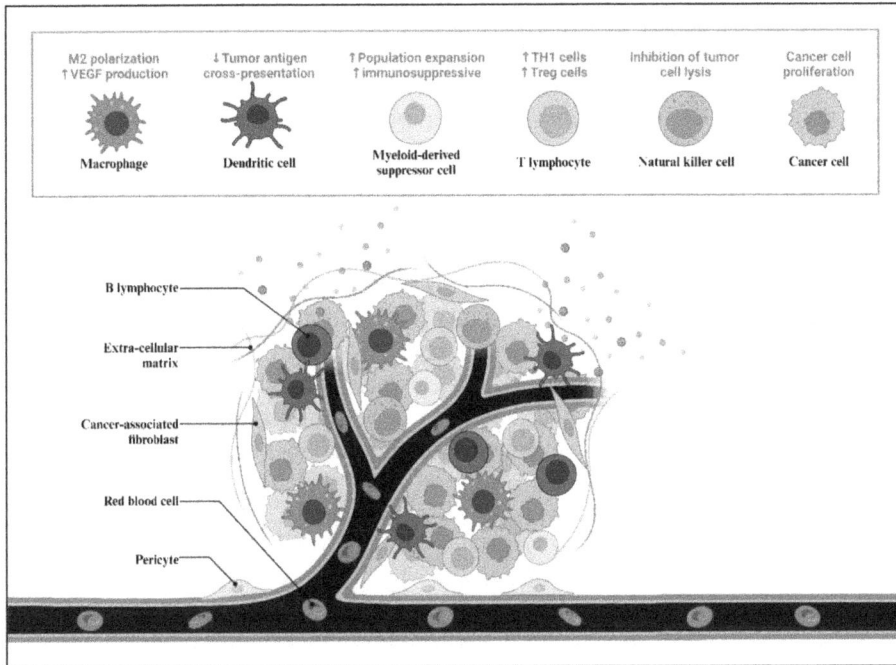

**Figure 1.2.** The tumor microenvironment. (Created with biorender.com.)

These cells have a variety of roles in immunological responses and actions, including inflammatory reactions that the tumor triggers in an attempt to prolong its life. The macrophage is the immune cell type that predominates in the TME. Macrophages have a variety of roles in the initiation and spread of cancer. They can inhibit the immune system's defenses against the tumor and encourage tumor cells to enter the bloodstream. Evidence from earlier research has demonstrated that macrophages may facilitate the extravasation of circulating cancer cells in remote locations, such as the lungs, which may contribute to the ongoing expansion of metastatic colonies. Tumor-associated macrophages have been shown in an increasing number of studies to enhance, mediate, or oppose the anti-cancer effect of cytotoxic drugs, checkpoint inhibitors, and radiation (Zhu *et al* 2021). The fibroblast is the last cell type found in the TME and it facilitates the migration of cancer cells into the bloodstream for systemic metastasis, moving them from the main tumor location. Moreover, endothelial cells undergoing angiogenesis in the tumor have a reliable pathway through fibroblasts (Arneth 2019). According to Lyssiotis and Kimmelman (2017), heterocellular interactions modify the metabolic makeup of the TME to promote tumor growth and elude immune elimination.

## 1.4 Tumor progression

The spread and metastasis of cancer are made possible by communication between cancer cells. Although chemical pathways have been the primary focus of research on cell-cell communication in cancer, new research indicates that mechanical communication via cell-cell junctions and cell–ECM connections is also a significant driver of cancer progression (Schwager *et al* 2019).

Tumorigenesis is a complex and multi-step process whereby oncogene and tumor-suppressor gene alterations lead to increases in cell proliferation and resistance to apoptosis. According to Yuan *et al* (2016), the majority of human tumor types have several characteristics in common, such as the ability to sustain proliferative signals, elude growth suppressors, resist cell death, replicate immortality, induce angiogenesis, activate invasion and metastasis, use energy metabolism, elude immune destruction, and cause genome instability and mutation, and tumor-promoting inflammation. It is becoming more widely recognized that the tumor microenvironment influences the intricate interactions between genetic and epigenetic changes within the cells, hence playing a role in the initiation and spread of cancer. Furthermore, recent studies have shown that physical signals can also significantly change cellular behavior, including proliferation, the characteristics of cancer stem cells, and the potential for metastatic spread, in addition to biochemical cues from the microenvironment (Spill *et al* 2016).

The primary cause of cancer-related death is metastasis. Neoplasia, or unchecked cell proliferation within a tissue, results in solid tumors at the site of origin. The tumor is usually considered benign and can be surgically removed if it gets too large or if it obstructs a vessel or nerve, indirectly causing ischemia, analgesia, and paralysis. On the other hand, metastasis occurs when cancerous cells penetrate the surrounding normal tissues of the original tumor mass. They also present malignant spread throughout the body, which is a defining feature of cancer. Malignant cells must have the ability to move to spread. They pass through the connective tissues thanks to the ECM protein meshwork. Furthermore, metastatic cancer cells must breach the barriers of various ECM components, including the sheet-like basement membrane, and pierce layers of closely spaced epithelial and endothelial cells. Furthermore, cancer cells must continue to proliferate throughout hematogenous and lymphatic spread, even when suspended. Cancer cells must come into contact with various ECM proteins and unique supramolecular ECM structures to attach, detach, and migrate. Furthermore, the ECM controls the location of cancer cells' metastases or places where they settle. Recent research has demonstrated that the ECM is qualitatively and quantitatively changed in a tumor-permissive manner even in the initial tumor mass, which influences cancer cell invasion and advances tumor growth (Eble and Niland 2019).

A century ago, metabolic reprogramming was identified as a marker of cancer. Reprogrammed metabolic processes may occasionally be used to detect, track, and treat cancer. The requirements of exponential growth and proliferation are supported by stereotyped metabolic activities in cultivated cancer cells, most notably aerobic glycolysis, glutamine catabolism, macromolecular synthesis, and redox homeostasis. Oncogenic signaling and transcriptional networks regulate these pathways in a cell-autonomous manner (Faubert *et al* 2020).

Tissues can adapt their cellular metabolism to fit their needs for growth and equilibrium. Malignant cells in cancer respond to both cell-intrinsic and cell-extrinsic signals by acquiring metabolic adaptations. A few of these modifications start the transformation process, while others encourage the proliferation of cancerous cells and make them more vulnerable to drugs that block important pathways (Faubert *et al* 2020).

One important mechanism for preserving cellular homeostasis is autophagy. Such homeostatic function provides a strong defense against malignant transformation in healthy cells. As a result, numerous oncoproteins inhibit autophagy, while many onco-suppressor proteins stimulate it. Furthermore, for the best anti-cancer immunosurveillance, autophagy is necessary. However, autophagic responses provide neoplastic cells with a way to deal with stress from the environment and within the cell, which promotes the growth of tumors. This suggests that, at least occasionally, autophagy may be temporarily inhibited or may acquire molecular roles that counteract autophagy's onco-suppressive effects as oncogenesis advances (Galluzzi *et al* 2015).

It has been shown that inflammation is intimately related to the majority of cancer types' malignant progression and all phases of development, as well as to the effectiveness of anti-cancer treatments. Specifically, immunosuppression caused by chronic inflammation creates a favorable environment for tumor initiation, growth, and metastasis. Moreover, anti-cancer treatments have the potential to trigger inflammatory reactions. By triggering an anti-tumor immune response, acute inflammation aids in the death of cancer cells, but chronic inflammation brought on by therapy encourages the development of therapeutic resistance and the spread of the disease. Rudolf Virchow first proposed the link between inflammation and cancer in the middle of the 1800s, drawing on data showing an abundance of inflammatory cells in tumor biopsies and the fact that cancer often began in areas of persistent inflammation.

These days, inflammation associated with cancer is thought to be a major feature of the disease, and a clear correlation has been shown between persistent inflammation and the growth of tumors. An elevated risk of cancers and the malignant course of most cancer types have been linked to chronic, dysregulated, persistent, and unresolved inflammation. Furthermore, an increasing body of research suggests that the inflammatory TME has a significant role in determining the therapeutic success of immunotherapy and conventional chemotherapy, including radiation and chemotherapy. On the other hand, acute inflammation brought on by external stimulants has been shown to improve anti-tumor immunity by encouraging dendritic cell maturation and activity as well as the start of effector T cell development (Zhao *et al* 2021). A general schematic representation of tumor progression is shown in figure 1.3 and the metastatic cascade is shown in figure 1.4.

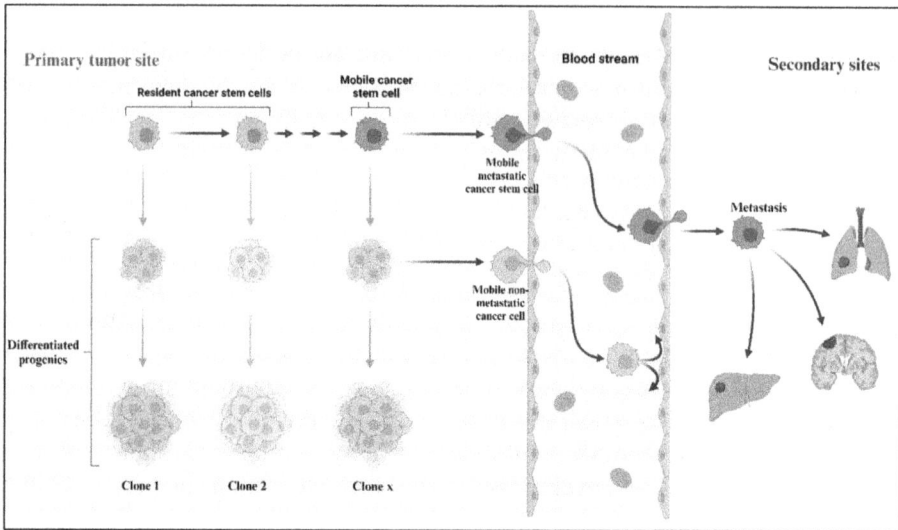

**Figure 1.3.** Tumor progression. (Created with biorender.com.)

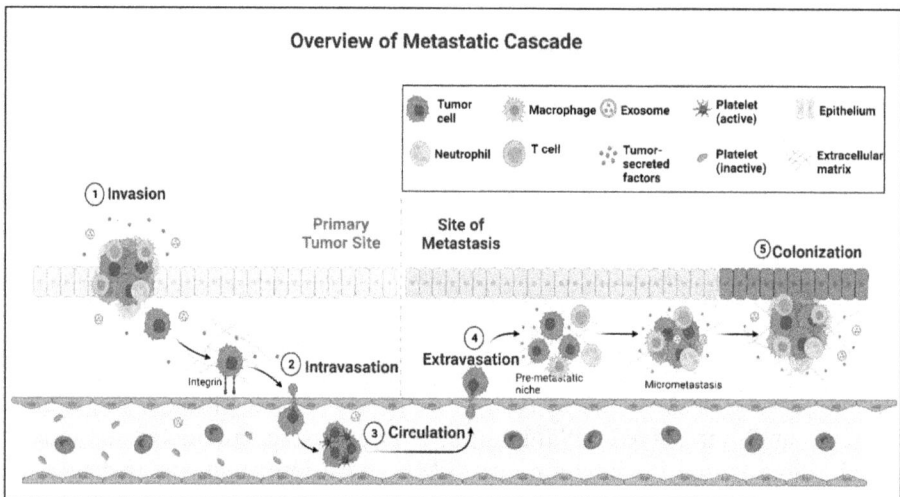

**Figure 1.4.** An overview of the metastatic cascade. The tumor microenvironment regulates cancer metastasis and contributes to every stage of tumor metastasis. (Created with biorender.com.)

## 1.5 Common cancers

### 1.5.1 Lung cancer

Lung cancer is the most common and deadly cancer in the world, and rising rates of tobacco use are expected to increase the disease's burden globally. Men, individuals over 60, African-Americans, and those with a family history of the disease are more likely to develop lung cancer. According to Thandra *et al* (2021), tobacco use is the primary preventable cause of death globally, contributing to nearly 80% of lung cancer occurrences. In North America and other affluent nations, lung cancer is the leading cause of cancer-related fatalities. Traditionally, lung cancers are classified as either small cell lung carcinoma (SCLC) or non-small cell carcinoma (NSCC), with the former accounting for 80% of cases and the latter for the remaining 20%. While NSCCs are addressed by a mix of surgery and adjuvant therapy, aggressive SCLCs are often treated non-surgically (Zheng 2016).

Lung cancer kills people because it is diagnosed when the disease has progressed to an advanced stage. Effective early detection, a thorough etiology, and the right medications all contribute to lung cancer treatment. Therefore, it is imperative to diagnose lung cancer as soon as possible, particularly when screening high-risk individuals and searching for new biomarkers. Additionally, the best course of action for each patient with lung cancer depends on a precise diagnosis (Nooreldeen and Bach 2021).

### 1.5.2 Breast cancer

Globally, breast cancer is the most frequent cancer to affect women and is the second most common cause of cancer-related fatalities in women. Breast cancer is a multi-step process that involves several cell types, and it is still difficult to prevent globally. One of the best ways to address breast cancer is to diagnose the condition as soon as possible (Sun *et al* 2017) as this increases the likelihood of successful treatment and survival. Researchers have looked into a variety of diagnostic techniques, such as mammography, magnetic resonance imaging (MRI), ultra-sonography, positron emission tomography (PET), and biopsy, to identify early-stage breast cancer (Wang 2017). Although mammogram screening has been utilized extensively for breast cancer screening, radiation from mammograms and high rates of false-positive and false-negative results have long been concerns. The accuracy and efficacy of mammography have long been questioned, as has its inability to identify small lesions, particularly in women with dense breast tissue. As a result, there is an unmet clinical need to provide a quick and easy diagnostic to address mammography's drawbacks. The examination of bodily fluids by liquid biopsy has garnered significant interest in the hunt for cancer biomarkers. Breast cancer can now be detected early thanks to recent advancements in analytical techniques, through a biomarker study of blood, sweat, urine, tears, or breath. As a biomarker for the early identification of breast cancer, a straightforward blood or breath test has a lot of promise (Li *et al* 2020).

### 1.5.3 Ovarian cancer

The deadliest type of gynecologic cancer is ovarian cancer. After diagnosis, less than half of patients live longer than five years. Women of various ages can be affected by ovarian cancer, however, the disease is typically discovered after menopause. Because early-stage disease is typically asymptomatic and late-stage disease symptoms are unclear, over 75% of affected women receive an advanced diagnosis.

Growing older and having a family history of breast and ovarian cancer are the biggest risk factors (Doubeni *et al* 2016).

### 1.5.4 Renal cancer

Renal cell carcinomas are a diverse category of malignancies that have various genetic and molecular changes that underlie the several histological subtypes that have been identified. Eighty-five to ninety percent of all renal malignancies are solid renal cell carcinomas, of which clear-cell, papillary (types 1 and 2), and chromo-phobe are the most common forms. Patients with renal cell carcinoma are more often being discovered by accident as routine imaging for numerous illnesses has expanded. Symptoms are used to diagnose only 30% of cases. While abdominal ultrasonography is often used to diagnose renal cell carcinoma, its sensitivity and accuracy are limited, necessitating the use of CT or MRI to confirm suspicious findings (Capitanio and Montorsi 2016).

### 1.5.5 Prostate cancer

With an estimated 1 600 000 cases and 366 000 deaths annually, prostate cancer is the most common noncutaneous cancer in men globally (Torre *et al* 2015). Prostate cancer is still a major medical issue for the men who are affected, even with recent advancements. Inadequate therapy for metastatic prostate cancer and overtreatment of an intrinsically benign illness are the main causes of this problem (Wang *et al* 2018). Prostate-specific antigen (PSA > 4 ng ml$^{-1}$) is a glycoprotein that is routinely expressed by prostate tissue, and increased plasmatic levels of this protein are used to detect several prostate malignancies. Nonetheless, a tissue biopsy is the recom-mended course of action to confirm the cancer's presence because males without the disease have also been shown to have increased PSA (Rawla 2019).

### 1.5.6 Pancreatic cancer

With a 10% five-year survival rate in the USA, pancreatic cancer is an extremely deadly disease that is rising in frequency as a cause of cancer death. Obesity, type 2 diabetes, tobacco use, and family history are risk factors for pancreatic cancer. Even when the cancer is still localized, patients usually show up with advanced disease because they have no symptoms or hazy ones. Multidetector CT angiography is the first imaging modality that is advised for the precise and prompt diagnosis of pancreatic cancer. With a sensitivity of 79%–81% and specificity of 82%–90% for the detection of the disease in symptomatic patients, CA 19-9 is a well-established and validated serum biomarker linked to pancreatic cancer (Mizrahi *et al* 2020).

### 1.5.7 Hepatocellular carcinoma

Globally, hepatocellular carcinoma (HCC) is the most prevalent primary liver cancer and the primary cause of cancer-related mortality. Viral hepatitis and excessive alcohol consumption are the most common risk factors globally for the development of HCC, with chronic liver disease and cirrhosis remaining the most significant risk factors. The identification of HCC is predicated on the elevation of contrast in the arterial phase (wash-in) and the subsequent elimination of contrast in the venous phase (washout). According to a recent meta-analysis comparing the diagnostic performance of CT and MRI for evaluating HCC, MRI is the preferred imaging modality for the diagnosis of HCC in patients with chronic liver disease because it has a higher per-lesion sensitivity than multidetector CT (Balogh *et al* 2016).

## 1.6 Cancer detection and diagnosis

Early cancer diagnosis is a public health and policy priority, and primary care is the ideal setting in which to do it. Better early detection tests for cancer are therefore needed, preferably ones that may be used in primary care. Prognostication and patient surveillance of those who have already received a diagnosis have primarily benefited from persistent and significant investment in the development of novel biomarkers and other tests (Walter *et al* 2019). There are currently only a few screening tests available for certain cancer types, such as cervical cytology, mammography, prostate-specific antigens, and colonoscopy. However, many people disregard medical recommendations for screening, and the effectiveness of certain tests has been questioned (Chen *et al* 2020). Early cancer detection leads to more effective therapy and a significant increase in survival, but about 50% of tumors are only found when they are already advanced. Enhancing early cancer detection has the potential to significantly raise survival rates. Even though recent improvements in early diagnosis have saved lives, more advancements and development of methods for early cancer detection are required. The discipline is changing quickly as a result of growing technical advancements and developments in our understanding of biology. The goal of early detection is to spot precancerous changes or subsequent cancer as soon as possible when a treatment could increase survival or lower morbidity (Pulumati *et al* 2023). A consequential disease will result in death or significant morbidity within the course of the person's anticipated remaining life. During the journey from normal cellular activity to dysregulation to cancer, there are multiple opportunities for early diagnosis. This includes not only identifying precursor abnormalities but also detecting the cancer at an earlier stage of development. One kind of early detection is screening, which is the proactive testing of asymptomatic individuals. Numerous early detection concepts intersect with various aspects of cancer care, including the identification of disease recurrence or minimal residual disease (Crosby *et al* 2022).

### 1.6.1 Detection and diagnosis techniques

#### 1.6.1.1 Imaging techniques

Numerous imaging modalities, including computed tomography (CT), positron emission tomography (PET), mammography, magnetic resonance imaging (MRI), and single-photon emission computed tomography (SPECT) have been demonstrated to be useful for the diagnosis and follow-up of patients with breast cancer at different stages (Jafari *et al* 2018). Chapter 2 provides a thorough overview of imaging methods and modern biosensors for cancer diagnosis.

### 1.6.1.2 Invasive techniques

The current gold standard for diagnosing cancer is tissue biopsy, which is only practical when the lump is visible and yields consistent results. Using a large needle, tissue samples from the lungs or any cancerous tissue are extracted during this process. Through the use of a microscope to examine the cellular architecture within this tissue, medical professionals can accurately and precisely identify any signs of cancer. The invasive techniques and their challenges in the early detection of cancer are discussed in detail in chapter 3.

### 1.6.1.3 Non-invasive techniques or liquid biopsy

A longitudinal study demonstrating asymptomatic cancer detection years before traditional diagnosis is necessary for an effective screening test to demonstrate its potential to reduce cancer mortality (Chen *et al* 2020). The identification of circulating tumor-derived components in biofluids, such as blood, via minimally invasive or non-invasive means is a novel method that holds great promise for the treatment of cancer. Compared to tissue biopsies alone, liquid biopsies offer a more thorough evaluation of the heterogeneous tumor profile and are more accurate in detecting genomic and transcriptome changes. Liquid biopsies have the potential to greatly enhance existing surveillance techniques by providing real-time monitoring of disease progression and therapy response. They could also help with diagnosis, prognosis, and treatment selection. Specifically, these methods are capable of identifying resistance mechanisms, predicting illness development, and detecting minimum residual disease, which enables timely reorientation of treatment tactics (Martins *et al* 2021).

In the last ten years, non-invasive procedures such as liquid biopsy have gradually supplanted invasive treatments for cancer diagnosis and surveillance. When compared to tissue samples, liquid biopsy's benefits include a shorter analysis time, a lower sample demand, and the absence of interpretation problems (Thenrajan *et al* 2023).

Clinical oncology has undergone a significant revolution thanks to liquid biopsies, which make tumor sampling simple and enable ongoing monitoring through recurrent sample collection, individualized treatment planning, and therapeutic resistance screening. Liquid biopsies involve removing tumor-derived materials from patient bodily fluids, such as extracellular vesicles (EVs), CTSs, and tumor DNA, and then analysing the proteome and genetic information found in those materials (Lone *et al* 2022). Chapter 4 covers the non-invasive approaches in early cancer detection.

### 1.6.2 Clinical or biological samples for diagnosis

Various sources are used for the diagnosis of cancer-associated biomarkers, as shown in figure 1.5 and discussed briefly in the following subsections.

### 1.6.2.1 Blood/serum

Whole blood and its parts, serum and plasma, are excellent sources for the detection of and diagnosis using cancer biomarkers. The use of protein biomarkers in liquid

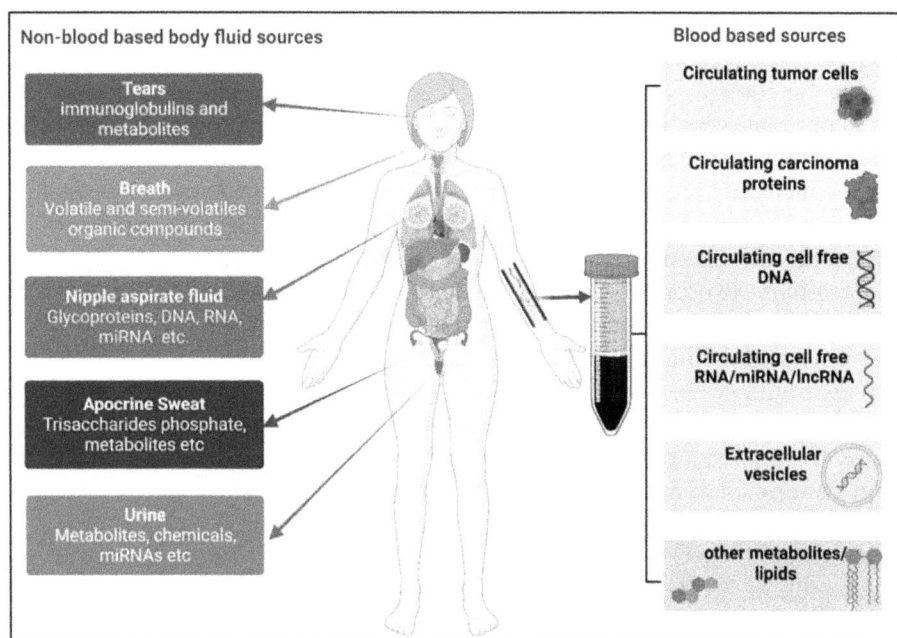

**Figure 1.5.** An overview of non-blood-based body fluid and blood-based sources of biomarkers for non-invasive diagnosis of cancer. (The idea for the figure was taken from Li *et al* (2020) and was recreated using biorender.com.)

biopsies offers promise for early cancer identification and disease progression tracking (Landegren and Hammond 2021). Blood-based biomarkers are not a novel concept. For many years, tumor protein biomarkers have been used to identify disease progression, recurrence, and response to therapy. Examples of these biomarkers include alpha-feto protein (AFP), carcinoembryonic antigen (CEA), cancer antigen 19-9 (CA 19-9) etc. These tumor markers have a well-established therapeutic value, however they are not totally specific and can occur in disorders other than cancer. Furthermore, they do not offer any prognostic data on therapeutic response, which makes the need for markers that can offer comprehensive details of tumor biology and direct treatment approaches necessary. Numerous such predictive blood-based biomarkers have made their way into the field of scientific study in the last few years. Tumor-derived exosomes, CTCs, circulating tumor DNA (ctDNA), tumor-educated platelets (TEPs), and microRNAs (miRNAs) are a few examples of these. Blood-based biomarkers are non-invasive and may be used to detect dynamically resistant clones and evaluate the tumor's response to therapy in real time. Technologies are becoming faster and more accurate as they develop (Mamdani *et al* 2017).

*1.6.2.2 Urine*
Because urine may be collected in significant amounts and is easily accessible, it is a valuable biological fluid for the identification of biomarkers. Urine is the model non-invasive sample. Its collection is inexpensive and typically free of problems or

negative effects. It therefore meets the criteria for being the perfect biomarker source for esophageal cancer (EC) detection. Urine contains a broad range of compounds that may function as EC biomarkers. These substances include malignant cells, peptides/proteins, genetic products including tumor DNA, endogenous metabolites, and secreted organelles such as EVs. Utilizing specialized methods based on platforms including spectroscopy, transcriptomics, proteomics, cytology/single-cell technologies, genomics, and metabolomics is necessary for the investigation of each of these targets for biomarker identification (Njoku *et al* 2020). According to Li *et al* (2021), urinary exosomal miRNAs can be used as innovative, non-invasive biomarkers to identify prostate cancer and track its progression.

The urine metabolite profile of breast cancer patients in one study differed from that of the healthy controls. Urine-based diagnostic screening is a cheap, simple, and non-invasive procedure. Urine metabolite concentration measurements may improve the survival rate by enabling early identification of breast cancer and prompt therapy administration (Park *et al* 2019).

*1.6.2.3 Saliva*
The recognition of the significance of bodily fluids, including saliva, in cancer diagnosis dates back to the late 1990s. Currently, numerous researchers are investigating the precision and effectiveness of this method for both localized and systemic tumors (Eftekhari *et al* 2019). Saliva provides a straightforward but intricate non-invasive method for determining blood analyte concentrations, which can be used to track a patient's immunological status (Ates *et al* 2021).

As a non-invasive biomarker, saliva may be able to distinguish breast cancer patients from healthy controls with high accuracy. Saliva-based diagnostics are now referred to as 'saliva omics' due to extensive study in this field. Saliva is easy to collect, requires little staff training, allows for quick samples, is hassle-free to store, is easy to transport, is less sensitive to clotting, and poses less risk to medical personnel. These are just some of the many benefits of using saliva for diagnosis. Despite these benefits, salivary biomarkers may differ from other bodily biofluids in terms of their presence or concentration, therefore it is important to identify which ones offer sufficient sensitivity and specificity for the diagnosis of cancer. While research has looked at salivary biomarkers in distant tumors, it is still unknown how these diseases affect salivary patterns pathophysiologically. There is some evidence to suggest that the pathology and function of mammary and salivary gland cells are comparable. Furthermore, salivary gland cells release microvesicles that resemble exosomes and contain proteins and mRNAs; they can be found in saliva (Koopaie *et al* 2022).

**1.6.3 Cancer diagnostic biomarkers**

A 'biological substance in body fluids or tissues that is indicative of a normal or abnormal process or a condition or disease' is what the National Cancer Institute defines as a biomarker. Proteins and peptides (such as an enzyme or receptor), nucleic acids (such as DNA, miRNA), antibodies, and metabolites can all be biomarkers. Biomarkers can consist of one or more components, such as specific proteins (e.g. CA-125) or signatures related to the genome, proteome, or metabolome. Tumor-derived entities that are thought to be breakaway products or entities released from cells within the primary tumor and are thought to play significant roles in metastasis include CTCs, ctDNA, and EVs (Vaidyanathan *et al* 2019). Novel insights for cancer identification can be obtained from multi-omics, which includes transcriptomics, glycomics/glycoproteomics, proteomics, genomics, epigenomics, and metabolomics. Further data suggests that ctDNAs and the epigenetic modifications they carry could serve as reliable biomarkers in the fields of genomics and epigenomics. Significant changes in mRNAs and non-coding RNAs (circular RNAs, miRNAs, and long non-coding RNAs (lncRNAs)) were found in transcriptomics. Glycosylation, phosphorylation, acetylation, and ubiquitination are examples of post-translational modifications (PTMs) that might be considered while looking for new biomarkers (Chen *et al* 2022).

### 1.6.3.1 Circulating tumor cells

Circulating tumor cells (CTCs) are a very readily obtained sample of cancer tissue that can reflect the true condition of cancer. Their evaluation can be repeated numerous times during therapy. CTCs are shed in the patient's bloodstream after becoming detached from the primary tumor or metastases. The assessment of CTCs as part of liquid biopsy yields a wealth of clinically significant data that represents the true, current state of the illness. CTCs can be employed for real-time long-term disease monitoring, cancer diagnosis or screening, and even therapy recommendations. Using immunocytochemistry and all '-omic' technologies, their number, morphology, and biological characteristics can all be analysed. The assessment of CTCs, as a liquid biopsy, offers a wealth of clinically significant data that represents the true, current state of the illness (Maly *et al* 2019). Chapter 5 highlights the detection of CTCs for early diagnosis of breast cancer.

### 1.6.3.2 Circulating DNA

The single- or double-stranded DNA that tumor cells release into the bloodstream is known as circulating tumor DNA (ctDNA), and it contains the original tumor's mutations. The DNA fragments produced by tumor cell necrosis, apoptosis, or secretion are known as ctDNA, a class of circulating free DNA (cfDNA). Generally speaking, point mutation amplification and rearrangement are among the gene abnormalities that are present in both the tumor DNA and the ctDNA. Since ctDNA has a short half-life in blood, it can serve as an indicator of tumor dynamics that are changing in real time (Wang *et al* 2021).

Liquid biopsy based on ctDNA analysis has provided new insights into cancer molecular diagnosis and surveillance in recent years. According to studies, ctDNA screening is a very sensitive and specific way to screen for genetic abnormalities. This suggests that ctDNA analysis could greatly enhance the current tumor diagnosis systems, even making early-stage identification easier. Furthermore, ctDNA analysis can help with targeted therapy by precisely predicting the prognosis and the rate at which a tumor is progressing. Thus, a revolution in the treatment of tumors may be brought about by the use of ctDNA through liquid biopsy (Cheng *et al* 2016).

### 1.6.3.3 miRNA

miRNA and lncRNA are the most common non-coding RNAs studied to date. A class of naturally occurring small non-coding RNA molecules that range in length from 18 to 22 nucleotides is known as miRNAs. To date, more than 48 000 miRNAs have been found, 2693 of which are human-derived. Most eukaryotic miRNAs have the role of post-transcriptionally controlling gene expression. They control the expression of post-transcriptional genes by either destabilizing mRNA or inhibiting translation. Since miRNAs play a crucial role in developmental processes, aberrant situations such as illnesses or poor growth may be linked to altered expression of miRNAs. As a result, miRNA expression under pathological circumstances can be utilized as a biomarker (Sohel 2020).

MiRNAs have gained attention as a new and promising class of biomarkers due to their ability to reflect the pathophysiologic state of the tissue of origin, be present in a variety of bodily fluids, and be stable. Because of their numerous qualities, circulating miRNAs are promising candidates for biomarkers in the detection of cancer and the tracking of therapeutic responses in patients. Biofluid sampling, in contrast to conventional tissue biopsies, is rapid, painless, and minimally invasive. The tumor does not even need to be localized, and the risk of related problems is minimal. MiRNAs can be identified individually with a resolution of just one nucleotide. Biomarkers such as proteins and mRNAs can discriminate between normal and cancerous samples (Valihrach *et al* 2020).

### 1.6.3.4 lncRNA

lncRNAs are a broad class of non-coding RNAs longer than 200 nucleotides. As regulatory factors, lncRNAs are involved in a variety of intricate biological processes, including growth, differentiation, proliferation, and death. Lately, numerous research findings have demonstrated their critical significance in the development of cancer. Tumor cells can exude endogenous lncRNAs into human bodily fluids in the form of protein complexes, exosomes, or microvesicles. This results in the formation of circulating lncRNAs that are stable and cannot be broken down. Cancer patients have been found to have aberrant lncRNA expression. In this case, endogenous lncRNAs can affect the expression of oncogenes linked to their oncogenic and suppressive properties, hence regulating the fundamental properties of cancer cells. Therefore, circulating lncRNAs can be excellent biomarkers in cancer as well (Beylerli *et al* 2022).

Since they are non-invasive indicators for better colorectal cancer (CRC) screening techniques, lncRNAs have drawn a lot of interest. All things considered, determining the expression of circulating lncRNA offers a novel and promising early diagnostic technique for CRC screening. Exosomes and microvesicles are two examples of EVs that store and protect circulating lncRNAs. Numerous studies have demonstrated distinct lncRNA expression profiles in serum or plasma in patients with different tumors. Peripheral blood has significant amounts of lncRNA in a very stable, cell-free form (Xu *et al* 2020).

Additionally, lncRNAs control the splicing of mRNA and function as precursors of other non-coding RNAs, including miRNAs. lncRNAs participate in a variety of signaling pathways and act as tumor suppressors or oncogenes. In terms of targeting lncRNAs, there are currently few therapeutic drugs and biomarkers available. The first and only lncRNA licensed for clinical usage at this moment is prostate cancer antigen 3 (PCA3), an early diagnostic biomarker for prostate cancer (Qian *et al* 2020). Chapters 6 and 7 discuss in detail the role of non-coding RNAs in breast cancer and lung cancer detection and diagnosis, respectively.

### 1.6.3.5 *Extracellular vesicles/exosomes*

Extracellular vesicles (EVs) produced by cancer have been found in cancer patients' blood and other biofluids. They contain a variety of chemicals that are specific to tumors, including oncoproteins, altered DNA and RNA fragments, miRNA, and protein signatures linked to different phenotypes. EVs' molecular cargo partly mirrors the intracellular state of the cells from whence they originate, but different sorting processes cause EVs to be enriched or depleted in particular proteins, lipids, or nucleic acids. Cancer-derived EVs are increasingly shown to modulate the anti-tumor immune response, remodel the tumor microenvironment, and create pre-metastatic niches in addition to acting in a paracrine and systemic manner to promote cancer progression by spreading aggressive phenotypic traits and drug-resistant phenotypes to other cancer cells. The possibility that cancer-derived EVs could be used as analytes in liquid biopsies to track tumor load and medication resistance in real time has been raised by these findings. Recently, EVs have become known as unique analytes for liquid biopsies. All types of naturally occurring particles that are confined by a lipid bilayer and incapable of replicating are referred to as EVs. The molecular makeup, size, morphological characteristics, biogenesis, and physiological roles of the many subtypes of EVs vary. The release of multi-vesicular endosome intraluminal vesicles into the extracellular environment and direct budding from the cell surface are the two primary mechanisms for EV formation in living cells. Exosomes, which are EVs formed from endosomes, are mostly 30–150 nm in diameter. On the other hand, vesicles derived from plasma membrane budding can reach up to 1000 nm in diameter and are also known as microvesicles, ectosomes, shedding vesicles, or microparticles. Additionally, bleb-bing of the apoptotic membrane and the development of membrane protrusions such microtubule spikes, apoptopodia, and beaded-apoptopodia can cause apop-totic cells to produce a range of EVs. The term 'apoptotic bodies' refers to EVs formed from apoptotic cells. These bodies are primarily 1–5 $\mu$m in diameter, while smaller vesicles have been shown to form as apoptosis progresses. Despite the fact that distinct EV subtypes have varying average sizes, it is presently not possible to accurately separate EV subtypes based on size, biochemical characteristics, or surface markers. Consequently, until their origin is clearly established, the International Society for Extracellular Vesicles (ISEV) advises utilizing operational words for EV subtypes such as size, density, marker profile, etc, instead of terminologies such as exosomes or microvesicles (Vasconcelos *et al* 2019).

Exosomes are membrane-bound phospholipid vesicles that circulate in bodily fluids and are released by all cell types. It is known that certain cellular components, such as cytoplasmic/membrane proteins, RNA, and DNA, are carried by these vesicles and are unique to the original cells. Exosomes have been used to monitor cancer in a less intrusive way than gold standard tissue biopsies since they are robust indicators of malignancy and are both plentiful and structurally stable (Kalishwaralal *et al* 2019).

The fact that exosomes, also known as small EVs, transport miRNAs linked to cancer processes such as angiogenesis and metastasis has piqued the interest of biomedical researchers. According to reports, tumor cells may release more exosomes than normal cells if they have a certain amount of cancer-specific biomarkers. Because exosomes are readily accessible and maintain stability *in vitro*, they have been identified as the most promising and fundamental indicators for patient diagnosis. Exosomal miRNAs are being used as non-invasive tumor markers because they have been found in all human physiological fluids, including plasma, serum, urine, saliva, bile, breast milk, and cerebrospinal fluids (Preethi *et al* 2022). Chapter 8 discusses the role of the exosomal bodies in cancer in detail.

### 1.6.3.6 Other metabolites

As a sensitive and high throughput profiling method, metabolomics keeps finding valuable candidate biomarkers that could be used to identify cancer. More and more metabolomic discoveries are anticipated to be converted into therapeutic cancer biomarkers as profiling methods advance and become more standardized (Wang *et al* 2016). Urine, blood, or tissue may include chemicals created by cancer cells throughout their growth, which raises the possibility of finding important bio-markers for an early diagnosis (Yang *et al* 2020).

The systematic identification and measurement of all metabolites in a specific organism or biological sample is known as metabolomics, and it is a new and promising scientific tool for examining the association between metabolites and disease, including cancer. These metabolites actually provide a link between genotype, environment and phenotype, are attractive biomarkers for the clinical diagnosis, prognosis, and diseases classification (Qiu *et al* 2023). Significantly, an individual's physiological and pathological status is immediately reflected in their metabolome, which is located downstream of the genome and proteome networks. Every attribute lends credence to the use of metabolomics as an effective method for locating cancer biomarkers and comprehending the mechanisms under-lying carcinogenesis. One of the main characteristics of cancer is dysregulated cellular metabolism. Normal metabolite levels fluctuate and aberrant metabolites are produced as a result of cancer cells' metabolic reprogramming, which promotes unchecked proliferation (Wang *et al* 2023).

By comparing the metabolomic profiles of individuals without cancer and those with non-small cell lung cancer, we could possibly able to detect notable changes in the concentration levels of metabolites mostly associated with the metabolism of amino acid metabolism and lipid metabolism. Furthermore, novel ratios of the metabolites that significantly separated the participants' considered groups were found using partial correlation network analysis (Shestakova *et al* 2023).

In the fields of medicine and the biological sciences, metabolomics which seeks and interprets the connections between metabolites and the pathogenic causes of disease is gaining popularity. It is a quick and precise technology that can provide fresh insights into biological processes on a local or global scale. Cancer metabolomics research can make use of a wide range of sample types. For instance, several studies have shown that biomarkers for cancer can be detected using blood, plasma, saliva, urine, sputum, and breath (Qi *et al* 2021). The primary approaches used in metabolomics have been based on mass spectrometry (MS) and nuclear magnetic resonance (NMR) spectroscopic techniques combined with either liquid chromatography (LC) or gas chromatography (GS), each having unique benefits and drawbacks (Xu *et al* 2023).

## 1.7 Applications of nanomaterials and nanotechnology in cancer diagnosis

Early detection is crucial for effective therapy in the fight against cancer. However, the inherent limitations of traditional cancer diagnostic techniques have made early cancer identification more difficult. Due to its high sensitivity, specificity, and multiplexed measuring capacity, nanotechnology has been studied for *in vivo* imaging as well as the detection of cancer cells and extracellular cancer biomarkers (Zhang *et al* 2019).

Global interest in using nanotechnology to cure cancer is growing. Combining medicines and diagnostics is facilitated by nanobiotechnology and is essential to a tailored approach to cancer treatment. Nanomedicine, which uses nanoparticles to diagnose and cure a variety of illnesses, including cancer, is now being employed. Because of their high surface-to-volume ratio, which makes them special in the field of nanomedicine, these particles may bind, absorb, and transport tiny biomolecules such as proteins, medicines, DNA, and RNA to the intended location, hence increasing the effectiveness of therapeutic agents (Chaturvedi *et al* 2019).

Gold nanoparticles (Sultana *et al* 2023), magnetic nanoparticles (Farzin *et al* 2020, Hosu *et al* 2019), polymeric nanoparticles (Perumal *et al* 2019, Hosseini *et al* 2023), quantum dots (Fang *et al* 2017), carbon nanotubes (Bura *et al* 2022, Singh and Kumar 2022), dendrimers (Bober *et al* 2022) and liposomes (Raza *et al* 2023, Mukherjee *et al* 2022) are the most common nanoparticles used in the development of biosensors for cancer detection; a few of them are listed in table 1.2. The applications of these nanoparticles in the development of biosensors are discussed in chapter 11.

Since biosensors can be used to evaluate clinical samples at home or in a doctor's office, they are regarded as point-of-care (POC) devices (POC diagnostic systems are discussed in chapter 10). Modern biomarker analysis platforms are

**Table 1.2.** Nanoparticles used in the development of nano biosensors for the detection of cancer-specific biomarkers.

| Nanocarrier | Biosensor | Target biomarker | Diagnosed cancer | References |
|---|---|---|---|---|
| Magnetic nanoparticle-based platform | Electrochemical sensor | Methylated septin9 gene/DNA | Colorectal cancer | Hanoglu et al (2022) |
| Graphene quantum dots | Electrochemiluminescence immunosensor | Carbohydrate antigen 19-9 | Tumor | Yang et al (2014) |
| $Fe_3O_4$@Ag magnetic nanoparticles | Surface-enhanced Raman scattering | MiRNA let-7b | Cancer cells | Pang et al (2016) |
| Nanoporous gold/chitosan | Paper based electrochemiluminescence | Carcinoembryonic antigen (CEA) | Cancer | Li et al (2014) |
| Carbon nanotubes | Electrochemical genosensor | CEACAM5, a tumor biomarker | Colorectal cancer | Gulati et al (2020) |
| Gold NPs | Optical biosensor | miRNA-155 | Breast cancer | Hakimian et al (2018) |
| Gold NPs | Optical fiber | CD44 protein marker | Cancer | Ashikbayeva et al (2023) |
| Gold NPs | Electrochemical bioassay | Prostate-specific antigen | Prostate cancer | Heydari-Bafrooei and Shamszadeh (2017) |
| Carbon QDs | FRET, optical biosensors | miRNA | Breast cancer | Khakbaz and Mahani (2017) |
| Carbon QDs | Electrochemiluminescence immunosensor | CA15-3 | Breast cancer | Qin et al (2019) |
| Carbon dots and $MnO_2$ nanosheets | Fluorometric | miRNA-155 | Breast cancer | Mohammadi and Salimi (2018) |
| Carbon dots and AuNPs | Immunoassay | Alpha-L-fucosidase | HCC | Mintz et al (2018) |
| ZnO@carbon quantum dots | Electrochemiluminescence device | K562 leukemia cells | Human chronic myelogenous leukemia | Zhang et al (2013) |

*(Continued)*

**Table 1.2.** (*Continued*)

| Nanocarrier | Biosensor | Target biomarker | Diagnosed cancer | References |
|---|---|---|---|---|
| Carbon dots and graphene oxide | FRET | Mucin 1 protein | Cancer marker | Ding *et al* (2015) |
| Carbon nanotubes | Electrochemiluminescence ELISA-like immunosensor | PSMA | Prostate cancer | Juzgado *et al* (2017) |
| Dendritic gold nanostructure | Electrochemical nano-genosensor | miR-21 biomarker | Prostate cancer | Sabahi *et al* (2020) |
| Carbon nanotubes and GQDs | Electrochemical immunoassay | Carcinoembryonic antigen (CEA) | Cancer | Luo *et al* (2018) |

provided by biosensors, which have the advantages of being easy to use, inexpensive, fast, reliable, and able to test multiple analytes at once (Lino *et al* 2022). It is commonly known that the majority of malignancies produce and secrete several biomarkers. Thus, the creation of biosensors with multiple analyte detection capabilities may prove beneficial for cancer diagnosis and tracking (Asci Erkocyigit *et al* 2023). In addition to helping with diagnosis, the simultaneous detection of many markers also reduces costs and saves time. Electrochemical biosensors are frequently reported to be used in the identification of cancer biomarkers. Table 1.3 shows the common biosensors according to their type, advantages and disadvantages. Nanostructured materials and nanocomposites are essential to the creation and design of many electrochemical biosensors, and their use has grown significantly (Hasan *et al* 2021). Optical biosensors have been extensively described as the preferable method for antibody detection. Additionally, optical imaging is better suited for *in vivo* sensing applications because of its direct signal translation process (Akgönüllü and Denizli 2022). Furthermore, because surface plasma resonance (SPR) allows for extremely sensitive real-time monitoring of analyte–analyte interactions, it has become a widely used sensing technology with a wide range of applications. SPR instruments often track variations in wavelength or resonance angle to obtain data regarding biomolecular interactions (Janith *et al* 2023). Microfluidic systems, albeit not yet employed in clinical settings, are expected to become an important tool for cancer prognosis and diagnostics (Garcia-Cordero and Maerkl 2020). All these techniques are evidence of biosensors' indispensable role in cancer diagnosis (Thenrajan *et al* 2023). The role and application of nanosensors in the cancer and biomedical domains are discussed in chapter 9, and chapter 12 discusses in detail the nano biosensors-based rapid detection of circulating biomarkers for cancer diagnosis. Challenges and future perspectives in the development of nano biosensors in the diagnosis of cancer are discussed in chapter 13.

## 1.8 Conclusion

Even with all of the advancements in detection and treatment, cancer is still one of the major global public health issues. People still suffer greatly from cancer, and early detection is crucial to treatment; in many situations, individuals can be fully cured if their cancer is discovered early. These days, non-coding RNAs, DNA, and RNA are receiving an increasing amount of attention thanks to high throughput sequencing technology and ongoing advancements in the field of molecular biology. Simultaneously, an abundance of research indicates that non-coding RNAs are crucial for controlling gene expression and for regulating cell growth, division, apoptosis, and intracellular communication. Furthermore, research has revealed that non-coding RNAs exhibit variable expression levels in tumors of all sizes. It has been discovered that circulating non-coding RNAs are stable in blood and other bodily fluids, making their detection simple and reliable.

**Table 1.3.** Biosensors, their type, advantages and disadvantages. The table contents was adopted and modified from Irkham *et al* (2023) and Suman (2008).

| Biosensors | Type | Principle | Advantages | Limitations |
|---|---|---|---|---|
| Electrochemical biosensors | Amperometric, conductometric, voltametric and potentiometric | Change in conductance/electric potential/oxidation and reduction | Excellent limit of detection, possible miniaturization | Unstable current and voltage |
| Optical biosensors | Surface plasmon resonance, Raman scattering and FTR | Change in wavelength and index of refraction; color development | High sensitivity | Susceptible to physical changes |
| Thermal/ colorimetric biosensors | Thermistors and thermopiles | Change in temperature | Easy to fabricate, easy to use/ colorimetric strip does not require any instruments | Lack of specificity; not quantitative |
| Piezoelectric biosensors | Quartz crystal microbalance, surface acoustic wave | Change in oscillation frequency and the electric charge under mechanical stress | Small size and high sensitivity | High temperature sensitivity |

# References

Akgönüllü S and Denizli A 2022 Recent advances in optical biosensing approaches for biomarkers detection *Biosens. Bioelectron.* X **12** 100269

Anderson N M and Simon M C 2020 The tumor microenvironment *Curr. Biol.* **30** R921–5

Arneth B 2019 Tumor microenvironment *Medicina* **56** 15

Asci Erkocyigit B, Ozufuklar O, Yardim A, Guler Celik E and Timur S 2023 Biomarker detection in early diagnosis of cancer: recent achievements in point-of-care devices based on paper microfluidics *Biosensors* **13** 387

Ashikbayeva Z, Bekmurzayeva A, Myrkhiyeva Z, Assylbekova N, Atabaev T S and Tosi D 2023 Green-synthesized gold nanoparticle-based optical fiber ball resonator biosensor for cancer biomarker detection *Opt. Laser Technol.* **161** 109136

Ates H C, Brunauer A, von Stetten F, Urban G A, Güder F, Merkoçi A, Früh S M and Dincer C 2021 Integrated devices for non-invasive diagnostics *Adv. Funct. Mater.* **31** 2010388

Balogh J, Victor D III, Asham E H, Burroughs S G, Boktour M, Saharia A, Li X, Ghobrial R M and Monsour H P 2016 Hepatocellular carcinoma: a review *J. Hepatocell. Carcinoma* **3** 41–53

Beylerli O, Gareev I, Sufianov A, Ilyasova T and Guang Y 2022 Long noncoding RNAs as promising biomarkers in cancer *Non-coding RNA Res.* **7** 66–70

Bober Z, Bartusik-Aebisher D and Aebisher D 2022 Application of dendrimers in anticancer diagnostics and therapy *Molecules* **27** 3237

Bura C, Mocan T, Grapa C and Mocan L 2022 Carbon nanotubes-based assays for cancer detection and screening *Pharmaceutics* **14** 781

Capitanio U and Montorsi F 2016 Renal cancer *Lancet* **387** 894–906

Chaturvedi V K, Singh A, Singh V K and Singh M P 2019 Cancer nanotechnology: a new revolution for cancer diagnosis and therapy *Curr. Drug Metab.* **20** 416–29

Chen F, Wang J, Wu Y, Gao Q and Zhang S 2022 Potential biomarkers for liver cancer diagnosis based on multi-omics strategy *Front. Oncol.* **12** 822449

Chen X *et al* 2020 Non-invasive early detection of cancer four years before conventional diagnosis using a blood test *Nat. Commun.* **11** 3475

Cheng F, Su L and Qian C 2016 Circulating tumor DNA: a promising biomarker in the liquid biopsy of cancer *Oncotarget* **7** 48832

Crosby D *et al* 2022 Early detection of cancer *Science* **375** eaay9040

Ding Y, Ling J, Wang H, Zou J, Wang K, Xiao X and Yang M 2015 Fluorescent detection of Mucin 1 protein based on aptamer functionalized biocompatible carbon dots and graphene oxide *Anal. Methods* **7** 7792–8

Doubeni C A, Doubeni A R and Myers A E 2016 Diagnosis and management of ovarian cancer *Am. Fam. Physician* **93** 937–44

Eble J A and Niland S 2019 The extracellular matrix in tumor progression and metastasis *Clin. Exp. Metastasis* **36** 171–98

Eftekhari A, Hasanzadeh M, Sharifi S, Dizaj S M, Khalilov R and Ahmadian E 2019 Bioassay of saliva proteins: the best alternative for conventional methods in non-invasive diagnosis of cancer *Int. J. Biol. Macromol.* **124** 1246–55

Fang M, Chen M, Liu L and Li Y 2017 Applications of quantum dots in cancer detection and diagnosis: a review *J. Biomed. Nanotechnol.* **13** 1–6

Fares J, Fares M Y, Khachfe H H, Salhab H A and Fares Y 2020 Molecular principles of metastasis: a hallmark of cancer revisited *Signal Transduct. Target. Ther.* **5** 28

Farzin A, Etesami S A, Quint J, Memic A and Tamayol A 2020 Magnetic nanoparticles in cancer therapy and diagnosis *Adv. Healthc. Mater.* **9** 1901058

Faubert B, Solmonson A and DeBerardinis R J 2020 Metabolic reprogramming and cancer progression *Science* **368** eaaw5473

Galluzzi L *et al* 2015 Autophagy in malignant transformation and cancer progression *EMBO* J. **34** 856–80

Garcia-Cordero J L and Maerkl S J 2020 Microfluidic systems for cancer diagnostics *Curr. Opin. Biotechnol.* **65** 37–44

Gulati P, Mishra P, Khanuja M, Narang J and Islam S S 2020 Nano-moles detection of tumor specific biomarker DNA for colorectal cancer detection using vertically aligned multi-wall carbon nanotubes based flexible electrodes *Process Biochem.* **90** 184–92

Hakimian F, Ghourchian H, Hashemi A S, Arastoo M R and Behnam Rad M 2018 Ultrasensitive optical biosensor for detection of miRNA-155 using positively charged Au nanoparticles *Sci. Rep.* **8** 2943

Hanahan D 2022 Hallmarks of cancer: new dimensions *Cancer Discov.* **12** 31–46

Hanoglu S B *et al* 2022 Magnetic nanoparticle-based electrochemical sensing platform using ferrocene-labelled peptide nucleic acid for the early diagnosis of colorectal cancer *Biosensors* **12** 736

Hasan M R, Ahommed M S, Daizy M, Bacchu M S, Ali M R, Al-Mamun M R, Aly M A, Khan M Z and Hossain S I 2021 Recent development in electrochemical biosensors for cancer biomarkers detection *Biosens. Bioelectron.* **8** 100075

Hassanpour S H and Dehghani M 2017 Review of cancer from perspective of molecular *J. Cancer Res. Pract.* **4** 127–9

Heydari-Bafrooei E and Shamszadeh N S 2017 Electrochemical bioassay development for ultrasensitive aptasensing of prostate specific antigen *Biosens. Bioelectron.* **91** 284–92

Hosseini S M, Mohammadnejad J, Salamat S, Zadeh Z B, Tanhaei M and Ramakrishna S 2023 Theranostic polymeric nanoparticles as a new approach in cancer therapy and diagnosis: a review *Mater. Today Chem.* **29** 101400

Hosu O, Tertis M and Cristea C 2019 Implication of magnetic nanoparticles in cancer detection, screening and treatment *Magnetochemistry* **5** 55

Irkham I, Ibrahim A U, Pwavodi P C, Al-Turjman F and Hartati Y W 2023 Smart graphene-based electrochemical nanobiosensor for clinical diagnosis *Sensors* **23** 2240

Jafari S H, Saadatpour Z, Salmaninejad A, Momeni F, Mokhtari M, Nahand J S, Rahmati M, Mirzaei H and Kianmehr M 2018 Breast cancer diagnosis: imaging techniques and biochemical markers *J. Cell. Physiol.* **233** 5200–13

Janith G I, Herath H S, Hendeniya N, Attygalle D, Amarasinghe D A, Logeeshan V, Wickramasinghe P M and Wijayasinghe Y S 2023 Advances in surface plasmon resonance biosensors for medical diagnostics: an overview of recent developments and techniques *J. Pharm. Biomed. Anal. Open* **2** 100019

Juzgado A, Soldà A, Ostric A, Criado A, Valenti G, Rapino S, Conti G, Fracasso G, Paolucci F and Prato M 2017 Highly sensitive electrochemiluminescence detection of a prostate cancer biomarker *J. Mater. Chem.* B **5** 6681–7

Kalishwaralal K, Kwon W Y and Park K S 2019 Exosomes for non-invasive cancer monitoring *Biotechnol. J.* **14** 1800430

Khakbaz F and Mahani M 2017 Micro-RNA detection based on fluorescence resonance energy transfer of DNA-carbon quantum dots probes *Anal. Biochem.* **523** 32–8

Koopaie M, Kolahdooz S, Fatahzadeh M and Manifar S 2022 Salivary biomarkers in breast cancer diagnosis: a systematic review and diagnostic meta-analysis *Cancer Med.* **11** 2644–61

Landegren U and Hammond M 2021 Cancer diagnostics based on plasma protein biomarkers: hard times but great expectations *Mol. Oncol.* **15** 1715–26

Li J, Guan X, Fan Z, Ching L M, Li Y, Wang X, Cao W M and Liu D X 2020 Non-invasive biomarkers for early detection of breast cancer *Cancers* **12** 2767

Li L, Li W, Ma C, Yang H, Ge S and Yu J 2014 Based electrochemiluminescence immunodevice for carcinoembryonic antigen using nanoporous gold-chitosan hybrids and graphene quantum dots functionalized Au@ Pt *Sens. Actuators B* **202** 314–22

Li Z, Li L X, Diao Y J, Wang J, Ye Y and Hao X K 2021 Identification of urinary exosomal miRNAs for the non-invasive diagnosis of prostate cancer *Cancer Manag. Res.* **13** 25–35

Lino C, Barrias S, Chaves R, Adega F, Martins-Lopes P and Fernandes J R 2022 Biosensors as diagnostic tools in clinical applications *Biochim. Biophys. Acta Rev. Cancer* **1877** 188726

Lone S N *et al* 2022 Liquid biopsy: a step closer to transform diagnosis, prognosis and future of cancer treatments *Mol. Cancer* **21** 79

Luo Y, Wang Y, Yan H, Wu Y, Zhu C, Du D and Lin Y 2018 SWCNTs@ GQDs composites as nanocarriers for enzyme-free dual-signal amplification electrochemical immunoassay of cancer biomarker *Anal. Chim. Acta* **1042** 44–51

Lyssiotis C A and Kimmelman A C 2017 Metabolic interactions in the tumor microenvironment *Trends Cell Biol.* **27** 863–75

Maly V, Maly O, Kolostova K and Bobek V 2019 Circulating tumor cells in diagnosis and treatment of lung cancer *In Vivo* **33** 1027–37

Mamdani H, Ahmed S, Armstrong S, Mok T and Jalal S I 2017 Blood-based tumor biomarkers in lung cancer for detection and treatment *Transl. Lung Cancer Res.* **6** 648

Martins I, Ribeiro I P, Jorge J, Gonçalves A C, Sarmento-Ribeiro A B, Melo J B and Carreira I M 2021 Liquid biopsies: applications for cancer diagnosis and monitoring *Genes* **12** 349

Mintz K, Waidely E, Zhou Y, Peng Z, Al-Youbi A O, Bashammakh A S, El-Shahawi M S and Leblanc R M 2018 Carbon dots and gold nanoparticles based immunoassay for detection of alpha-L-fucosidase *Anal. Chim. Acta* **1041** 114–21

Mizrahi J D, Surana R, Valle J W and Shroff R T 2020 Pancreatic cancer *Lancet* **395** 2008–20

Mohammadi S and Salimi A 2018 Fluorometric determination of microRNA-155 in cancer cells based on carbon dots and $MnO_2$ nanosheets as a donor-acceptor pair *Microchim. Acta* **185** 1–0

Mukherjee A, Bisht B, Dutta S and Paul M K 2022 Current advances in the use of exosomes, liposomes, and bioengineered hybrid nanovesicles in cancer detection and therapy *Acta Pharmacol. Sin.* **43** 2759–76

Njoku K, Chiasserini D, Jones E R, Barr C E, O'Flynn H, Whetton A D and Crosbie E J 2020 Urinary biomarkers and their potential for the non-invasive detection of endometrial cancer *Front. Oncol.* **10** 559016

Nooreldeen R and Bach H 2021 Current and future development in lung cancer diagnosis *Int. J. Mol. Sci.* **22** 8661

Pang Y, Wang C, Wang J, Sun Z, Xiao R and Wang S 2016 $Fe_3O_4$@ Ag magnetic nanoparticles for microRNA capture and duplex-specific nuclease signal amplification based SERS detection in cancer cells *Biosens. Bioelectron.* **79** 574–80

Park J, Shin Y, Kim T H, Kim D H and Lee A 2019 Urinary metabolites as biomarkers for diagnosis of breast cancer: a preliminary study *J. Breast Dis.* **7** 44–51

Patel A 2020 Benign vs malignant tumors *JAMA Oncol.* **6** 1488

Perumal V, Sivakumar P M, Zarrabi A, Muthupandian S, Vijayaraghavalu S, Sahoo K, Das A, Das S, Payyappilly S S and Das S 2019 Near infra-red polymeric nanoparticle based optical imaging in cancer diagnosis *J. Photochem. Photobiol.* B **199** 111630

Preethi K A, Selvakumar S C, Ross K, Jayaraman S, Tusubira D and Sekar D 2022 Liquid biopsy: exosomal microRNAs as novel diagnostic and prognostic biomarkers in cancer *Mol. Cancer* **21** 1–5

Pulumati A, Pulumati A, Dwarakanath B S, Verma A and Papineni R V 2023 Technological advancements in cancer diagnostics: improvements and limitations *Cancer Rep.* **6** e1764

Qi S A *et al* 2021 High-resolution metabolomic biomarkers for lung cancer diagnosis and prognosis *Sci. Rep.* **11** 11805

Qian Y, Shi L and Luo Z 2020 Long non-coding RNAs in cancer: implications for diagnosis, prognosis, and therapy *Front. Med.* **7** 902

Qin D, Jiang X, Mo G, Feng J, Yu C and Deng B 2019 A novel carbon quantum dots signal amplification strategy coupled with sandwich electrochemiluminescence immunosensor for the detection of CA15-3 in human serum *ACS Sens.* **4** 504–12

Qiu S, Cai Y, Yao H, Lin C, Xie Y, Tang S and Zhang A 2023 Small molecule metabolites: discovery of biomarkers and therapeutic targets *Signal Transduct. Target. Ther.* **8** 132

Rankin E B and Giaccia A J 2016 Hypoxic control of metastasis *Science* **352** 175–80

Rawla P 2019 Epidemiology of prostate cancer *World J. Oncol.* **10** 63

Raza F *et al* 2023 Liposome-based diagnostic and therapeutic applications for pancreatic cancer *Acta Biomater.* **157** 1–23

Sabahi A, Salahandish R, Ghaffarinejad A and Omidinia E 2020 Electrochemical nano-genosensor for highly sensitive detection of miR-21 biomarker based on SWCNT-grafted dendritic Au nanostructure for early detection of prostate cancer *Talanta* **209** 120595

Schwager S C, Taufalele P V and Reinhart-King C A 2019 Cell–cell mechanical communication in cancer *Cell. Mol. Bioeng.* **12** 1–4

Shestakova K M *et al* 2023 Targeted metabolomic profiling as a tool for diagnostics of patients with non-small-cell lung cancer *Sci. Rep.* **13** 11072

Siegel R L, Miller K D, Wagle N S and Jemal A 2023 Cancer statistics, 2023 *CA: Cancer J. Clin.* **73** 17–48

Singh R and Kumar S 2022 Cancer targeting and diagnosis: recent trends with carbon nanotubes *Nanomaterials* **12** 2283

Sohel M M 2020 Circulating microRNAs as biomarkers in cancer diagnosis *Life Sci.* **248** 117473

Spill F, Reynolds D S, Kamm R D and Zaman M H 2016 Impact of the physical microenvironment on tumor progression and metastasis *Curr. Opin. Biotechnol.* **40** 41–8

Sultana R, Yadav D, Puranik N, Chavda V, Kim J and Song M 2023 A review on the use of gold nanoparticles in cancer treatment *Anti-Cancer Agents Med. Chem.* **23** 2171–82

Suman A K 2008 Recent advances in DNA biosensor *Sens. Transducers* J. **92** 122–33

Sun Y S, Zhao Z, Yang Z N, Xu F, Lu H J, Zhu Z Y, Shi W, Jiang J, Yao P P and Zhu H P 2017 Risk factors and preventions of breast cancer *Int. J. Biol. Sci.* **13** 1387

Thandra K C, Barsouk A, Saginala K, Aluru J S and Barsouk A 2021 Epidemiology of lung cancer *Contem. Oncol.* **25** 45–52

Thenrajan T, Alwarappan S and Wilson J 2023 Molecular diagnosis and cancer prognosis—a concise review *Diagnostics* **13** 766

Torre L A, Bray F, Siegel R L, Ferlay J, Lortet-Tieulent J and Jemal A 2015 Global cancer statistics 2012 *CA: Cancer J.* **65** 87–108

Vaidyanathan R, Soon R H, Zhang P, Jiang K and Lim C T 2019 Cancer diagnosis: from tumor to liquid biopsy and beyond *Lab Chip* **19** 11–34

Valihrach L, Androvic P and Kubista M 2020 Circulating miRNA analysis for cancer diagnostics and therapy *Mol. Aspects Med.* **72** 100825

Vasconcelos M H, Caires H R, Ābols A, Xavier C P and Linē A 2019 Extracellular vesicles as a novel source of biomarkers in liquid biopsies for monitoring cancer progression and drug resistance *Drug Resist. Updat.* **47** 100647

Walter F M *et al* 2019 Evaluating diagnostic strategies for early detection of cancer: the CanTest framework *BMC Cancer* **19** 1

Wang G, Zhao D, Spring D J and DePinho R A 2018 Genetics and biology of prostate cancer *Genes Dev.* **32** 1105–40

Wang L 2017 Early diagnosis of breast cancer *Sensors* **17** 1572

Wang W, Rong Z, Wang G, Hou Y, Yang F and Qiu M 2023 Cancer metabolites: promising biomarkers for cancer liquid biopsy *Biomark. Res.* **11** 66

Wang X, Chen S and Jia W 2016 Metabolomics in cancer biomarker research *Curr. Pharmacol. Rep.* **2** 293–8

Wang Y H, Song Z, Hu X Y and Wang H S 2021 Circulating tumor DNA analysis for tumor diagnosis *Talanta* **228** 122220

Xu W, Zhou G, Wang H, Liu Y, Chen B, Chen W, Lin C, Wu S, Gong A and Xu M 2020 Circulating lncRNA SNHG11 as a novel biomarker for early diagnosis and prognosis of colorectal cancer *Int. J. Cancer* **146** 2901–12

Xu Y *et al* 2023 Metabolic biomarkers in lung cancer screening and early diagnosis *Oncol. Lett.* **25** 1

Yang H, Liu W, Ma C, Zhang Y, Wang X, Yu J and Song X 2014 Gold–silver nanocomposite-functionalized graphene based electrochemiluminescence immunosensor using graphene quantum dots coated porous PtPd nanochains as labels *Electrochim. Acta* **123** 470–6

Yang L, Wang Y, Cai H, Wang S, Shen Y and Ke C 2020 Application of metabolomics in the diagnosis of breast cancer: a systematic review *J. Cancer* **11** 2540

Yuan Y, Jiang Y C, Sun C K and Chen Q M 2016 Role of the tumor microenvironment in tumor progression and the clinical applications *Oncol. Rep.* **35** 2499–515

Zhang M, Liu H, Chen L, Yan M, Ge L, Ge S and Yu J 2013 A disposable electro-chemiluminescence device for ultrasensitive monitoring of K562 leukemia cells based on aptamers and ZnO@ carbon quantum dots *Biosens. Bioelectron.* **49** 79–85

Zhang Y, Li M, Gao X, Chen Y and Liu T 2019 Nanotechnology in cancer diagnosis: progress, challenges and opportunities *J. Hematol. Oncol.* **12** 1–3

Zhao H, Wu L, Yan G, Chen Y, Zhou M, Wu Y and Li Y 2021 Inflammation and tumor progression: signaling pathways and targeted intervention *Signal Transduct. Target. Ther.* **6** 263

Zheng M 2016 Classification and pathology of lung cancer *Surg. Oncol. Clin.* **25** 447–68

Zhu S, Yi M, Wu Y, Dong B and Wu K 2021 Roles of tumor-associated macrophages in tumor progression: implications on therapeutic strategies *Exp. Hematol. Oncol.* **10** 1–7

# Chapter 2

# Imaging techniques in current biosensor advancements in cancer diagnosis

**Vikas Pitre, Megha Srivastava and Gayatri Rai**

Imaging techniques are advanced techniques in cancer diagnosis. There are six imaging modalities accessible for the clinical diagnosis and treatment of cancer. Imaging technology works based on different concepts of physics, and include optical imaging, positron emission tomography (PET), single photon emission computed tomography (SPECT), computed tomography (CT), ultrasound (US), magnetic resonance imaging (MRI), and x-rays. Only four are capable of identifying cancer in any part of the human body in three dimensions (3D). Imaging methods identify the fewest number of cancer cells. To view inside soft tissues and examine the findings in the form of a picture, US uses sound waves that range from 1 to 10 MHz. The basic idea behind x-ray and CT scans is to measure the attenuation of an x-ray beam as it passes through the body. To reassemble the recorded data into a three-dimensional image, CT rotates a pair of detectors around the subject. The small excess in the nuclear spin's Boltzmann distribution inside a magnetic field is imaged by MRI. The protons, which are the source of the MRI signal, are present in a concentration of only about 80 $\mu$mol l$^{-1}$. Increasing the magnetic field strength from 1.5 to 3 T and higher has been shown to increase the signal-to-noise ratio in MRI. SPECT is an effective method for measuring a radioactive compound's dispersion. Only 1/100 000 of the photons emitted at the cancer location are detected by SPECT, and its maximum resolution is 12 × 12 × 12 mm. PET measures a form of antimatter, positrons, that emits electrons from nuclei rich in protons, although it has the opposite charge. This chapter describes the use of new imaging techniques to develop biosensor technology for cancer diagnosis and therapy.

## 2.1 Introduction

With more than 200 different forms of the disease and more than 1500 deaths from cancer every day, it is the most common cause of death worldwide. The unchecked development, multiplication, and penetration of malignantly altered cancer cells beyond normal limits into neighboring tissues are what defines cancer. Conventional methods such as MRI, US, and biopsy are not useful for early cancer detection since they depend on the phenotypic features of the tumor [1]. Del Sol *et al* state that cancer is a multistage illness whose origins and progression are connected to a wide range of complicated genetic or epigenetic alterations [2] that interfere with cellular signaling, result in tumorigenic transformation, and eventually induce malignancy. From a therapeutic perspective, the molecules that undergo major changes throughout cancer are called biomarkers, and they are crucial. Biomarkers can be classified as prognostic, predictive, diagnostic, or metabolites. They can be isoenzymes, proteins, metabolites, nucleic acids, or hormones. Whereas diagnostic biomarkers are linked to the detection of a disease, prognostic biomarkers offer information about the probability of a disease recurrence, while therapy response is measured by predictive biomarkers [3]. A specific biomarker's existence, absence, or change in a cell's level is often a sign that cancer is developing, according to Chatterjee and Zetter [4]. The discovery and identification of these cancer-specific biomarkers may help with the early diagnosis and monitoring of the course of the illness [5, 6].

Rusling *et al* report that the traditional techniques for identifying biomarkers, the enzyme-linked immunosorbent assay (ELISA) and or polymerase chain reaction (PCR),have certain technological shortcomings, including slow detection and expensive reagent consumption for each assay [7]. These methods—which are also manual—cannot keep a patient under constant observation while they are undergoing treatment.

Cancer will be the world's biggest cause of death by 2020, accounting for 10 million deaths and 19.3 million new diagnoses. Due to continued research into the disease and advancements in technology that make more precise diagnostic techniques possible, the field of cancer diagnosis is always evolving. Early cancer detection rates have been made possible by the application of currently available cancer diagnostic techniques, such as magnetic resonance spectroscopy (MRS), PET, x-ray CT, and molecular diagnostic techniques. These techniques are essential for both early cancer detection and the therapeutic management of cancer patients. The effectiveness of these cancer screening programs depends critically on the accuracy of precursor lesion detection; a higher identification rate allows for earlier treatment initiation, which reduces the long-term incidence of invasive cancer and improves overall prognosis. These diagnostic methods have several benefits, including being non-invasive and easily accessible in a clinical setting, despite their high cost. Nevertheless, several disadvantages, such as poor target definition, high signal-to-noise ratios, and related artifacts, make it challenging to diagnose some deep-seated tumor types [8].

The purpose of this chapter is to provide a summary of the most recent developments in biosensors for cancer detection and treatment, including modalities such as PET, SPECT, MRI, optical, x-ray, and CT scan imaging.

## 2.2 Advanced imaging techniques in cancer diagnosis

Cancer management requires reliable diagnosis to identify the primary tumor and assess its dissemination to surrounding tissues, as well as to other organs and structures throughout the body. This procedure, which is referred to as 'staging' in technical terms, is crucial in determining the treatment strategy to be used because staging determines prognosis and, by extension, therapy. Radiation medicine imaging is typically the initial step in clinical management. Nuclear medicine and diagnostic radiology studies are crucial for cancer patient screening, staging, therapy monitoring, and long-term follow-up. Clinicians now have access to powerful diagnostic tomographic (cross-section view) modalities, including nuclear medicine procedures such as PET and SPECT, as well as MRI and x-ray CT (figure 2.1 and table 2.1).

### 2.2.1 X-rays

Probably the most common type of imaging is x-ray imaging. The majority of adults have undergone a chest x-ray to check for infections or perhaps just as part of a job health examination. Some people have had x-rays taken of their hands or feet in an attempt to find metallic splinters or fractures. Different tissues absorb radiation at different rates, which results in the images that x-rays produce. Because calcium in bones absorbs x-rays more than any other material, bones look white on a radiograph or film capture of the x-ray image. Fat and other soft tissues seem gray because they absorb less radiation [9]. Air absorbs the least on a radiograph, giving the appearance of black lungs. X-rays are frequently used to check for fractures but it is also possible to look for cancer with x-rays and x-rays are used in the diagnosis of cancer. Mammography and chest radiography, for example, are commonly used to identify cancer at an early stage or to assess if the disease has

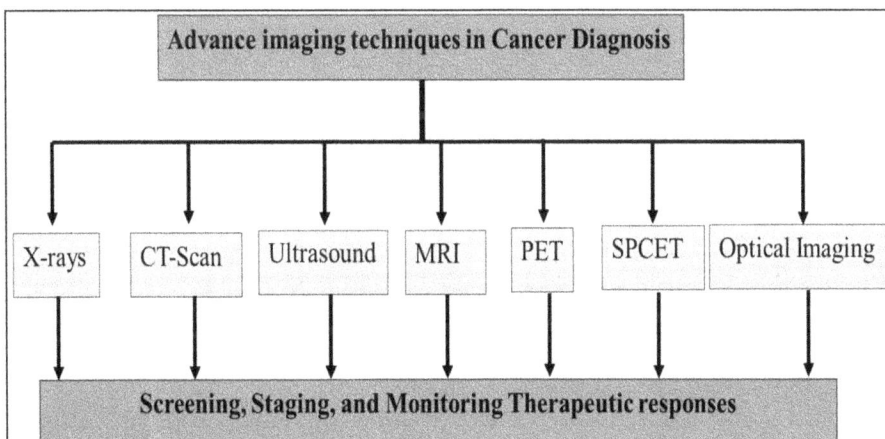

**Figure 2.1.** Flow chart of advanced imaging techniques in cancer diagnosis.

Table 2.1. Advanced imaging techniques in cancer diagnosis.

| Imaging techniques | Action | Cancer types detected | Advantages | Disadvantages | References |
|---|---|---|---|---|---|
| X-rays | X-rays are a form of electromagnetic that can pass through the body to generate images of tissues and structures inside the body. | Bones, lungs | 1. X-rays can also be used to search for cancer. 2. X-rays are used in mammograms to search the breasts for abnormal regions or tumors. | 1. Radiation is introduced to your body when you are exposed to x-rays. Although generally harmless, excessive exposure may have negative effects. 2. X-rays are great for viewing bones, but they struggle to clearly show soft tissues such as muscles or organs. This can limit their diagnostic use. | [9, 10] |
| CT scan | To create cross-sectional images of the bones, blood vessels, and soft tissues throughout the body, a sequence of x-ray images are acquired at various angles. | Tumors of the colon, stomach, head and neck, kidney, bone, bladder, and ovaries. | 1. A quick scan that may help reduce motion artifacts. 2. Radiographs that have been digitally recreated using cortical bone information. 3. Precise spatial data. | 1. Inadequate imaging of soft tissues. 2. Radiation exposure. 3. Less functional information. | [11–15] |

| | | | | |
|---|---|---|---|---|
| Ultrasound | By utilizing a transducer to introduce sound waves into the body, which are then reflected from tissues and organs, an internal organ image can be produced. | Lungs, brain, or the entire abdomen or pelvis. | 1. Able to detect tumors.<br>2. Can help physicians treat or guide biopsies on the disease. | 1. The greatest risk associated with high-frequency ultrasonography during fetal imaging is the possibility of microscopic mechanical damage or thermal heating of tissue.<br>2. Ultrasonography cannot assess the internal structure of tissues that have a high acoustical impedance. Its evaluation of structures embedded in bone is likewise restricted. [18] |
| MRI | Utilizes radio waves and a magnetic field to create intricate images of tissues and organs. | Brain, main bone, spinal cord, prostatic, bladder, uterine, and ovarian tumors; soft tissue sarcomas. | 1. In-depth imaging of soft tissues.<br>2. Ionizing radiation exposure is absent.<br>3. Compared to the iodine-based contrast agents used in CT and x-ray scans, gadolinium, the contrast agent used in MRIs, is less likely to result in an allergic reaction. | 1. Because of magnetic field interference, it is contraindicated when there are metal items present, both within and outside the body.<br>2. Expensive.<br>3. Time-consuming.<br>4. Must stay in an enclosed machine, which some patients with claustrophobia may find difficult. [19] |

(*Continued*)

**Table 2.1.** (*Continued*)

| Imaging techniques | Action | Cancer types detected | Advantages | Disadvantages | References |
|---|---|---|---|---|---|
| PET | Measures the blood flow to different parts of a given organ, making it possible to create an image that shows the parts of the organ that are busier at a given moment. | Cancers of the brain, breast, neck, esophagus, colon, lung, pancreas, lymphatic system, skin, and thyroid. | 1. Can be carried out in addition to a CT scan to offer anatomical and functional data. 2. Could be useful for diagnosing malignant tumors that traditional imaging may have missed. 3. Examines lymph node metastases with greater accuracy compared to traditional imaging. | 1. Low spatial resolution and detectability of malignant lesions. 2. Radiation exposure through the injection of radioactive substances intravenously. | [14, 20–22] |

spread to the lungs or other areas of the chest. Mammograms employ x-rays to look for abnormal areas or tumors in the breasts [10].

## 2.2.2 CT

Computed tomography is another imaging method that can be used to identify cancer. For the detection of several cancers, including those of the breast, lungs, colon, and head and neck, CT has been shown to be an effective screening method, offering accurate tumor imaging in both space and time, assisting with radio-chemotherapy, surgery, and follow-up biopsy procedures [11, 12]. Numerous device advancements, such as low kilovoltage, dual-energy, iterative reconstruction, increased scan speed, perfusion imaging, and lower radiation dosage, have demon-strated the therapeutic usefulness of CT-based cancer imaging [13]. Spiral multi-detector CT with a multi-fan measurement strategy has improved spatial resolution and eliminated artifacts thanks to superior reconstruction and noise reduction techniques. Reducing radiation exposure and artifacts as well as reconstructing high-resolution CT images has been made possible using artificial intelligence and photon counting, which is the counting and measurement of incoming photons. A CT scan is frequently used in conjunction with a PET scan to precisely localize the lesions found by PET [14, 15]. The PET scan relies on the biochemical processes taking place within the cells to provide an image with a poor spatial resolution, whereas the CT scan produces an image with a high spatial resolution that highlights the structural and morphological aspects of the tumor [14]. Additionally, by compensating for the intrinsic attenuation seen in PET scans, the concurrent CT scan enhances the sensitivity and specificity of the image [16]. In a study by Shawky *et al* comparing PET/CT versus CT alone in the identification of breast cancer, the sensitivity of the former was 100%, specificity was 95.4%, Positive Predictive Value (PPV) was 88.9%, and Negative Predictive Value (NPV) was 100%. On the other hand, CT alone had a sensitivity of 81.2%, specificity of 90%, PPV of 76.4%, and NPV of 93%. However, it is important to note that there is a considerable probability that the PET overlay will be obscured by artifacts from the add-on CT, in particular if contrast agents are being employed. Additionally frequently utilized in tandem with CT scans are SPECT scans. SPECT/CT hybrid imaging is frequently used to detect metastases in cancers with a higher affinity for bone, such as lung, prostate, and breast carcinomas [14]. Two types of SPECT/CT are used in practice today: targeted and whole body. Whole-body SPECT/CT imaging was found to be highly beneficial in the detection of extra-axial skeletal lesions in research by Rager *et al* Moreover, in 5.7% of study participants, the diagnosis was changed following whole-body imaging as opposed to targeted CT [17].

## 2.2.3 Ultrasound

Ultrasound (US) uses sound waves that have frequencies higher than human hearing. By utilizing a transducer to introduce sound waves into the body, which are then reflected from tissues and organs, an internal organ picture can be produced. In addition to being able to detect tumors, ultrasound can help physicians treat or guide biopsies on the disease. Like diagnostic MRI, diagnostic US produces no hazardous radiation. Although it is quite rare now, both MRI and US can be utilized for treatment under specific circumstances. Regrettably, although US is highly beneficial for imaging specific body areas, it is not as effective as other imaging modalities when examining the lungs, brain, or the entire abdomen or pelvis. To locate suspected tumor spread locations, we typically need to employ CT, MRI, and/or PET because lumps can occasionally be small and far below the skin's surface [18].

### 2.2.4 MRI

To induce tissues to emit radio waves of their own, magnetic resonance imaging (MRI) uses radio waves in the presence of a strong magnetic field that surrounds the MRI machine's opening where the patient rests. Organ images can be viewed on a computer screen because different tissues—including tumors—emit powerful signals based on their chemical makeup. Both MRI and CT scans have the potential to produce three-dimensional images of bodily parts, while MRI is occasionally more sensitive than CT scans in identifying between soft tissues. The noise level of MR scanners is well known, and almost all MRI technologists carry a large supply of earplugs or over-the-ear headphones for patients to utilize. Some people become claustrophobic in MRI units. Medical professionals and medical technicians are used to assisting patients with this. Additionally, MRI is showing great promise for revealing not only the body's structure and architecture, but also its functioning and inner workings. There are further advances in MRI, such as fast acquisition methods with several new pulse sequences and new MRI contrast agents [19].

### 2.2.5 PET

Positron emission tomography (PET), as well as x-ray absorbance, magnetic resonance characteristics, and US reflection, are used to create tomographic images based on the structural features of the tumor. PET scanning could end up being the most popular imaging technique now utilised in cancer detection, depending on how the tumour tissue functions. Similar to a camera, a PET scan gathers simultaneous gamma rays from the annihilation of two positrons from a drug that is distributed differently across the tumor tissue and associated with the functional state of the tissue. With this technique, an image is created without the need for visible light [20, 21]. First, particular isotopes of oxygen, nitrogen, and carbon created in a cyclotron —a device that accelerates the particles—replace a hydrogen atom in a target molecule that produces a positron. When an electron and positron meet inside the tissue, gamma rays are generated, which are detected by a PET scan [20]. The National Oncologic PET Registry (NOPR) conducted a prospective cohort study that found that the complex mechanism used by this diagnostic tool forms the foundation for the clinical decision-making process for treatment as well as the three principles of cancer detection [22].

One study collected data on a cancer treatment plan using questionnaires, both before and after the PET scan results were analysed. The results of the study showed that 48% of the patients received therapy, and 37% of the patients had their post-PET care plan changed to monitoring and observation. Moreover, around 70% of patients who had initially intended to undergo a biopsy were told not to go ahead with that plan once the PET scan was completed. Last but not least, in 8.7% of cases, the post-PET management strategy included a significant change to the type of treatment, and in 5.6% of cases, the patients whose management plan included treatment both before and after the PET scan had their goals changed. Overall, 36.5% of cases had clinicians changing their original treatment plan according to the results of the PET scan, indicating the substantial benefits this imaging modality provides in oncologic settings. Additional variations have been developed since PET imaging was first developed. One of the most commonly used drugs is 2-fluoro-2-deoxy-D-glucose (FDG), also known as positron-labeled [20]. The PET scan image is based on the Warburg effect, which postulates that increased glucose utilization to sustain continuous cell growth and division is the source of heightened metabolic activity in cancer cells [14]. This property allows the antimetabolite glucose analogue 2-deoxy D-glucose (2-DG), connected to the positron-emitting 18 F molecule, to accumulate as a tracer in the area of the tumor, facilitating imaging.

### 2.2.6 SPCET

Using radioactive tracers and a scanner, single photon emission computed tomography (SPECT) captures data that a computer converts into two- or three-dimensional images. A small dose of a radioactive medication is injected into a vein, and the body parts where the radioactive material is absorbed by the cells are precisely photographed using a scanner. SPECT can provide information on the body's metabolic processes and blood flow to various tissues. In this procedure, the radioactive material is bound to antibodies, which are proteins that bind to and identify tumor cells. If a tumor is present, the antibodies will bind to it. Subsequently, the location of the tumor and the radioactive material can be determined with a SPECT scan [23].

### 2.2.7 Optical imaging

The application of light as a research imaging technique for medical purposes is known as optical imaging, and it was created by American physical chemist Britton Chance. Examples include optical coherence tomography, laser Doppler imaging, optical microscopy, spectroscopy, endoscopy, and scanning laser ophthalmoscopy. Since light is an electromagnetic wave, radio waves, microwaves, and x-rays all exhibit similar behaviors.

The emphasis on optical imaging techniques for molecular imaging is largely due to the sensitivity of imaging optical contrast agents and reporter molecules *in vivo*. The lower limits of detection for optical imaging may approach picomolar or even femtomolar concentrations when employing an optical reporter or contrast agent. In addition to the low background of techniques such as bioluminescence imaging and near-infrared fluorescence imaging, the signal-to-noise ratio for chemical signal identification is comparable to or superior to other molecular imaging modalities.

One of the biggest challenges facing optical imaging probes and equipment, particularly those geared towards possible therapeutic applications, is overcoming tissue attenuation and light scattering. The absorption of visible light by components such as hemoglobin can reduce optical signals by approximately ten times for each centimeter of tissue [24]. In order to observe fluorescence in deeper tissues, scientists have developed techniques for imaging near-infrared fluorescence (NIRF), which has emission wavelengths between 650 and 900 nm. Light, at least at these wavelengths, is absorbed by water, lipids, and hemoglobin; tissue autofluorescence is thus markedly reduced. As a result, NIRF imaging agents become much more sensitive, potentially making it possible to detect tomographic optical imaging signals at depths of 7–14 cm [25]. The tissues' varying light absorption also results in images that are biased towards optical reporters and probes that are positioned closer to a subject's surface. While this limitation is being overcome by three-dimensional imaging and analysis techniques such as fluorescent molecular tomography (FMT) [26], optical techniques typically allow relative quantification of imaging signals rather than the absolute quantification that PET can accomplish. The application of optical techniques in molecular imaging research and clinical translation is growing despite these challenges.

## 2.3 Functions of imaging techniques

Cancer is detected through anatomical abnormalities or structural alterations using anatomical imaging modalities such as CT and conventional MRI. However, there are times when this is insufficient, and misleading negative results could be discovered. Metastatic illness involving lymph nodes is a common case. When using CT or MRI in these circumstances, nodal invasion by cancer cells may be suspected, but only if nodes are shown to be larger and so stand out as aberrant. This is not always the case, though, as cancer can spread to lymph nodes of normal size. Functional imaging approaches, on the other hand, rely on molecular and metabolic processes occurring within the tumor tissue to identify malignant involvement. It involves displaying changes in the turnover of biomolecules at different tissue levels, and this data is closely related to the biochemistry of the tissue [27]. The recent significant developments in imaging, along with the integration of the imaging sciences and molecular biology, have given rise to a brand-new area of study called 'molecular imaging'. All imaging modalities utilized in cancer imaging are included, and new applications are always being created. Among the technologies in use are dynamic CT, dynamic SPECT, MR spectroscopy, functional MRI, and dynamic MRI [28].

Although the study focuses on nuclear imaging techniques, magnetic resonance is a significant component in the field of molecular imaging. Dynamic MR imaging, comprising spectroscopic imaging, diffusion-weighted imaging, and perfusion imaging, has recently progressed to the point where all of these techniques can offer quantitative cellular, hemodynamic (blood dynamic), and metabolic data that could potentially enhance treatment response assessment, improve understanding of tumor biology, more precisely determine tumor activity during therapy, and differentiate between recurrent tumors and treatment side effects. The two most widely used MR spectroscopy techniques involve collecting resonance signals from non-water molecules with hydrogen-1 or phosphorus-31 nuclei. Functional magnetic resonance imaging (fMRI) is a tool used to examine brain diseases as well as healthy brain function by examining the brain's response to different stimuli [29].

## 2.4 Precautions for patients and operators when using imaging techniques

Radiation safety is a problem for patients, physicians, and staff in several areas, including radiology, interventional cardiology, and surgery. During fluoroscopic operations, medical workers are exposed to the maximum radiation exposure. The radiation dose that healthcare personnel are exposed to overall is mostly unaffected by the radiation from diagnostic imaging modalities including computed tomography, nuclear imaging, and mammography. Nonetheless, radiation exposure of any kind poses a risk to both patients and medical staff [30].

Today, ionizing radiation is a vital tool in medicine, utilized for both the diagnosis and treatment of a broad variety of ailments. Alongside its expanding use, the lifetime radiation doses to patients and healthcare providers have also increased. The main source of radiation exposure in medical settings is fluoroscopic imaging, which uses x-rays to create dynamic and visually stunning functional imaging. Formal radiation protection training reduces radiation exposure to patients and medical personnel [31].

However, applying radiation safety guidelines can be a lengthy undertaking, and many interventionists do not receive formal training in radiation dose reduction during their residency or fellowship. When using fluoroscopic imaging outside of radiology or interventional departments, doctors and other medical personnel do not always adhere to strict radiation safety regulations. Fluoroscopy is used in many different medical specialties, including vascular surgery, gastrointestinal medicine, interventional radiology, orthopedics, and urology. As radiation exposure rises in frequency, a thorough understanding of the risks associated with it as well as techniques for dosage reduction will be essential.

Physical shielding, distance from the radiation source, and duration of radiation exposure are the three most crucial variables in reducing exposure. There are several ways to shorten the exposure period. The technician or physician should plan the required images in advance of exposing the patient to radiation in order to avoid unnecessary and repetitive radiation exposure. Since magnification significantly increases the patient's exposure, it should only be utilized in very limited circumstances [32]. There are several precautions that must be followed both before and after these scanning procedures, including MRI, CT, US, PET, and x-rays. For example, patients should refrain from eating or drinking anything 6 h prior to a PET scan, but they are still allowed to drink water. They should also avoid doing any intense exercise a day before the visit. Patients should consume a lot of water following the scan to aid in the removal of the radioactive material from their bodies. Patients may be instructed to stay away from close contact with infants, young children, and pregnant women for a few hours following a PET scan as a precaution. There are no after-effects precautions for an x-ray scan. For each type of scan, a healthcare professional will provide particular recommendations that the patient should follow to ensure accurate results and reduce any potential hazards. There are no particular restrictions for SPECT imaging, but physicians should carefully weigh the hazards of radiation exposure when referring patients, according to a review of research. Patients who are obese may weigh more than the scanner's weight capacity. [33]. Given the advantages CT scans offer in terms of medical condition diagnosis and treatment, the dangers involved are usually deemed tolerable. Nonetheless, before undergoing any imaging process, it is vital to comprehend the possible hazards and advantages.

- *X-ray scans*: These scans provide images of the inside of the body using ionizing radiation. An x-ray scan has a comparatively modest radiation dosage, and the advantages typically exceed the hazards [9].
- *CT scans*: Compared to x-ray scans, computed tomography scans subject patients to greater radiation doses. Radiation exposure from a CT scan of the abdomen and pelvis is around 10 mSv. Although there are frequently substantial advantages to CT scans, patients should carefully weigh the dangers, particularly if they are pregnant or have other health issues [17].
- *PET scans*: Positron emission tomography scans use radioactive isotopes to image physiological processes, including blood flow. A PET/CT scan is a combination of PET and CT scans that is frequently performed. A PET/CT scan produces radiation at a dose of around 25 mSv or the same as eight years' worth of background radiation exposure [20].
- *MRI scans*: Ionizing radiation is not used during a magnetic resonance imaging scan. Rather, they produce images of the inside of the body using radio waves and magnetic fields. Although MRI scans are usually thought to be safe, not all hospitals may be able to provide them, and they can be costly [19].
- *US*: High-frequency sound waves are used in ultrasound scans to provide images of the interior of the body. They are thought to be safe for the majority of applications and do not employ ionizing radiation [14].

Before undertaking any procedure, it is imperative to discuss with the healthcare professional the advantages and disadvantages of each imaging approach. Depending on the circumstances, different imaging procedures such as MRI or US might frequently be utilized in place of CT, PET, or x-ray scans [15].

## 2.5 Current biosensors and their advantages over imaging techniques

Biosensors use a transducer to link a biocomponent to an electrical component (see figure 2.2). This method aids in the identification of changes and the qualitative and quantitative analysis of biological changes. Different kinds of sensors that examine biological reactions, their products, or reaction responses are produced by integrating an electronic component called a transducer. Biosensors are used in medicine at

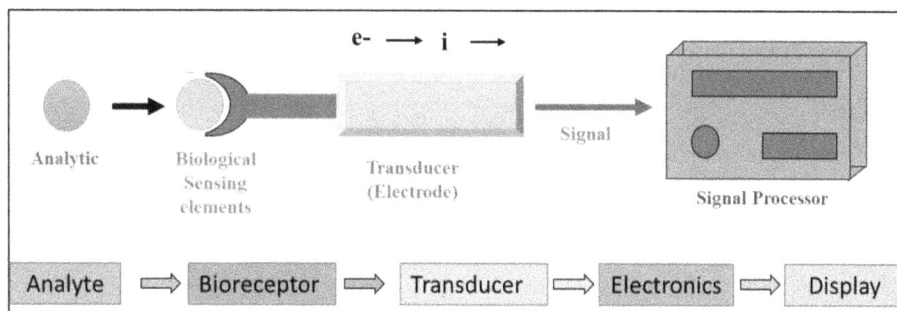

**Figure 2.2.** Mechanism of a biosensor.

several stages for both diagnosis and treatment. Biosensing in food technology, biotechnology, genetic engineering, nanotechnology, medical diagnostics (including cancer detection), and enzyme, antibody, and DNA research are just a few of the numerous applications for biosensors.

The development of biosensors must take these aspects into account as they improve the sensitivity, specificity, and precision of readings. Utilizing a transducing device, biosensor technology takes advantage of a biological recognition event's special characteristics. In this scenario, the analyte's interaction with the bioreceptor results in an appropriate output that the user can easily read. This strategy not only makes use of the chemical binding event but also connects scientists and engineers to share expertise. Comparable methods have had a significant impact on early-career biosensor researchers. It has paved the way for new directions in scientific research, with a focus on developing technology that would improve a variety of fields, including healthcare. Working in an interdisciplinary field encourages creative problem-solving and collaboration with diverse professions, where ideas are integrated to produce meaningful results. A simple example is a pregnancy test biosensor, where engineers and biologists collaborated to design the electronics of the device for the read-out while biologists focused on the biological components. Finally, clients around the world can access laboratory research because of management specialists. The dramatic increase in biosensors available on the market in recent years is proof that biosensor development is not confined to any particular niche. Globally, there has been a steady rise in biosensor based start-up businesses in recent years, which is significantly affecting the healthcare industry. Broadly speaking, biosensors have become indispensable in modern society because they seek to enhance living standards in a variety of fields, including ecology, pharmacology, food safety, agriculture, homeland security, and medicine (table 2.2).

Biosensors have been developed for around 50 years, and within the past ten years, academic research in this area has greatly advanced the subject. However, very few biosensors have achieved widespread commercial success at the retail level worldwide, except for lateral flow pregnancy tests and electrochemical glucose biosensors. The industry's difficulties in translating research from academic institutions into commercially viable prototypes, the complexity of regulatory issues in

**Table 2.2.** Types of biosensors including applications and principles.

| S. No. | Type | Principle | Application | References |
|---|---|---|---|---|
| 1. | Biosensor based on glucose oxidase electrodes | Electrochemistry with the oxidation of glucose. | Examination of a biological sample's glucose | [34] |
| 2. | Biosensor of uric acid | Electrochemistry | To identify clinical anomalies in illnesses | [35] |
| 3. | Biosensor based on acetylcholinesterase inhibition | Electrochemistry | Recognizing the effects of pesticides | [36] |
| 4. | Biosensor of silicon | Visual, optical, and fluorescent methods | Cancer therapy, biosensing, and bioimaging | [37, 38] |
| 6. | Biosensor of nanomaterials | Optical, visual, or fluorescent methods | For a variety of uses, including biomedical ones, such as diagnostic instruments | [39] |

clinical applications, and the difficulty in locating researchers with experience in biosensor technology or collaborating with researchers from other scientific and engineering disciplines are some of the reasons for this. The reliance on sophisticated imaging methods in clinical settings affects the education of the next generation as well. The younger generation of doctors and radiologists has less expertise in using US and x-rays, and they are also less confident in their ability to diagnose certain illnesses using those imaging modalities. Understanding that not all imaging modalities are appropriate in all circumstances is crucial. One of the most accessible, affordable, and patient-friendly imaging modalities is US. It has no serious negative effects and is safe to use during pregnancy and pediatric imaging. Because of its non-invasiveness, enhanced sensitivity, and repeatability, ultrasound is also increasingly important in emergencies. Diagnosis is possible with ultrasonography, even at the patient's bedside. Additionally, it shields the patient from ionizing radiation. Even though simple x-rays and ultrasound are more affordable and widely accessible imaging modalities, their ability to capture fine details is sometimes compromised. The high resolution provided by a CT scan allows for information that an ultrasound would miss [39].

## 2.6 Conclusion

Imaging techniques related to radiation medicine continue to be important for managing cancer, achieving earlier diagnosis, more precise staging, and consequently more precise treatment planning and decisions, as well as monitoring the effects of treatment. CT scanning and, when suitable, MRI will continue to be the first-choice modalities among these. One of the developments in this field over the past ten years is PET. The development of PET from a strictly scientific means of examining significant physiological variables to an imaging modality with established utility in clinical practice was a long and winding road. In recent years, the introduction of hybrid devices—such as PET-CT scanners—has rendered this approach vital for the treatment of cancer. Because of cost and resolution issues, it will not replace CT as the first-line investigation, but it appears to be very useful when CT scans cannot reveal all the information clinical oncologists need to distinguish between tumor masses and benign lesions, identify cancerous cells invading lymph nodes, distinguish residual tumor from scarring and necrosis, and find undiscovered distant metastases that could influence a patient's prognosis and course of treatment. The 'molecular imaging revolution' will be sparked by PET's capacity to study diseases at the molecular level, which will facilitate early cancer detection, the characterization of medical problems, and the efficient treatment of a wide range of illnesses. Furthermore, it serves as a useful instrument for tracking the efficacy of treatment plans in a more customized approach to patient care.

# References

[1] Altintas Z, Uludag Y, Gurbuz Y and Tothill I E 2011 Surface plasmon resonance based immunosensor for the detection of the cancer biomarker carcinoembryonic antigen *Talanta* **86** 377–83

[2] Del Sol A, Balling R, Hood L and Galas D 2010 Diseases as network perturbations *Curr. Opin. Biotechnol.* **21** 566–71

[3] Fong Z V and Winter J M 2012 Biomarkers in pancreatic cancer: diagnostic, prognostic, and predictive *Cancer J.* **18** 530–8

[4] Chatterjee S K and Zetter B R 2005 Cancer biomarkers: knowing the present and predicting the future *Future Oncol.* **1** 37–50

[5] Kumar S, Mohan A and Guleria R 2006 Biomarkers in cancer screening, research and detection: present and future: a review *Biomarkers* **11** 385–405

[6] Verma M and Srivastava S 2003 New cancer biomarkers deriving from NCI early detection research *Tumor Prevent. Genetics* **163** 72–84

[7] Rusling J F, Kumar C V, Gutkind J S and Patel V 2010 Measurement of biomarker proteins for point-of-care early detection and monitoring of cancer *Analyst* **135** 2496–511

[8] Pulumati A, Pulumati A, Dwarakanath B S, Verma A and Papineni R V 2023 Technological advancements in cancer diagnostics: improvements and limitations *Cancer Rep.* **6** e1764

[9] Keetile T P 2019 Image quality optimization and radiation dose minimization in bone x-ray radiography *Doctoral Dissertation* North-West University, South Africa

[10] Lewis R 1997 Medical applications of synchrotron radiation x-rays *Phys. Med. Biol.* **42** 1213

[11] Zhou Y, Han Z, Dou F and Yan T 2021 Pre-colectomy location and TNM staging of colon cancer by the computed tomography colonography: a diagnostic performance study *World J. Surg. Oncol.* **19** 1–13

[12] Wang X, Liu D, Zeng X, Jiang S, Li L, Yu T and Zhang J 2021 Dual-energy CT quantitative parameters for evaluating immunohistochemical biomarkers of invasive breast cancer *Cancer Imaging* **21** 1–10

[13] Booij R, Budde R P, Dijkshoorn M L and van Straten M 2020 Technological developments of x-ray computed tomography over half a century: user's influence on protocol optimization *Eur. J. Radiol.* **131** 109261

[14] Bockisch A, Freudenberg L S, Schmidt D and Kuwert T 2009 Hybrid imaging by SPECT/CT and PET/CT: proven outcomes in cancer imaging *Semin. Nucl. Med.* **39** 276–89

[15] Jadvar H, Colletti P M, Delgado-Bolton R, Esposito G, Krause B J, Iagaru A H and Griffeth L 2017 Appropriate use criteria for 18F-FDG PET/CT in restaging and treatment response assessment of malignant disease *J. Nucl. Med.* **58** 2026–37

[16] Lu R C, She B, Gao W T, Ji Y H, Xu D D, Wang Q S and Wang S B 2019 Positron-emission tomography for hepatocellular carcinoma: current status and future prospects *World J. Gastroenterol.* **25** 4682

[17] Rager O, Nkoulou R, Exquis N, Garibotto V, Tabouret-Viaud C, Zaidi H and Ratib O 2017 Whole-body SPECT/CT versus planar bone scan with targeted SPECT/CT for metastatic workup *BioMed Res. Int.* **2017**

[18] Krasil'nikov V A 1963 *Sound and Ultrasound Waves* (Washington, DC: NASA)

[19] Hanson L G and Groth T 2009 Introduction to magnetic resonance imaging techniques. In Clinical and research applications of diagnostic imaging techniques: MR, PET, SPECT, CT and ultrasound *PhD Course* University of Copenhagen, Copenhagen, Denmark

[20] Gambhir S S 2002 Molecular imaging of cancer with positron emission tomography *Nat. Rev. Cancer* **2** 683–93

[21] Vaquero J J and Kinahan P 2015 Positron emission tomography: current challenges and opportunities for technological advances in clinical and preclinical imaging systems *Annu. Rev. Biomed. Eng.* **17** 385–414

[22] Hillner B E, Siegel B A, Liu D, Shields A F, Gareen I F, Hanna L and Coleman R E 2008 Impact of positron emission tomography/computed tomography and positron emission tomography (PET) alone on expected management of patients with cancer: initial results from the National Oncologic PET Registry *J. Clin. Oncol.* **26** 2155–61

[23] Holly T A, Abbott B G, Al-Mallah M, Calnon D A, Cohen M C, DiFilippo F P and Soman P 2010 Single photon-emission computed tomography *J. Nucl. Cardiol.* **17** 941–73

[24] Luker G D and Luker K E 2008 Optical imaging: current applications and future directions *J. Nucl. Med.* **49** 1–4

[25] Weissleder R and Ntziachristos V 2003 Shedding light onto live molecular targets *Nat. Med.* **9** 123–8

[26] Montet X, Ntziachristos V, Grimm J and Weissleder R 2005 Tomographic fluorescence mapping of tumor targets *Cancer Res.* **65** 6330–6

[27] Torigian D A, Huang S S, Houseni M and Alavi A 2007 Functional imaging of cancer with emphasis on molecular techniques *CA: Cancer J. Clin.* **57** 206–24

[28] Fass L 2008 Imaging and cancer: a review *Mol. Oncol.* **2** 115–52

[29] Logothetis N K, Pauls J, Augath M, Trinath T and Oeltermann A 2001 Neurophysiological investigation of the basis of the fMRI signal *Nature* **412** 150–7

[30] Mitchell E L and Furey P 2011 Prevention of radiation injury from medical imaging *J. Vasc. Surg.* **53** 22S–7S

[31] ICRP 2007 The 2007 recommendations of the International Commission on Radiological Protection. ICRP publication 103 *Ann. ICRP* **37** 1–332

[32] Srinivasan D, Than K D, Wang A C, La Marca F, Wang P I, Schermerhorn T C and Park P 2014 Radiation safety and spine surgery: systematic review of exposure limits and methods to minimize radiation exposure *World Neurosurg.* **82** 1337–43

[33] Greuter M, Meijne E, de Jong J R and Tukker W 2017 Radiation safety in patients *Quality in Nuclear Medicine* (Berlin: Springer) pp 131–50

[34] Clark L C and Lyons C 1962 Electrode systems for continuous monitoring in cardiovascular surgery *Ann. N. Y. Acad. Sci.* **102** 29–45

[35] Kim J *et al* 2015 Wearable salivary uric acid mouthguard biosensor with integrated wireless electronics *Biosens. Bioelectron.* **74** 1061–8

[36] Pundir C S and Chauhan N 2012 Acetylcholinesterase inhibition-based biosensors for pesticide determination: a review *Anal. Biochem.* **429** 19–31

[37] Peng F, Su Y, Zhong Y, Fan C, Lee S T and He Y 2014 Silicon nanomaterials platform for bioimaging, biosensing, and cancer therapy *Acc. Chem. Res.* **47** 612–23

[38] Shen M Y, Li B R and Li Y K 2014 Silicon nanowire field-effect-transistor based biosensors: from sensitive to ultra-sensitive *Biosens. Bioelectron.* **60** 101–11

[39] Sang S, Wang Y, Feng Q, Wei Y, Ji J and Zhang W 2015 Progress of new label-free techniques for biosensors: a review *Crit. Rev. Biotechnol.* **15** 1–17

**IOP** Publishing

Nano Biosensors for Non-Invasive Diagnosis of Cancer

**Nidhi Puranik and Shiv Kumar Yadav**

# Chapter 3

# Invasive and non-invasive techniques and their challenges in the early detection of cancer

**Rashmi Gupta, Bimal Prasad Jit, Alisha Behara, Rohit Kumar Singh and Ashok Sharma[1]**

Cancer is a leading cause of mortality worldwide. The phenotype is the second leading cause of death before 70 years of age. Identification of aggressive tumors at an earlier stage can enable more effective treatment as well as a better survival rate. At later disease stages, surgery is less effective, radiotherapy and chemo-therapeutic drugs are often more toxic, and late diagnosis results in a poorer patient outcome. The current clinical detection techniques, such as blood markers CA-125, HE4, CT-45, ultrasound, mammography, colonoscopy, bronchoscopy, magnetic resonance imaging (MRI), positron emission tomography/computer tomography (PET/CT) scans, x-ray, biopsy, and other potential tumor-specific biofluids (liquid biopsy) are used routinely for determining patient's treatment protocol, and some of these are invasive. The widespread availability of CT and MRI has allowed the incidental detection of lesions within the body and contributed to the detection of many malignancies. Evidence suggests that the implementation of radiographic procedures may contribute to tumor aggressiveness and be associated with excessive bleeding, infection, and scarring. Moreover, these techniques are more expensive and can increase patient expenditure. Therefore, it is highly crucial to adopt, develop, and implement a non-invasive technological approach for the detection of cancer malignancy. Furthermore, the multi-cancer detection assay (MCD), a precision medicine approach, needs to be implemented for better diagnostic outcomes in the clinical setting.

## 3.1 Introduction

Half the battle in the fight against cancer is won through early diagnosis. Identifying cancer in its initial stages substantially improves the five-year survival rate and often

---

[1] Corresponding author.

allows for a less aggressive treatment approach [1]. However, conventional imaging techniques and morphologic analysis of tissues or cells have limitations when it comes to achieving early cancer diagnosis. Numerous cancer types are often identified at a later stage, which results in few options for therapy and a poor prognosis [2]. The early detection of cancer holds the potential to significantly enhance survival rates. Conversely, this approach poses certain difficulties, which include the risk of overtreatment and overdiagnosis, potentially causing harm to patients who may not have developed apparent malignancy. The effectiveness of cancer treatment and the likelihood of survival drastically improve in the early phases of cancer detection. However, approximately half of all cancers are identified at a later stage [3]. Improving early detection techniques could increase survival rates by a significant margin. While recent advancements in early detection have already achieved better efficiency, ongoing development and the innovations of new approaches for early cancer detection remain imperative [4]. The field is evolving rapidly, due to the acceleration of technological advancements and improvements in our understanding of biological processes. Research and development efforts in early cancer detection have yielded significant health benefits, as evidenced by established screening approaches for colorectal, breast, and cervical cancers. These screening methods have contributed to a notable decrease in the frequency of later stage diagnoses compared to cancers without established screening protocols. Despite these successes, certain cancers, including esophageal, pancreatic, and ovarian cancers, continue to be frequently diagnosed at advanced stages, leading to exceptionally poor prognoses [5]. Even though early identification increases survival in all populations, around 70% of cancer fatalities occur in low- and middle-income countries, frequently as a result of delayed diagnosis.

Even though there are efficient early detection tests for several cancers, the mortality rates from these diseases are significantly higher in low-human development index (HDI) countries than in high-HDI countries. For example, cervical cancer shows a substantial disparity in mortality rates (19.8 versus 3.1 deaths per 100 000) between low and high-HDI countries. In contrast, cancers without reliable early detection tests, such as stomach cancer, demonstrate smaller differences in mortality rates (5.0 versus 4.0 deaths per 100 000) [6]. Moreover, advanced-stage cancer detection is a worldwide issue, intensified in countries with limited resources, emphasizing major equity concerns [6]. Late-stage diagnoses can lead to missed opportunities for curative interventions, and the subsequent expensive systemic treatments can have negative side effects and poorer outcomes.

## 3.2 Early detection strategies in cancer

### 3.2.1 Breast cancer

Breast cancer holds the unfortunate distinction of being the most lethal among all cancer types globally, with the highest mortality rate among women in the Arabic region. This critical issue can be mitigated through prevention and improved patient survival, particularly with early diagnosis [7]. This form of cancer develops when certain breast cells start growing abnormally [8]. Currently, due to advancements in early detection, survival rates have increased and the number of deaths attributed to this disease is consistently decreasing. Until now mammography has been the paramount imaging method for detecting breast alterations, boasting a sensitivity close to 90%. However, it is crucial to recognize that the majority of breast lumps are benign (non-cancerous), while only some are cancerous. Malignant tumors can spread throughout the body, and damage nearby normal tissues, but benign tumors typically grow slowly and do not spread. However, problems occur when individuals have dense breasts or are young, which reduces the quality of mammograms [9]. On the other hand, women's breasts that are going through parenchymal tissue involution as they approach menopause provide better image quality and definition. In the medical field, a significant portion of diagnoses relies on imaging. Also image processing is dedicated to developing procedures for extracting information from images suitable for computational processing. Radiology, which encompasses a spectrum from the conventional approach to the latest approaches such as nuclear medicine, positron emission tomography, mammography, computed tomography, ultrasound, magnetic resonance, and radiotherapy, provides better prognosis and therapeutic support in cancer diagnosis [10].

As early breast lesions are identified, fewer mastectomies are performed, and survival rates rise. Despite being the 'gold standard' for identifying breast cancer, mammography has limited specificity and high sensitivity, which can result in false-positive results and needless biopsies.

### 3.2.2 Ovarian cancer

Ovarian cancer (OC) is one of the most common causes of gynecological cancer-related death worldwide in women. Most often OC affects post-menopausal women who present abdominal discomfort and bloating over a few months before detection [11]. Because the disease is usually asymptomatic in its early stages, the majority of individuals are diagnosed when the disease has progressed. Among all types of OC, epithelial ovarian cancer (EOC) accounts for around 90% of overall cases. Cancer antigen-125 (CA-125) analysis and transvaginal imaging such as ultrasound, MRI imaging, and CT scans are standard components of ovarian cancer diagnosis [13]. CA-125, a blood biomarker, is widely used, but its lack of sensitivity or specificity prevents it from being used alone as a screening test. This biomarker is not particularly useful for early diagnosis as its expression levels are often too low for accurate detection at early stages [14]. Additionally, high CA-125 levels can be connected with several other conditions, such as endometriosis, gall bladder disease, and liver cancer, leading to false-positive results. Transvaginal imaging also faces challenges in detecting small early-stage tumors [15]. Consequently, the diagnosis of ovarian cancer often necessitates invasive techniques such as laparoscopy and tissue biopsies. In treatment, the primary and most widely used approach to treating OC is a combination of surgery and chemotherapy [12]. Usually, surgery is performed to remove the cancer mass after a diagnosis, but in cases where the cancer has reached an advanced stage, surgery may not be as effective as in the early stages.

To address the limitations of current techniques, various approaches have been proposed. Recently research has focused on smaller molecules, such as circulating microRNA (miRNA) and cell-free DNA (cfDNA), which have garnering significant attention. These molecules are potential cancer biomarkers [16, 17].

### 3.2.3 Lung cancer

Lung cancer, or bronchogenic carcinoma, specifically refers to tumors that originate in the lung parenchyma (the tissue of the lung) or within the bronchi (the main air passages in the lungs). Lung cancer is a type of cancer that can be broadly classified into two main types: small cell lung cancer (SCLC) and non-small cell lung cancer (NSCLC), each with different subtypes [20]. It is a leading cause of cancer-related deaths worldwide, and early detection is crucial for improving treatment outcomes. Less than 15% of cases of lung cancer are cured, and the morbidity rate is significantly high. If a tumor is excised without any lymph nodes or distant metastases, surgery may be the best option for the treatment of lung cancer [18]. However, many patients are still at risk for local relapse, distant metastasis, and the formation of successive primary tumors after complete resection. The majority of individuals with lung cancer are diagnosed at a late stage. Smoking-related issues, such as chronic obstructive pulmonary disease (COPD) and poor cardiovascular status, can limit the ability to implement the best treatment strategies due to unacceptable morbidity and mortality [19].

The utilization of biomolecular markers, techniques such as autofluorescence bronchoscopy, low-dose spiral and high-resolution computed tomography, endobronchial ultrasonography, optical coherence tomography, confocal micro-endoscopy, and positron emission tomography in combination with video-assisted thoracic surgery, and intraluminal bronchoscopic treatments represent a diverse set of modalities that may offer new approaches to managing lung cancer at its earliest stage. These advanced diagnostic and imaging technologies play a crucial role in early detection, accurate diagnosis, and the development of effective treatment strategies for lung cancer [21, 22].

The combined use of more accurate and minimally invasive diagnostic and treatment techniques may justify screening efforts and contribute to reducing the mortality associated with lung cancer. Advances in these technologies offer the potential for earlier detection, which is critical for improving outcomes and increasing the effectiveness of interventions in lung cancer. Fundamental to cancer development are alterations in DNA, encompassing mutational and copy-number changes. These alterations include driver mutations that play a significant role in regulating passenger mutations and tumor biology that are phenotypically silent, yet common in lung cancer. The mutation rate is further accelerated by smoking, the primary risk factor for lung cancer. Mutational and epigenetic alterations in DNA lead to changes in messenger RNA (mRNA), miRNA (a non-coding RNA that regulates gene expression), and proteins. Detection of mRNA is challenging due to its instability in circulation caused by the presence of RNase, making miRNA more promising for the early detection of lung cancer [23, 24].

### 3.2.4 Prostate cancer

The second most prevalent cause of cancer-related deaths in males is prostate carcinoma, which is not always fatal. From being asymptomatic to quickly progressing systemic cancer, PC has a diverse form of heterogeneity [25]. Because of its extreme prevalence, prostate cancer may just be viewed as a typical aging condition. Despite its high prevalence, the incidence and mortality rates of prostate cancer exhibit distinct patterns [26]. Epidemiological estimates suggest that one in six men will receive a diagnosis of prostate cancer, yet the anticipated mortality rate is considerably lower at one in 36. This divergence could be attributed to the predominant diagnosis of prostate cancer among the elderly population [27]. Furthermore, the generally favorable prognosis associated with this malignancy may contribute to the observed lower mortality rate, as individuals often succumb to other causes before symptomatic manifestations of prostate cancer become apparent [28]. Conventional methods such as ultrasound, the prostate-specific antigen (PSA) test, MRI, CT, and nuclear medicine are unable to identify early-stage disease and offer limited insights into disease staging. However, there is ongoing research into several promising emerging techniques, either as standalone approaches or in combination with conventional imaging methods [29].

To address the challenge of prostate cancer, the integration of new biomarkers capable of offering prognostic insights into disease severity and predicting treatment responses is essential. Consequently, initiatives have been undertaken to enhance our understanding of the genetic aspects of prostate cancer and to find new prognostic biomarkers using assays based on tissue and serum. Imaging probes can also be used to target some of these biomarkers. Prostate cancer patients have been found to have notable genetic abnormalities, such as TMPRSS2-ERG gene fusion and CpG hypermethylation of GSPT1. As prospective techniques for detection and prognostication, assessments are ongoing which include the detection of RNA biomarkers (e.g. PCA3) in blood and urine and the examination of prostate cancer tissue-specific proteins using antibodies (e.g. EPCA). As a result, it is still difficult to forecast the biological ferocity of prostate cancer [30, 31]. However, because of the disease's high incidence, ease of diagnosis, aging population, and treatment-related side effects, it is crucial to be able to identify aggressive forms from benign forms of cancer.

### 3.2.5 Endometrial cancer

Endometrial cancer (EC) is one of the most prevalent cancers of the female reproductive system, and its global rate of incidence is on the rise [32]. Despite the poor prognosis associated with advanced EC, early diagnosis could significantly enhance long-term patient outcomes [33]. In 2020 there were 417 367 new diagnoses of EC, resulting in 97 370 mortalities worldwide [34]. Globally, there has been a noticeable increase in the incidence and fatality rates of EC, and over the next ten years, this trend is anticipated to continue. If detected early on, EC is thought to have a good prognosis. Patients with stage I EC may have a five-year survival rate of 80%–90%, whereas it drops to 50%–65% for stage III and further to 15%–17% for stage IV. Given the correlation between early diagnosis and improved prognosis, early detection and precise therapeutics play pivotal roles in EC management. Furthermore, early detection can significantly decrease the necessity for widespread invasive procedures or adjuvant treatments during follow-up therapy, which can reduce the costs, mortality, and morbidity associated with the disease [35].

The primary focus of early detection efforts for EC is on high-risk individuals, such as those with obesity, Lynch syndrome, metabolic syndrome, lifetime exposure to unopposed estrogen, and those displaying indications indicative of EC (e.g. persistent or recurrent uterine bleeding, abnormal post-menopausal bleeding). Sadly, no precise and trustworthy early screening test for EC exists at this time that can be used to prioritize high-risk women who may have EC [36]. With an elevated negative predictive accuracy (99%), transvaginal ultrasonography (TVU), the widely used technology, is a reasonable first step towards early EC detection. For conclusively ruling out endometrial cancer, however, its rather low specificity requires further testing. Although endometrial biopsy is a cost-effective procedure, common risks include pain and false-negative results. Endometrial biopsy under hysteroscopy, while considered less aggressive, can be associated with vasovagal episodes and pain, contributing to potential disappointment in the procedure. As a result, there is an urgent need for precise and less invasive methods for EC early diagnosis. Promising directions for investigation include uterine lavage, the least-invasive extraction of peripheral blood, cervicovaginal fluid, and other possible tumor-specific biofluids. Gene sequencing applied to these biofluids can enable the detection of tumorigenic DNA, potentially leading to the early identification of tumors and facilitating early diagnosis of EC. The integration of minimally invasive methods with gene sequencing technologies represents a current research hotspot and a future developmental direction to address the challenges associated with early diagnosis of EC [37].

Using blood samples is a well-established and widely acknowledged method for early cancer diagnosis. However, the search for an appropriate serum biomarker for the diagnosis of an early form of EC has been challenging due to low concentrations of samples and unsatisfactory accuracy. As of now, HE4 can offer some guidance when diagnosing EC. As a result, scientists are now more interested in the gene data about circulating tumor components in the blood, such as circulating tumor cells, circulating miRNAs, plasma cfDNA, and circulating tumor DNA (ctDNA) [38]. Numerous investigations with the density of cfDNA in individuals with EC and benign gynecologic disorders have shown that ECs typically have higher amounts of cfDNA than patients with benign problems. Furthermore, in high-grade EC, the rise in cfDNA levels is more noticeable [39–41]. Two possible options for detecting EC early have emerged: plasma cfDNA, which is released into the bloodstream by dying cells, and ctDNA, which is the cfDNA fraction produced from tumors. In one study, 48 EC patients had their ctDNA tested using a four-gene panel (KRAS, CTNNB1, PTEN, and PIK3CA); in 33 of the patients, somatic mutations consistent with tumor tissue were found. This implies that ctDNA testing may play a potential role in the early identification of EC [42].

However, there is currently no agreement on efficient early detection methods for EC, and the diagnostic procedures that are already in use, such as hysteroscopy, transvaginal ultrasound, and endometrial biopsy, are invasive, expensive, and have low specificity. As a result, the need for precise and minimally invasive screening technologies that can identify EC early on is critical. Research is still ongoing and has produced breakthroughs in new approaches to early EC identification in a variety of domains.

### 3.2.6 Oral cancer

Oral cancer is a prevalent type of cancer, particularly in countries with low- and middle-incomes, characterized by a significant effect on patients' quality of life after treatment. This kind of cancer affects the lips, cheeks, tongue, neck, and other areas of the mouth. Improving results and lessening the impact of cancer of the oral cavity on afflicted persons depend heavily on early detection and timely treatment [43]. The World Health Organization (WHO) 2020 report states that the global age-standardized incidence rate of cancer in the oral cavity, which includes the lips, is 4.1 per 100 000 irrespective of gender and age. In India, approximately 135 000 new instances and 75 000 fatalities from oral cancer were recorded in 2020 (roughly one-third of all cases and deaths worldwide) and thus oral cancer poses a serious public health concern [44]. Substantial prevalence of tobacco use, with nearly one-third of all adults in India consuming tobacco, according to the most recent Global Adult Tobacco Survey—contributes to the endemic character of oral cancer in the vicinity [45]. Organized screening initiatives are missing in many parts of India, despite evidence showing that monitoring for oral cancer can considerably reduce fatalities, especially in high-risk populations such as tobacco users and excessive alcohol consumers. The conventional methods of assessing risk involve histology, unstimulated and stimulated morning saliva, brush biopsy, and ctDNA, which is an non-invasive procedure that has a strong prognostic correlation [46]. Thus, fewer intrusive methods are necessary. The aided optical examination of the oral cavity may provide a rapid, painless, and economical assessment that can be incorporated into standard medical procedures, either in place of or in addition to sample-based diagnosis. Optical approaches stand out among other procedures because they are simple to use, safe, and have already been used in dentistry. Within this framework, optical coherence tomography (OCT), Raman techniques, and fluorescence are regarded as the most promising technologies. These optical methods can offer insightful information about oral cancer, facilitating initial identification and enhancing results [47].

### 3.2.7 Pancreatic cancer

Pancreatic cancer is commonly detected as an advanced condition, often with symptoms indicative of late-stage disease. As a result, only 10%–20% of patients with newly discovered pancreatic ductal adenocarcinoma (PDAC) qualify for a potentially effective upfront resection. In pancreatic cancer studies, early identification is regarded as a vital goal since it would greatly influence and enhance survival rates [49]. By 2030, PDAC is expected to rank second in terms of cancer-related deaths due to its increasing occurrence. Significant improvements in peri-operative

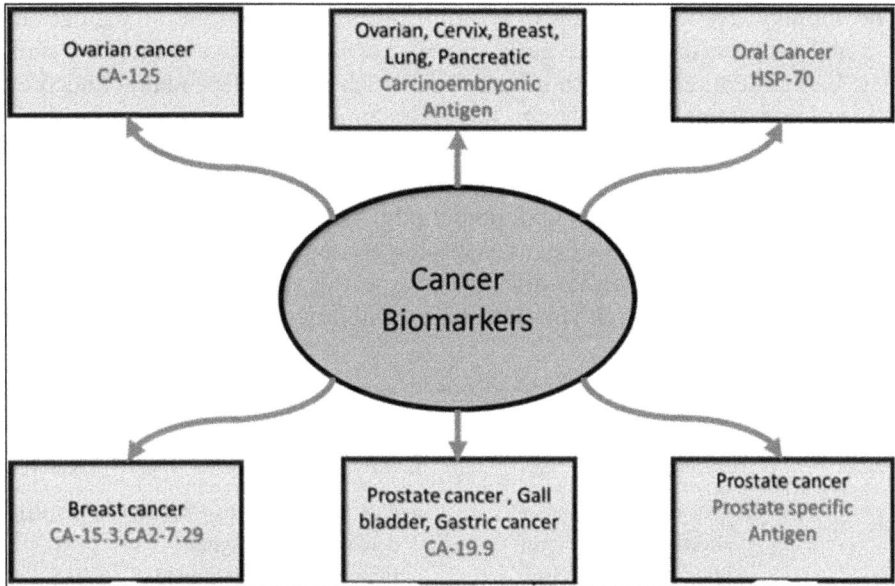

**Figure 3.1.** Potential biomarker expression associated with different cancers.

care and surgical technique over the past few decades have helped to lower the incidence of significant morbidity and death after pancreatic resection [50].

An excellent test with high specificity and sensitivity that is non-invasive, reproducible, and inexpensive would be ideal for the early identification of PDAC. A test like this could be used to identify pre-malignant high-grade dysplasia or even early-stage PDAC that is treatable [51]. Widespread CT surveillance is not feasible since the initial stages of pancreatic cancer are difficult to detect with conventional imaging. On the other hand, new developments in the domains of machine learning and radiomics—the extraction of particular data from imaging scans—have shown encouraging outcomes. Serum carbohydrate antigen (CA) 19-9 sampling was utilized in high-grade dysplasia or pancreatic cancer, according to a recent investigation. For patients with PDAC, the most often used blood-based protein marker at the moment is CA 19-9 (figure 3.1). Conversely, benign diseases and extra-pancreatic cancer patients may also have increased levels of this marker [52].

## 3.3 Invasive approaches and their implication in cancer

Early cancer diagnosis involves a variety of indicators that may not always be directly related to the cancer cells themselves, and this can be accomplished through the use of innovative technology and numerous screening methods that are currently in use. The biochemical signals of a malignant tumor change as the lesion develops. In the early stages, sources not directly linked to the tumor, such as the immune response, play a dominant role [53].

The immune response significantly contributes to the initiation regulation of tumor and progression. Because early tumors are small, there are very few tumor-related biomarkers released into circulation, which makes dependable and precise identification extremely difficult. On the other hand, systemic, non-tumor-derived biomarkers are more frequent in cancer [54]. Existing imaging methods, such as MRI, PET, and CT, possess sensitivities that only allow detection once thousands of cancer cells have proliferated and potentially spread (table 3.1). The ongoing development and translation of nanotechnology-based imaging contrast agents for conventional imaging modalities offer the prospect of specifically targeting tumors and significantly enhancing *in vivo* detection capabilities [55]. Additionally, current

**Table 3.1.** A summary of imaging techniques with their advantages and disadvantages.

| Invasive technique | Advantages | Disadvantages | References |
|---|---|---|---|
| PET | • Can be carried out in addition to a CT scan to offer anatomical and functional data.<br>• Has the potential to be useful in diagnosing malignant lesions that traditional imaging may have missed.<br>• Analyzes metastases more correctly through lymph nodes than traditional imaging does. | • Can be difficult to effectively detect small malignant tumors due to its limited spatial resolution.<br>• Radiation exposure from intravenous radioactive compound injection. | [57–60] |
| MRI | • In-depth imaging of soft tissues.<br>• Absence of exposure to ionizing radiation.<br>• Can gather data on biology, anatomy, physiology, and metabolism. | • Takes a lot of time.<br>• Expensive.<br>• Insufficient information on anatomy. | [57, 58, 61] |
| Mammography | • The gold standard for identifying patients with breast cancer.<br>• Adequate as a breast cancer screening technique.<br>• Mammary gland calcification can be discovered. | • Not appropriate for anyone under 40.<br>• Not appropriate for individuals with high gland density.<br>• A maximum of twice a year. | [62, 63] |

*(Continued)*

**Table 3.1.** (*Continued*)

| Invasive technique | Advantages | Disadvantages | References |
|---|---|---|---|
| X-rays | • Often entail only little ionizing radiation.<br>• A preliminary screening instrument that aids in locating questionable lesions. | • Lacks specificity in differentiating between benign and malignant abnormalities, and may be insensitive to tiny or early-stage lesions. | [64] |
| Ultrasound | • Provides effective real-time imaging of soft tissues.<br>• Detecting inflammation of the mammary glands. | • Unsuitable for unusual tissues and tiny masses.<br>• Influenced by the medical examiner.<br>• There is not much definition or resolution. | [62, 65] |
| CT scan | • A quick scan that may help reduce motion artefacts.<br>• Radiographs that have been digitally rebuilt using cortical bone information.<br>• Precise spatial data. | • Inadequate imaging of soft tissues.<br>• Radiation exposure.<br>• Absence of functional information. | [57, 58] |

nanoscale imaging platforms are facilitating the utilization of innovative imaging techniques not traditionally employed in cancer diagnosis and treatment, including Raman spectroscopic imaging, photoacoustic tomography (PAT), and multimodal imaging—utilizing contrast agents designed for multiple imaging techniques simultaneously [56]. Furthermore, nanotechnology plays a pivotal role in creating nanoparticles with the ability to transport several components (such as traditional contrast agents) and compounds targeted tumor cells, hence enabling these imaging systems.

### 3.3.1 Positron emission tomography

Tomographic images, derived from x-ray absorbance, magnetic resonance properties, and ultrasound reflection, employ structural characteristics of tumors for imaging. Of them, positron emission tomography (PET) is a popular approach for the diagnosis of cancer since it focuses on the tumor tissue's functional state. By simultaneously recording two positrons that are annihilated by a pharmaceutical substance that is specifically localized in the tumor tissue and represents the functional condition of the tissue, PET creates images [66–68]. The procedure includes substituting specific nitrogen, oxygen, and carbon isotopes produced in a cyclotron for a hydrogen atom in a target molecule. These isotopes release positrons, and the PET scan records the measurable gamma rays that are released when they collide with tissue electrons [69]. The foundation for clinical decision-making is this complex mechanism, which also supports the three fundamentals (clinical evaluation, imaging studies, and pathological examination to accurately identify, stage, and characterize tumors for effective treatment planning) of cancer diagnosis: 1) physical examination; 2) laboratory tests; 3) imaging/biopsy tests. The National Oncologic PET Registry (NOPR) looked at a prospective cohort study to see how the results of PET scans affected cancer treatment. The Warburg phenomenon, which states that increased glucose utilization is the reason for the elevated metabolic activity seen in cancer cells in order to support ongoing cell growth and division, is the basis for the image produced by the PET scan [70]. This characteristic makes it possible for the positron-emitting 18F to accumulate in the tumor area and function as a tracer for the antimetabolite glucose analogue 2-deoxy-D-glucose (2-DG), which facilitates imaging. Recently introduced hybrid PET-MR systems combine the advantages of both MR and PET imaging modalities in one system. Ongoing instrumentation developments are intended to reduce cross-interference between the MR and PET signals. Furthermore, state-of-the-art PET technologies, including INSIDE in-beam PET scanning for monitoring carbon ion beam therapy, are being developed as novel approaches to cancer treatment. Prominent developments in radiation oncology include the use of PET scans with certain tracers to diagnose and stage different forms of cancer. The use of 18 kDa translocator protein (TSPO) in neurodegenerative diseases and glioblastoma is one instance. By using tracers unique to the TSPO protein, TSPO PET can detect inflammatory hotspots in the brain and provide an early diagnosis of cancer. The identification of the enzyme specific to tissue, i.e. PSMA is useful for prostate cancers. Even with low PSA levels, PSMA PET scans, which use radioactive tracers labeled with gallium or fluorine to target this enzyme, show significant sensitivity in the screening of prostate cancer. Elevated amino acid synthesis, a sign of widespread proliferation of tumor cells, is evaluated with PET imaging agents such as L-methyl-11C-methionine (11C-MET), which quantifies the build-up of methionine in leptomeningeal metastases, gliomas, and breast cancer. However, time limits for PET imaging are imposed by the short half-life of the of 11C-MET. On the other hand, longer half-lives of fluorine-18-labeled amino acids, such as O-18F-fluoromethyl-D-tyrosine (18F-FMT), L-3, 4-dihydroxy-6-18F-fluoro-phenylalanine (18F-DOPA), anti-1-amino-3-18F-fluoro-cyclobutane-1carboxylic acid (18F-FACBC), and O-(2-18F-fluoroethyl)- L-tyrosine (18F-FET), are utilized in clinical settings for PET imaging of different tumors. For instance, 18F-DOPA PET reliably identifies glioblastoma and predicts survival without progression. Research suggests that 18F-FET PET/CT offers supplementary diagnostic data for spinal cord and brain stem gliomas. 18F-FACBC's slow metabolism, which prevents fast accumulation in the bladder, makes it an effective PET imaging agent for prostate tumors. Analogues of thymidine, such as 11C-thymidine, 1-(2'-deoxy-2'-fluoro-1-$\beta$-D-arabinofuranosyl)-thymine (FMAU) and 3'-deoxy-3-18fluorothymidine (18F-FLT), are employed in PET imaging to measure tumor cell proliferation by targeting thymidine uptake during DNA synthesis. This approach offers insights into tumor prognosis and aggressiveness [71].

### 3.3.2 Magnetic resonance spectroscopy

Magnetic resonance spectroscopy (MRS) is a commonly used technique of imaging and employed for the diagnosis of cancers. The difference between MRS and conventional MRI is that the former focuses on the measurement of signals from specific compounds, such as lactate, N-acetylaspartatecarbon, hydrogen, and creatinine, instead of water signals. The introduction of the idea of Larmor frequencies emphasizes that protons in various compounds display multiple frequencies according to the arrangement of the surrounding electrons [72, 73]. The charged particles within the electrons create a magnetic field in response to an external magnetic force, which shifts the frequency of the molecule. Unlike traditional MRI, which produces images of soft tissues, MRS goes beyond by quantifying numerous compounds, including inorganic phosphates, nucleotide triphosphate (NTP) lactate, phosphocreatine (PCr), and phosphate monoesters, Furthermore, MRS provides the information to determine the presence and variable concentrations of these compounds in various target tissues, offering insights that may indicate abnormalities [74]. MRS plays a crucial role in identifying metabolic changes within tumors, including assessing choline proportion with other metabolites. These measurements offer insights into the proliferative abilities and aggressiveness of the cancers. Additionally, MRS can aid in distinguishing between tumor necrosis and tumor reappearances by examining the proportions of these metabolites [73].

### 3.3.3 X-ray computed tomography

Computed tomography (CT) uses a spiral multi-detector with a multi-fan measurement technique that has led to enhanced spatial resolution, eliminating artifacts through high-end reconstruction and noise reduction algorithms. The facilitation of high-resolution CT image reconstruction using photon counting along with artificial intelligence has resulted in a reduction of radiation dose and decreased artifacts. CT scans are often used concurrently with PET scans, resulting in increased accuracy-driven identification and anatomical localization of lesions [75, 76]. While PET scans rely on biochemical reactions within cells to form images with low spatial resolution, CT scans generate high-resolution images that delineate the structural and morphological characteristics of tumors. Additionally, the concurrent use of CT scans corrects for the inherent attenuation observed in PET scans, enhancing both the sensitivity and specificity in the imaging process. CT scans are commonly conducted in conjunction with SPECT scans, a combination known as SPECT/CT hybrid imaging [77].

This fusion of the imaging SPECT/CT hybrid method is implemented for detecting metastasis in cancers with greater affinity for the skeletal system, such as lung, breast, prostate, and carcinomas. Further, a drastic change was observed in the diagnosis of study participants (5.7%) subjected to targeted SPECT/CT imaging. This underscores the enhanced diagnostic capability of whole-body SPECT/CT, particularly in identifying skeletal lesions beyond the axial region [78].

### 3.3.4 Mammography

A mammogram is an x-ray imaging technique used to identify both benign and malignant abnormalities in the breast. This procedure involves applying a small dose of radiation to the compressed breast between two plates, producing detailed x-ray images. Mammograms serve dual purposes for screening and diagnosis [79]. A low-dose energy x-ray process called a mammography, or mastography creates radiographic images of the breast using ionizing radiation. This diagnostic method is employed for both screening and diagnosing individuals, whether they exhibit symptoms (symptomatic) or not (asymptomatic). Approximately 0.4 millisieverts (mSv) or 30 peak kilovoltages (kVp) are administered during mammography for two images of each breast. Traditional two-dimensional mammograms involve compacting the breast and capturing images from both the front and side [80]. Tomosynthesis, also known as three-dimensional mammography, produces x-ray images by capturing several images across the breast in an arc. Several researches have shown that combining 2D and 3D mammography results in noticeably better detection. In mammography, a radiologist reviews the mammogram, looking for abnormal patterns that differ from normal tissues. These patterns may indicate various conditions, including cancerous tumors, non-cancerous masses, or cysts. During the procedure, the breasts are compressed between two firm surfaces to separate overlapping breast tissue and reduce breast thickness [81]. X-ray images are then produced, presenting black-and-white pictures of the breasts on a computer screen. A radiologist examines these images, searching for signs of cancer or other abnormalities. In screening, mammograms aim to detect early signs of breast cancer before symptoms manifest, contributing to decreased mortality through early diagnosis. On the other hand, diagnostic mammograms are used when a woman experiences symptoms, such as a palpable lump in her breast, aiding in the detection and evaluation of breast cancer. After curative treatment of breast cancer, mammography plays an important role as the primary method for examination imaging, detecting 8%–50% of ipsilateral reappearance and 18%–80% of contralateral metachronous cancer through just one scan. According to the clinical procedure, patients should undergo their first post-treatment mammogram one year after the initial mammogram leading to diagnosis, but no earlier than six months after definitive radiation therapy [82].

Recently the US Preventive Services Task Force (USPSTF) issued new mammography screening guidelines, and advised routine screening for women under the age of 50. This marks a departure from its earlier stance, which aligned with American Cancer Society guidelines that advocated for mammography every 1–2 years for all women aged 40 and older. Many researchers concur that regular screening for women diagnosed with initial-stage breast cancer contributes to prolonged survival [83]. Digital mammography, a recent advancement in breast screening, employs the detection of tumor angiogenesis to identify breast cancer. It is utilized as an adjunct tool alongside traditional mammography. This technique involves higher exposure compared to the standard technique because it requires intravenous iodinated contrast injections. When compared to mammography and ultrasound, contrast-enhanced (CE) mammography improves sensitivity and overall performance, which improves detection accuracy [84].

### 3.3.5 Ultrasound

Ultrasound imaging, also known as sonography, is a technique that uses high-frequency sound waves (echoes) to take real-time images of the body's internal structures or tissue [85]. Notably, ultrasound avoids the use of ionizing radiation, distinguishing it from MRI and mammography. The frequency range commonly utilized in medical ultrasound spans from 2 to 18 mHz, significantly surpassing the human hearing range by hundreds of times [85]. During an ultrasound, a transducer is utilized to glide across the skin that is being investigated. Sometimes it fails to pick up on small masses, which could result in false-positive and false-negative readings. It assists in determining the size, shape, and location of the mass, allowing healthcare professionals to assess whether the growth is malignant or benign. By precisely locating the tumor or suspicious mass, ultrasound helps clinicians obtain tissue samples for pathological analysis [62]. It is often used to assess the liver, kidneys, ovaries, and other structures, providing detailed images that aid in the diagnosis and monitoring of cancer.

Doppler ultrasound, a specific type of ultrasound, is used to assess blood flow within vessels. It is a specific method for assessing blood flow in blood arteries using sound waves [86]. In the context of cancer detection, Doppler ultrasound plays a crucial role in assessing the vascularity of tumors, providing valuable information about the blood supply to cancerous tissues [87, 88].

### 3.3.6 X-rays

The chest x-ray (CXR) serves as the initial diagnostic step in the evaluation of suspected lung and breast bone cancer. Its historical significance lies in its widespread availability, technical feasibility, low risk, and cost-effectiveness. CXR has traditionally been a valuable tool in the early detection of lung abnormalities, prompting further investigation when suspicious lesions are identified. Traditional x-ray radiography involves the use of x-ray beams to create two-dimensional images of internal structures. X-rays are directed through the body, and the amount of radiation absorbed by tissues is detected on the other side, creating a shadow-like image on x-ray film or a digital detector. Radiography is commonly used for detecting abnormalities in bones, such as fractures or bone tumors [64, 89].

### 3.3.7 Biopsy

A biopsy is a crucial diagnostic procedure in cancer detection, providing definitive information about the nature of a suspicious mass or lesion. It involves the removal of small tissue from the suspected area for microscope assessment. Biopsies are essential for determining whether a tumor is benign (non-cancerous) or malignant (cancerous), identifying the specific type of cancer, and guiding treatment decisions [90]. Biopsies are typically performed after the identification of a suspicious mass through imaging studies such as ultrasound, CT scans, or MRI. There are several types of biopsies, each tailored to the location and characteristics of the suspected cancer:

### 3.3.7.1 Needle biopsy

#### 3.3.7.1.1 Fine needle aspiration
A thin, hollow needle is used to take out a small tissue sample or fluid from the suspected area. Fine needle aspiration (FNA) is commonly used for accessible masses, such as those in the breast, thyroid, or lymph nodes.

#### 3.3.7.1.2 Core needle biopsy
A larger, hollow needle is used to extract a core of tissue from the tumor. Core needle biopsy is often used for breast and prostate cancers [91].

### 3.3.7.2 Surgical biopsy

#### 3.3.7.2.1 Incisional biopsy
A portion of the tumor is surgically removed for examination. This type of biopsy is often performed when the entire tumor cannot be safely or practically removed.

#### 3.3.7.2.2 Excisional biopsy
The entire tumor, along with a margin of healthy tissue, is surgically removed. Excisional biopsy is more common for smaller tumors that are easily accessible.

#### 3.3.7.2.3 Endoscopic biopsy
A thin tube with a light and camera, is inserted into a body cavity or organ to visualize and collect tissue samples. This type of biopsy is commonly used for gastrointestinal and respiratory cancers [92].

### 3.3.7.3 Bone marrow biopsy

#### 3.3.7.3.1 Bone marrow aspiration and biopsy
A needle is used to withdraw a sample of bone marrow from the hipbone. This procedure is often performed to diagnose blood cancers, such as leukemia and lymphoma [93].

## 3.4 Limitations associated with invasive techniques

### 3.4.1 Positron emission tomography

PET scans are typically more adept at identifying the initial stages of cancer. However, this technique is also frequently employed to assess relapse, particularly in cases of colorectal and lung cancers, melanomas, breast cancer, ovarian cancer and lymphomas. Whole-body PET scans are commonly used to identify metastases in melanomas; nevertheless, they have drawbacks primarily stemming from their restricted field of view (FOV). This significantly contributes to the imaging modality's poor sensitivity. PET scans have demonstrated utility in various types of cancers, including gastrointestinal cancers, head and neck cancers, lung cancers, and pancreatic, esophageal, rectal, and anal cancers. In staging these cancers, PET scans have a potential role in lymph node involvement and identifying areas of malignancy. This information aids in determining the extent of the cancer and guides decisions on the course of treatment. Additionally, PET scans are useful for defining the target volume, determining the size and form of the affected area, and giving a precise picture of the tumor so that treatment may be administered [57, 75].

PET-based imaging faces several clinical limitations, including potential unpredictability between measurements, logistical constraints, inadequate training in machine learning and computational methods, and the absence of suitable statistical procedures for collecting repeatable and reproducible large datasets [66].

### 3.4.2 Magnetic resonance spectroscopy

MRS and MRI are widely utilized imaging techniques for diagnosing various cancers, with their primary application in brain tumor, diagnosis. However, its scope has expanded to include pancreatic, prostate, breast, cervical, and gastrointestinal cancers. MRI and MRS have disadvantages of high false-positive rate, high cost, and time consumption [57, 58, 72].

### 3.4.3 X-ray computed tomography

CT is a valuable imaging method employed for cancer diagnosis, demonstrating effectiveness in screening for colon, lung, head and neck, breast cancers, and prostate cancer. Its ability to provide accurate spatial and temporal tumor imaging proves beneficial for subsequent biopsy procedures, surgery, and radio-chemo-therapy. Technological advancements in CT instrumentation, such as enhanced scan speed, dual-energy, iterative reconstruction, low kilovolt, perfusion imaging, and reduced radiation dose, have heightened its clinical utility in tumor imaging. In a study conducted by Shawky *et al* comparing PET/CT to CT alone in the detection of breast cancer, the sensitivity of PET/CT examinations was 100%, specificity while the sensitivity of CT alone was 81.2%, specificity [57, 58].

### 3.4.4 Mammography

The sensitivity of mammography is influenced by factors such as age, ethnicity, personal history, the experience of the radiologist, and the quality of the imaging technique. Reduced sensitivity may be observed in individuals with high breast density and premenopausal women. Mammography has many drawbacks such as the use of ionizing radiation, not being suitable for subjects with dense breasts, relatively high false-positive and false-negative rates, and uncomfortable examination. Mammography only reduced breast cancer death rates by 0.0004% [62, 63, 79].

### 3.4.5 Ultrasound

Ultrasonography is a cost-effective and widely used screening technique, which detects tumors by reflecting sound waves off tissues. It provides concurrent imaging, enabling clinician to examine dynamic processes within the body, such as organ motion and blood flow. This real-time capability is particularly valuable during interventions, biopsies, and procedures requiring immediate feedback. Ultrasound is generally more cost-effective compared to MRI or CT scans. This makes it a practical choice for routine screening, follow-up assessments, and imaging in resource-limited settings. Ultrasound does not use ionizing radiation, which is a significant advantage over x-ray-based imaging methods. This absence of radiation exposure is particularly beneficial for certain patient populations, including pregnant women and individuals who require frequent imaging. Ultrasound is versatile and can be used to assess various organs and tissues in the body. Its applications range from abdominal and pelvic imaging to breast, thyroid, and musculoskeletal evaluations. This versatility makes it a valuable tool for detecting cancers in different anatomical regions [62, 65, 85]. Additionally, early-stage tumors, especially those smaller than a few millimeters, may be difficult for an ultrasound to identify. This restriction may be important for breast or prostate cancer, which respond best to treatment when found early [62].

### 3.4.6 X-rays

X-ray imaging is widely available in various healthcare settings, making it easily accessible for initial screening and diagnostic purposes. As compared to some advanced imaging modalities, x-ray examinations are generally more cost-effective, making them a practical choice for routine screenings and initial assessments. X-rays are effective in detecting abnormalities in dense structures such as bones and bone metastases (figure 3.2). X-ray imaging may lack sensitivity for detecting small or early-stage lesions, and its specificity in distinguishing between benign and

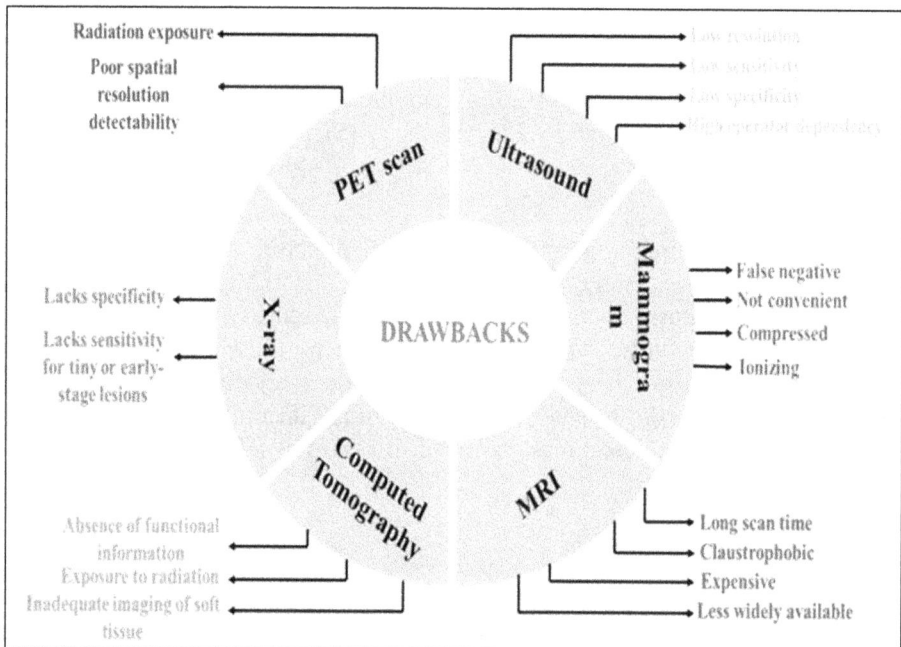

**Figure 3.2.** Disadvantages associated with invasive techniques in cancer.

malignant abnormalities and may not provide detailed morphological information about tumors, such as their size, shape, or precise location [64, 89].

### 3.4.7 Biopsy

Biopsy provides a definitive diagnosis of whether a suspicious mass is benign or malignant, and if malignant, it identifies the specific type of cancer. This information is crucial for determining appropriate treatment strategies, tumor grading, and staging. Biopsies help in grading the tumor (assessing its aggressiveness) and staging cancer (determining the extent of spread). This information is vital for treatment planning and predicting the prognosis. Biopsies are invasive procedures that involve the removal of tissue from the body. Biopsies carry a risk of complications, including bleeding, infection, damage to surrounding structures, or in rare cases, the spread of cancer cells along the biopsy tract. The accuracy of biopsy results depends on the quality and representativeness of the tissue sample collected. There is a possibility of sampling error, where the obtained tissue may not fully represent the entire tumor [90, 91].

## 3.5 Future directions

It is worth considering that, despite the significant advancement in cancer research, the treatment outcomes and survival have not been improved significantly in the last decades for several types of cancer. Early detection, quality healthcare services, and timely diagnosis have been shown to play a significant role in the improvement of prognosis and quality of life with cancer. Early cancer diagnosis involves a variety of indicators that may not always be directly related to the cancer cells themselves, however, can be accomplished through the use of innovative technology and numerous screening methods. Because early tumors are small, there are very few tumor-related biomarkers released into circulation, which makes dependable and precise identification extremely difficult. It is also important to consider that existing imaging methods such as MRI, PET, and CT have sensitivities that only can allow detection once thousands of cancer cells have proliferated and potentially spread [94]. In the last decades, MRI, PET, and CT, histopathology, bioimaging, and ELISA have been shown to possess immense potential in the detection of several malignancies such as cancer and contributed significantly to clinical practice. Given the disadvantages of these techniques, several novel detection strategies have been put forward which exhibit potential clinical benefits.

In the realm of cancer therapeutics, non-invasive technologies are being harnessed for disease treatment and supportive care. In recent years, research has been focused on the development of point-of-care devices to improve and resolve the diagnosis problems for better and easily accessible detection of cancer malignancies. Recently it has been observed that scalp cooling is as a safe and efficient method for targeting chemotherapy-induced alopecia and is regarded as a non-invasive intervention approach in supportive healthcare [95]. Cryotherapy-induced vaso-constriction is a non-invasive approach against chemotherapy-induced side toxicities. Currently, liquid biopsy and circulating tumor biomarkers have been shown to be ideal candidates for identifying several cancers. In addition to the detection of changes specific to tumors, the implementation of digital droplet PCR (ddPCR) and sequencing approaches to detect the ctDNA at a very low level will be an ideal strategy [96]. In addition to this, ctDNA has been shown to predict tumor relapse, suggesting the detection of minimal residual disease. It is also worth noting that cfDNA analysis for chromosomal instability has been proposed as a specific marker for malignancy for patients with adnexal masses over CA-125 and a cancer risk of malignancy index (RMI). For example, it has been observed that detection of TP3 mutation by ddPCR and the next-generation sequencing (NGS) approach is possible in plasma cfDNA in blood and peritoneal fluid [97]. Currently, new alternative techniques,, such as the cancer SEEK multi-analyte blood test which combines ctDNA mutations with traditional biomarkers and growth factors have improved sensitivity [95]. In addition to this, the potential of nanomaterials for the detection of oral and lung cancer it has been observed. Several studies have highlighted the role of different nanomaterials such as metal oxides, graphenes, and polymers. Conducting nanoparticles can be used to improve the optical and electrochemical properties [98]. Further, the integration of nanoparticles with different sensors can show higher stability, sensitivity, and specificity for the detection of ctDNA, cfDNA, circulating tumor cells, mMRA, and miRNA as well as extracellular vesicles (EVs) in several cancer types including ovarian and endometrial cancer [99].

The implication of the epigenetic process is shown to contribute to cancer phenotype [100–104], therefore, deeper insight into the epigenetic-based biomarker approach needs to be explored. In addition to this, a strong foundation should be built up to understand the basic biology and mechanistic understanding of carcinogenesis and risk factor prediction in cancer. Furthermore, a multi-cancer detection (MCD) assay system needs to be developed to detect the multiple signals for several cancers from a single blood sample. Furthermore, more randomized clinical trials need to be carried out that can implicate wearable technology for patient self-monitoring in cancer patients. Ongoing efforts to delve deeper into the biology and genetics of cancer are underway, to develop an effective precision medicine approach. This approach may encompass targeted therapies and immune-based treatments, holding promise for improving outcomes in pancreatic and other cancer patients. Furthermore, more studies should be focused on detecting different malignancies by taking insight from the mechanistic underpinning governing the immunology of cancer.

# References

[1] Loud J T and Murphy J 2017 Cancer screening and early detection in the 21st century *Semin. Oncol. Nurs.* **33** 121–8

[2] Byers T, Wender R C, Jemal A, Baskies A M, Ward E E and Brawley O W 2016 The American Cancer Society challenge goal to reduce US cancer mortality by 50% between 1990 and 2015: results and reflections *CA: Cancer J. Clin.* **66** 359–69

[3] Shieh Y, Eklund M, Sawaya G F, Black W C, Kramer B S and Esserman L J 2016 Population-based screening for cancer: hope and hype *Nat. Rev. Clin. Oncol.* **13** 550–65

[4] Fleshner K, Carlsson S V and Roobol M J 2017 The effect of the USPSTF PSA screening recommendation on prostate cancer incidence patterns in the USA *Nat. Rev. Urol.* **14** 26–37

[5] Esserman L J, Thompson I M, Reid B, Nelson P, Ransohoff D F, Welch H G and Srivastava S 2014 Addressing overdiagnosis and overtreatment in cancer: a prescription for change *Lancet Oncol.* **15** e234–42

[6] Klugman J 2011 Sustainability and equity: a better future for all *UNDP-HDRO Human Development Report*

[7] He Z *et al* 2020 A review on methods for diagnosis of breast cancer cells and tissues *Cell Prolif.* **53** e12822

[8] Ayer T 2015 Inverse optimization for assessing emerging technologies in breast cancer screening *Ann. Oper. Res.* **230** 57–85

[9] Ginsburg O *et al* 2020 Breast cancer early detection: a phased approach to implementation *Cancer* **126** 2379–93

[10] Monticciolo D L, Newell M S, Hendrick R E, Helvie M A, Moy L, Monsees B and Sickles E A 2017 Breast cancer screening for average-risk women: recommendations from the ACR commission on breast imaging *J. Am. Coll. Radiol.* **14** 1137–43

[11] Hossain K R, Escobar Bermeo J D, Warton K and Valenzuela S M 2022 New approaches and biomarker candidates for the early detection of ovarian cancer *Front. Bioeng. Biotechnol.* **10** 819183

[12] Jayson G C, Kohn E C, Kitchener H C and Ledermann J A 2014 Ovarian cancer *Lancet* **384** 1376–88

[13] Nisenblat V, Bossuyt P M, Shaikh R, Farquhar C, Jordan V and Scheffers C SCochrane Gynaecology and Fertility Group 1996 Blood biomarkers for the non-invasive diagnosis of endometriosis *Cochrane Database Syst. Rev.* **2016** CD012179

[14] Wang Y F, Feng F L, Zhao X H, Ye Z X, Zeng H P, Li Z and Peng Z H 2014 Combined detection tumor markers for diagnosis and prognosis of gallbladder cancer *World J. Gastroenterol.: WJG* **20** 4085

[15] Ling H, Fabbri M and Calin G A 2013 MicroRNAs and other non-coding RNAs as targets for anticancer drug development *Nat. Rev. Drug Discov.* **12** 847–65

[16] Peng Y and Croce C M 2016 The role of MicroRNAs in human cancer *Signal Transduct. Target. Ther.* **1** 1–9

[17] Jorgensen M, Bæk R, Pedersen S, Søndergaard E K, Kristensen S R and Varming K 2013 Extracellular vesicle (EV) array: microarray capturing of exosomes and other extracellular vesicles for multiplexed phenotyping *J. Extracell. Vesicles* **2** 20920

[18] Feld R, Rubinstein L V and Weisenberger T H 1984 Sites of recurrence in resected stage I non-small-cell lung cancer: a guide for future studies *J. Clin. Oncol.* **2** 1352–8

[19] Woolner L B, Fontana R S, Cortese D A, Sanderson D R, Bernatz P E, Payne W S and Taylor W F 1984 Roentgenographically occult lung cancer: pathologic findings and frequency of multicentricity during a 10-year period *Mayo Clinic Proceedings* vol **59** (Amsterdam: Elsevier) pp 453–66

[20] Sutedja G 2003 New techniques for early detection of lung cancer *Eur. Respir. J.* **21** 57s–66s

[21] Hayata Y, Kato H, Furuse K, Kusunoki Y, Suzuki S and Mimura S 1996 Photodynamic therapy of 168 early stage cancers of the lung and oesophagus: a Japanese multi-centre study *Lasers Med. Sci.* **11** 255–9

[22] van Boxem T J, Venmans B J, Postmus P E and Sutedja T G 1999 Curative endobronchial therapy in early-stage non-small cell lung cancer *J. Bronchol. Interv. Pulmonol.* **6** 198–206

[23] Bota S, Auliac J B, Paris C, Métayer J, Sesboue R, Nouvet G and Thiberville L 2001 Follow-up of bronchial precancerous lesions and carcinoma *in situ* using fluorescence endoscopy *Am. J. Respir. Crit. Care Med.* **164** 1688–93

[24] Bardelli A and Pantel K 2017 Liquid biopsies, what we do not know (yet) *Cancer Cell* **31** 172–9

[25] Catalona W J 2014 History of the discovery and clinical translation of prostate-specific antigen *Asian J. Urol.* **1** 12

[26] Grossman D C, Curry S J, Owens D K, Bibbins-Domingo K, Caughey A B and Davidson K WUS Preventive Services Task Force 2018 Screening for prostate cancer: US Preventive Services Task Force recommendation statement *JAMA* **319** 1901–13

[27] Kehinde E O, Sheikh M, Mojimoniyi O A, Francis I, Anim J T, Nkansa-Dwamena D and Al-Awadi K A 2003 High serum prostate-specific antigen levels in the absence of prostate cancer in Middle-Eastern men: the clinician's dilemma *BJU Int.* **91** 618–22

[28] Schröder F H, Hugosson J, Roobol M J, Tammela T L, Zappa M, Nelen V and Auvinen A 2014 Screening and prostate cancer mortality: results of the European Randomised Study of Screening for Prostate Cancer (ERSPC) at 13 years of follow-up *Lancet* **384** 2027–35

[29] Ghai S and Haider M A 2015 Multiparametric-MRI in diagnosis of prostate cancer *Indian J. Urol.* **31** 194

[30] Lein , Koenig , Jung , Mcgovern , Skates , Schnorr and Loening 1998 The percentage of free prostate specific antigen is an age-independent tumour marker for prostate cancer: establishment of reference ranges in a large population *Br. J. Urol.* **82** 231–6

[31] Hong S K 2014 Kallikreins as biomarkers for prostate cancer *BioMed Res. Int.* **2014** 526341

[32] Siegel R L, Miller K D, Fuchs H E and Jemal A 2022 Cancer statistics, 2022 *CA: Cancer J. Clin.* **72** 7–33

[33] Sung H, Ferlay J, Siegel R L, Laversanne M, Soerjomataram I, Jemal A and Bray F 2021 Global cancer statistics 2020: GLOBOCAN estimates of incidence and mortality worldwide for 36 cancers in 185 countries *CA: Cancer J. Clin.* **71** 209–49

[34] Sheikh M A, Althouse A D, Freese K E, Soisson S, Edwards R P, Welburn S and Linkov F 2014 USA endometrial cancer projections to 2030: should we be concerned? *Future Oncol.* **10** 2561–8

[35] Makker V, MacKay H, Ray-Coquard I, Levine D A, Westin S N, Aoki D and Oaknin A 2021 Endometrial cancer *Nat. Rev. Dis. Primers* **7** 88

[36] Urick M E and Bell D W 2019 Clinical actionability of molecular targets in endometrial cancer *Nat. Rev. Cancer* **19** 510–21

[37] Dijkhuizen F P H, Mol B W, Brölmann H A and Heintz A P M 2003 Cost-effectiveness of the use of transvaginal sonography in the evaluation of postmenopausal bleeding *Maturitas* **45** 275–82

[38] Morganti S, Tarantino P, Ferraro E, D'Amico P, Viale G, Trapani D, Duso B A and Curigliano G 2019. Complexity of genome sequencing and reporting: next generation sequencing (NGS) technologies and implementation of precision medicine in real life *Crit. Rev. Oncol. Hematol.* **133** 171–82

[39] Bagaria M, Shields E and Bakkum-Gamez J N 2017 Novel approaches to early detection of endometrial cancer *Curr. Opin. Obstet. Gynecol.* **29** 40–6

[40] Lin B, Lei Y, Wang J, Zhu L, Wu Y, Zhang H and Yang C 2021 Microfluidic-based exosome analysis for liquid biopsy *Small Methods* **5** 2001131

[41] Jiang N, Pan J, Fang S, Zhou C, Han Y, Chen J and Gong Z 2019 Liquid biopsy: circulating exosomal long noncoding RNAs in cancer *Clin. Chim. Acta* **495** 331–7

[42] Bolivar A M, Luthra R, Mehrotra M, Chen W, Barkoh B A, Hu P and Broaddus R R 2019 Targeted next-generation sequencing of endometrial cancer and matched circulating tumor DNA: identification of plasma-based, tumor-associated mutations in early stage patients *Mod. Pathol.* **32** 405–14

[43] Gupta B, Bray F, Kumar N and Johnson N W 2017 Associations between oral hygiene habits, diet, tobacco and alcohol and risk of oral cancer: a case–control study from India *Cancer Epidemiol.* **51** 7–14

[44] Laprise C, Shahul H P, Madathil S A, Thekkepurakkal A S, Castonguay G, Varghese I and Nicolau B 2016 Periodontal diseases and risk of oral cancer in Southern India: results from the HeNCe Life study *Int. J. Cancer* **139** 1512–9

[45] Sharma S, Satyanarayana L, Asthana S, Shivalingesh K K, Goutham B S and Ramachandra S 2018 Oral cancer statistics in India on the basis of first report of 29 population-based cancer registries *J. Oral Maxillofac. Pathol.* **22** 18

[46] Borse V, Konwar A N and Buragohain P 2020 Oral cancer diagnosis and perspectives in India *Sens. Int.* **1** 100046

[47] Mangalath U, Aslam S A, Khadar A H K A, Francis P G, Mikacha M S K and Kalathingal J H 2014 Recent trends in prevention of oral cancer *J. Int. Soc. Prev. Community Dent.* **4** S131

[48] Venmans B J, van Boxem T J, Smit E F, Postmus P E and Sutedja G 2000 Outcome of bronchial CIS *Chest* **117** 1472–6

[49] Siegel R L, Miller K D and Jemal A 2020 Cancer statistics, 2020 *CA: Cancer J. Clin.* **70** 7–30

[50] Shakeel S, Finley C, Akhtar-Danesh G, Seow H Y and Akhtar-Danesh N 2020 Trends in survival based on treatment modality in patients with pancreatic cancer: a population-based study *Curr. Oncol.* **27** 1–8

[51] Andrén-Sandberg Å 2012 Prognostic factors in pancreatic cancer *N. Am. J. Med. Sci.* **4** 9

[52] Corral J E, Das A, Bruno M J and Wallace M B 2019 Cost-effectiveness of pancreatic cancer surveillance in high-risk individuals: an economic analysis *Pancreas* **48** 526–36

[53] Pulumati A, Pulumati A, Dwarakanath B S, Verma A and Papineni R V L 2023 Technological advancements in cancer diagnostics: improvements and limitations *Cancer Rep. (Hoboken, N.J.)* **6** e1764

[54] Bi W L, Hosny A, Schabath M B, Giger M L, Birkbak N J, Mehrtash A and Aerts H J 2019 Artificial intelligence in cancer imaging: clinical challenges and applications *CA: Cancer J. Clin.* **69** 127–57

[55] Crosby D, Bhatia S, Brindle K M, Coussens L M, Dive C, Emberton M and Balasubramanian S 2022 Early detection of cancer *Science* **375** eaay9040

[56] Pal S and Singh R K 2023 An overview of phytochemicals under clinical trials for various cancers *Phytochemicals as an Epigenetic Modifier in Cancer Prevention* (Bristol: IOP Publishing) pp 10–1

[57] Frangioni J V 2008 New technologies for human cancer imaging *J. Clin. Oncol.* **26** 4012

[58] Fass L 2008 Imaging and cancer: a review *Mol. Oncol.* **2** 115–52

[59] Padma M V, Jacobs M, Kraus G, Collins M, Dunigan K and Mantil J 2001 11C-methionine PET imaging of leptomeningeal metastases from primary breast cancer—a case report *J. Neurooncol.* **55** 39–44

[60] Lopci E, Nanni C, Castellucci P, Montini G C, Allegri V, Rubello D and Fanti S 2010 Imaging with non-FDG PET tracers: outlook for current clinical applications *Insights Imaging* **1** 373–85

[61] Yoon J, Shin M, Lim J, Lee J Y and Choi J W 2020 Recent advances in MXene nanocomposite-based biosensors *Biosensors* **10** 185

[62] Wang L 2017 Early diagnosis of breast cancer *Sensors* **17** 1572

[63] Lobbes M B I, Smidt M L, Houwers J, Tjan-Heijnen V C and Wildberger J E 2013 Contrast enhanced mammography: techniques, current results, and potential indications *Clin. Radiol.* **68** 935–44

[64] Schulze-Rath R, Hammer G P and Blettner M 2008 Are pre- or postnatal diagnostic x-rays a risk factor for childhood cancer? A systematic review *Radiat. Environ. Biophys.* **47** 301–12

[65] Lee C H, Dershaw D D, Kopans D, Evans P, Monsees B, Monticciolo D and Burhenne L W 2010 Breast cancer screening with imaging: recommendations from the Society of Breast Imaging and the ACR on the use of mammography, breast MRI, breast ultrasound, and other technologies for the detection of clinically occult breast cancer *J. Am. Coll. Radiol.* **7** 18–27

[66] Singh R K, Bhol P, Mandal D and Mohanty P S 2019 Stimuli-responsive photolumines-cence soft hybrid microgel particles: synthesis and characterizations *J. Phys. Condens. Matter* **32** 044001

[67] Gambhir S S 2002 Molecular imaging of cancer with positron emission tomography *Nat. Rev. Cancer* **2** 683–93

[68] Hillner B E, Siegel B A, Liu D, Shields A F, Gareen I F, Hanna L and Coleman R E 2008 Impact of positron emission tomography/computed tomography and positron emission tomography (PET) alone on expected management of patients with cancer: initial results from the National Oncologic PET Registry *J. Clin. Oncol.* **26** 2155–61

[69] Jadvar H, Colletti P M, Delgado-Bolton R, Esposito G, Krause B J, Iagaru A H and Griffeth L 2017 Appropriate use criteria for 18F-FDG PET/CT in restaging and treatment response assessment of malignant disease *J. Nucl. Med.* **58** 2026–37

[70] Qi Y, Liu X, Li J, Yao H and Yuan S 2017 Fluorine-18 labeled amino acids for tumor PET/CT imaging *Oncotarget* **8** 60581

[71] Van de Wiele C, Ustmert S, De Spiegeleer B, De Jonghe P J, Sathekge M and Alex M 2021 Apoptosis imaging in oncology by means of positron emission tomography: a review *Int. J. Mol. Sci.* **22** 2753

[72] Sabbih G, Kulabhusan P K, Singh R K, Jeevanandam J and Danquah M K 2021 Biocomposites for the fabrication of artificial organs *Green Biocomposites for Biomedical Engineering* (Cambridge: Woodhead) pp 301–28

[73] Verma A, Kumar I, Verma N, Aggarwal P and Ojha R 2016 Magnetic resonance spectroscopy—revisiting the biochemical and molecular milieu of brain tumors *BBA Clin.* **5** 170–8

[74] Elmogy S A, Mousa A E, Elashry M S and Megahed A M 2011 MR spectroscopy in post-treatment follow up of brain tumors *Egypt. J. Radiol. Nucl. Med.* **42** 413–24

[75] Zhou Y, Han Z, Dou F and Yan T 2021 Pre-colectomy location and TNM staging of colon cancer by the computed tomography colonography: a diagnostic performance study *World J. Surg. Oncol.* **19** 1–13

[76] Evangelista L, Baretta Z, Vinante L, Sotti G and Muzzio P C 2012 Tumour markers and molecular imaging with FDG PET/CT in breast cancer: their combination for improving

the prediction of disease relapse *Positron Emission Tomography-Current Clinical and Research Aspects* (London: IntechOpen)

[77] Wang X, Liu D, Zeng X, Jiang S, Li L, Yu T and Zhang J 2021 Dual-energy CT quantitative parameters for evaluating immunohistochemical biomarkers of invasive breast cancer *Cancer Imaging* **21** 1–10

[78] Lu R C, She B, Gao W T, Ji Y H, Xu D D, Wang Q S and Wang S B 2019 Positron-emission tomography for hepatocellular carcinoma: current status and future prospects *World J. Gastroenterol.* **25** 4682

[79] Kesh M 2021 Technological advancements in the screening and detection of breast tissue malignancies *Reason-A Tech. J.* **20** 62–83

[80] Mandelblatt J S, Cronin K A, Bailey S, Berry D A, De Koning H J and Draisma GBreast Cancer Working Group of the Cancer Intervention and Surveillance Modeling Network (CISNET) 2009 Effects of mammography screening under different screening schedules: model estimates of potential benefits and harms *Ann. Intern. Med.* **151** 738–47

[81] Nelson H D, Tyne K, Naik A, Bougatsos C, Chan B K and Humphrey L 2009 Screening for breast cancer: an update for the US Preventive Services Task Force *Ann. Intern. Med.* **151** 727–37

[82] Sprague B L, Conant E F, Onega T, Garcia M P, Beaber E F and Herschorn S DProspr Consortium 2016 Variation in mammographic breast density assessments among radiologists in clinical practice: a multicenter observational study *Ann. Intern. Med.* **165** 457–64

[83] Yala A, Lehman C, Schuster T, Portnoi T and Barzilay R 2019 A deep learning mammography-based model for improved breast cancer risk prediction *Radiology* **292** 60–6

[84] Singh R K, Mishra S, Jena S, Panigrahi B, Das B, Jayabalan R, Parhi P K and Mandal D 2018 Rapid colorimetric sensing of gadolinium by EGCG-derived AgNPs: the development of a nanohybrid bioimaging probe *Chem. Commun.* **54** 3981–4

[85] Al-Dhabyani W, Gomaa M, Khaled H and Fahmy A 2020 Dataset of breast ultrasound images *Data in Brief* **28** 104863

[86] Ha R, Kim H, Mango V, Wynn R and Comstock C 2015 Ultrasonographic features and clinical implications of benign palpable breast lesions in young women *Ultrasonography* **34** 66

[87] Signore G, Nifosi R, Albertazzi L, Storti B and Bizzarri R 2010 Polarity-sensitive coumarins tailored to live cell imaging *JACS* **132** 1276–88

[88] Wang X and Yang M 2021 The application of ultrasound image in cancer diagnosis *J. Healthc. Eng.* **2021** 8619251
Journal of Healthcare Engineering 2023 Retracted: The application of ultrasound image in cancer diagnosis *J. Healthc. Eng.* **2023** 9789783 (retraction)

[89] Gillies R J and Schabath M B 2020 Radiomics improves cancer screening and early detection *Cancer Epidemiol. Biomarkers Prev.* **29** 2556–67

[90] Yang G, Wei L, Thong B K S, Fu Y, Cheong I H, Kozlakidis Z, Li X, Wang H and Li X 2022 A systematic review of oral biopsies, sample types, and detection techniques applied in relation to oral cancer detection *Biotech* **11** 5

[91] Ito Y *et al* 2021 Use of core-needle biopsy for the diagnosis of malignant lymphomas in clinical practice *Acta Haematol.* **144** 641–8

[92] Rogalla S and Contag C H 2015 Early cancer detection at the epithelial surface *Cancer J.* **21** 179–87

[93] Singh R K, Panigarhi B and Suryakant U 2023 Development of paper-based assay for detection of miRNA in various diseases *Paper-Based Diagnostic Devices for Infectious Diseases* (Bristol: IOP Publishing) p 8-1

[94] Pulumati A, Pulumati A, Dwarakanath B S, Verma A and Papineni R V 2023 Technological advancements in cancer diagnostics: improvements and limitations *Cancer Rep.* **6** e1764

[95] Wang Y *et al* 2018. Evaluation of liquid from the Papanicolaou test and other liquid biopsies for the detection of endometrial and ovarian cancers *Sci. Transl. Med.* **10** eaap8793

[96] Hudecova I 2015 Digital PCR analysis of circulating nucleic acids *Clin. Biochem.* **48** 948–56

[97] Jahr S *et al* 2001 DNA fragments in the blood plasma of cancer patients: quantitations and evidence for their origin from apoptotic and necrotic cells *Cancer Res.* **61** 1659–65

[98] Mandal D, Singh R K, Maharana U S, Panigrahi B and Mishra S 2021 Microbial gold nanoparticles and their biomedical applications *Microbial Interactions at Nanobiotechnology Interfaces* ed R N Krishnaraj and R K Sani. (Hoboken, NJ: Wiley)

[99] Openshaw M R and McVeigh T P 2020 Non-invasive technology advances in cancer—a review of the advances in the liquid biopsy for endometrial and ovarian cancers *Front. Digit. Health* **2** 573010

[100] Gupta R *et al* 2022 Leveraging epigenetics to enhance the efficacy of cancer-testis antigen: a potential candidate for immunotherapy *Epigenomics* **14** 865–86

[101] Jit B P, Qazi S, Arya R, Srivastava A, Gupta N and Sharma A 2021 An immune epigenetic insight to COVID-19 infection *Epigenomics* **13** 465–80

[102] Jit B P, Bera R and Sharma A 2022 Mechanistic basis of regulation of host epigenetic landscape and its association with immune function: a COVID19 perspective *Epigenetics and Anticipation* (Cham: Springer International) pp 59–75

[103] Gupta R, Jit B P and Sharma A 2022 Epigenetic mediated regulation of cancer-testis/germline antigen and its implication in cancer immunotherapy: a treasure map for future anticipatory medicine *Epigenetics and Anticipation* (Cham: Springer International) pp 149–66

[104] Qazi S, Jit B P, Das A, Karthikeyan M, Saxena A, Ray M D and Sharma A 2022 BESFA: bioinformatics based evolutionary, structural and functional analysis of prostate, placenta, ovary, testis, and embryo (POTE) paralogs *Heliyon* **8** e10476

# Chapter 4

## Insights into noninvasive approaches for the early detection of cancer with a special focus on nanodiagnostics

**Rahul Kumar, Pankaj Keshari, Abhinav Kant, Ajay Kumar, Rohit Gupta and Subhash Chandra Yadav**

The early detection of cancer involves downstaging and screening. Downstaging is the early diagnosis of symptomatic patients and screening involves assessing healthy individuals for cancer before the appearance of symptoms. The early detection of cancer maximizes the success rate of treatment. This chapter provides an illustrative account of important non-invasive methods used for the early detection of cancer with a special focus on nanotechnology-based interventions. Most non-invasive methods rely upon the detection of specific biomarkers. A comprehensive list of important biomarkers that are useful for early cancer detection has been also provided. Nanotechnology has enabled scientists to develop diagnostic methods with enhanced specificity and high sensitivity. Nanotechnology based non-invasive diagnostic tools have great potential in the early diagnosis of cancer, with shorter testing time and lower cost.

## Abbreviations

| | |
|---|---|
| AgNPs | silver nanoparticles |
| CT | computed tomography |
| CTC | circulating tumor cells |
| ctDNA | circulating tumor DNA |
| GNPs | gold nanoparticles |
| LOH | loss of heterozygosity |
| MRI | magnetic resonance imaging |
| PET | positron emission tomography |
| QDs | quantum dots |
| SNPs | single nucleotide polymorphisms |

## 4.1 Introduction

'Because there is no glory in illness. There is no meaning to it. There is no honor in dying of.'

—John Green, *The Fault in Our Stars*, 2012

Diseases are the major cause of human misery. Cancer is one of the most dreaded diseases globally. Over ten million cancer related deaths were reported in 2020. It is the second leading cause of death worldwide. With respect to mortality rates, breast cancer, lung cancer, colon and rectum cancer, and prostate cancer form the top five cancer types. Most cancers are curable if detected early and treated properly (World Health Organization 2022). The early detection of cancer has two components. The first is early diagnosis (or downstaging) and the second is screening. Early diagnosis focuses on discovering symptomatic patients as soon as possible, whereas screening involves evaluating healthy people to identify those who have cancer before symptoms develop (Ananth 2000, Yip 2019). The early diagnosis of patients necessitates prompt patient presentation, timely diagnosis, and therapy upon the onset of initial symptoms. This holds significance across various forms of cancer. In contrast, screening is applicable solely to a certain group of cancer types, specifically cervical, colorectal, and breast cancers (Ananth 2000, Yip 2019, Law *et al* 2022). Whether it is downstaging or screening, most non-invasive early cancer detection methods involve clinical imaging techniques or the detection of molecular bio-markers or both. At present, there are only a few screening tests available for certain types of cancer, including colonoscopy, prostate specific antigens, mammography, and cervical cytology. The diagnostic procedures employed for cancer detection encompass a range of imaging methods, such as computed tomography (CT) scans, bone scans, magnetic resonance imaging (MRI), positron emission tomography (PET) scans, ultrasound, and x-rays, but these methods detect cancer when cancer-ous tissue has already started growing and even after there is a possibility of metastasis. During a biopsy procedure a medical professional procures a cellular sample from the affected body part for further laboratory analysis; this process is invasive in nature (Mayo Clinic 2022, Zhang *et al* 2019). The majority of cancer types currently do not have a reliable non-invasive methods for early detection (Chen *et al* 2020). Of this limited number of tests, most non-invasive cancer detection techniques utilize the principles of cancer cell biology. These methods operate by identifying several metabolites produced by cancer cells, such as cell-free DNA (cfDNA), microRNA (miRNA), and circulating tumor cells (CTCs). This chapter provides an account of important diagnostic and prognostic biomarkers used in the early detection of cancer followed by the basic principles behind some of the important diagnostic tools, with a special focus on nano-diagnostics.

## 4.2 Biomarkers in non-invasive early cancer detection

The term 'biomarker' denotes a quantifiable variable that is linked to the outcome of an illness (Ballman 2015). A cancer biomarker refers to a specific attribute that is measured as a reliable indicator of the likelihood of developing cancer, the occurrence of cancer, or the patient outcome (Sarhadi and Armengol 2022). These attributes may be morphological, physiological, cytological or chemical. Chemical attributes include molecular and genetic components. Molecular and genetic attributes can be detected before the presentation of other attributes. This feature makes molecular biomarkers suitable targets for the early detection of cancer. In the present chapter 'molecular biomarker' will refer to both the molecular and genetic components.

### 4.2.1 Diagnostic biomarkers

Table 4.1 provides a comprehensive list of some of the important potential and established biomarkers for cancer detection. Molecular biomarker testing in cancer includes the analysis of normal cells or cancerous cells or body fluids to identify alterations in DNA, RNA, proteins, or other biomolecules (Sarhadi and Armengol 2022). Circulating cells are also useful for early cancer detection (Lawrence *et al* 2023). These biomarkers offer valuable insights for several purposes, including cancer diagnosis, prognosis, precision medicine, cancer treatment guidance, drug response prediction, and cancer monitoring.

Biomarkers in cancer detection have been in use for a long time. The following discussion presents some examples of such strategies that are being explored. The detection of epigenetic alterations and microRNAs have been used in the early detection of gastric cancer. DNA methylation offers potential diagnostic biomarkers for gastric cancer screening, particularly in noninvasive forms such as peripheral blood, saliva, gastric wash, or urine. The detection of DNA hypermethylation in these body fluids may be clinically significant, serving as a valuable biomarker for early gastric cancer detection and facilitating noninvasive screening methods (Qu *et al* 2013). Gastric cancer diagnosis benefits from circulating microRNA (miRNA) analysis. Elevated serum miRNA-21 levels outperformed the traditional markers CA19-9 and CEA, showing an 88% positive prediction rate (PPR) for gastric cancer, reaching 89% for stage I gastric cancer. Plasma miR-196a and miR-376c demonstrated diagnostic potential, with urine-based miR-376c offering noninvasive detection. A panel of plasma miRNAs, including miR-16, miR-25, miR-92a, miR-451, and miR-486-5p, exhibited high diagnostic ability for early-stage gastric cancer. Additionally, six up-regulated miRNAs, including miR10b-5p and miR20a-3p, showed diagnostic accuracy for gastric cancer, and exosomal miR-19b-3p and miR-106a-5p distinguished gastric cancer with high sensitivity and specificity. Notably, miRNA alterations in *Helicobacter pylori*-infected gastric cancer patients, such as increased miR-21 and miR-19, and decreased let-7, miR-146, and miR-375, suggest their potential as early detection biomarkers. Recent insights highlight the involvement of miRNAs in regulating gastric cancer stem cells, offering promising avenues for understanding molecular mechanisms and developing strategies for early gastric cancer detection. Continued validation of these findings may lead to noninvasive and effective miRNA-based biomarkers for diagnosing gastric cancer at various stages (Hanke *et al* 2010, Arroyo *et al* 2011, Zhu *et al* 2014, Zhou *et al* 2015,

**Table 4.1.** Some of the potential and established biomarkers for cancer detection are categorized by tissue/organ type based on a literature survey.

| Cancer type | Protein | References | DNA | References | miRNA/circulating cells/mRNA | References |
|---|---|---|---|---|---|---|
| Breast cancer | Alphafeto protein (AFP) | Luo et al (2023) | Methylated promoters of adenomatous polyposis coli (APC) and retinoic acid receptors-2 (RARb2) | Afzal et al (2022) | miR-10b, miR-125b, miR145 (down-regulated) miR-21, and miR-155 (up-regulated) | Lorio et al (2005) |
| | Carcinoembryonic antigen (CEA) | | | | | |
| | Carbohydrate antigen/cancer antigen (CA) 153,125,199 k/a Mucin | | BRCA1/2 translocation | | | |
| | Estrogen receptor (ER) | Kabel (2017) | | | | |
| | Progesteron receptor (PR) | | | | | |
| | Human epidermal growth factor receptor 2 (HER2) | | | | | |
| | Urokinase plasminogen activator (uPA) | | | | | |
| | Plasminogen activator inhibitor 1 (PAI-1) | | | | | |
| | P53 | | | | | |
| | Cathepsin D | | | | | |
| | Cyclin E | | | | | |
| | Nestin | | | | | |
| | Human epididymis protein 4 (HE4) | Afzal et al (2022) | | | | |
| | Triple negative breast cancer | NCCN (2024) | | | | |
| | Microsatellite instability high (MSI-H), NTRK, RET, TMB-H | | | | | |

| Cancer type | Biomarkers | Reference | Genes | Reference | miRNA | Reference |
|---|---|---|---|---|---|---|
| Gastrointestinal cancer | CEA, CA 19-9, CA 72-4, CA 125, SLE, BCA-225, hCG, Pepsinogen I/II | Cäinap et al (2015), Matsuoka and Yashiro (2018) | HER2, ADAM23, MINT25, GDNF, PRDM5, MLF1, Roar | Garcia-Alfonso et al (2021) | miR-650, 126 (over-expression), miR-663 (down-regulation), miR-1, miR-20a, miR-27a, miR-34 and miR-423-5p | Yin et al (2012) |
| Endocrine cancer | Chromogranin A, Chromogranin B, Secretogranin II, Keratin proteins (CD8, CK18, CK19, AE1/AE3), Ki67, p27Kip1, Synaptophysin, PGP9.5, Thyroglobulin | Ericksson and Lloyd (2004), Ericksson et al (2000) | RET point mutations, PAX8-PPAR gamma translocation | Erickson and Lloyd (2004) | miR-96-5p, miR-22-3p, miR-1290, miR-193b, miR-222 and miR-21-5 (up-regulation), miR-150-5p, miR-129-5p and miR-133a (down-regulation), miR-7-5p and miR-96-5p, miR-137, miR-196a and miR-1290, miR-1 and miR-143 | Geisler et al (2021), Korotaeva et al (2021) |

*(Continued)*

**Table 4.1.** (*Continued*)

| Cancer type | Protein | References | DNA | References | miRNA/circulating cells/mRNA | References |
|---|---|---|---|---|---|---|
| | Thyroid transcription factor-1 | | | | | |
| Genitourinary cancer | Nuclear matrix protein-22 | Jeong and Ku (2022) | Aneuploidy of chromosomes (3, 7, and 17) and deletion of the 9p21 locus | Jeong and Ku (2022) | Let-7c, miR-135a, miR-135b, miR-148a, miR-204, miR-345 | Jeong and Ku (2022) |
| | Bladder tumor antigen (BTA) | | Hypermethylation | Santoni et al (2018) | miR-152, miR-148b-3p, miR-3187-3p, miR-15b-5p, miR-27a-3p, and miR-30a-5p | Santoni et al (2018) |
| | CK20 and insulin like growth factor II (IGFII) | Santoni et al (2018) | HS3ST2, SEPTIN9 and SLIT2 genes combined with FGFR3 mutation | | miR-146a-5p | Santoni et al (2018) |
| | Human complement factor H-related protein (hCFHrp) and complement factor H | Schmitz-Dräger et al (2015) | HAK20me3 | | Increase in isoleucine glutamine motif-containing GTAase-activating proteins (IQGAP3) mRNA | Bratu et al (2021) |
| | Cytokeratin (CK) 8 and 18 fragments | | H3K27me3 | | | |
| | Survivin | | Adenomatous polyposis coli (APC) | Bratu et al (2021) | | |
| | CYFRA 21-1 | | Glutathione S-transferase π1 (GSTP1) | | | |
| | BLCA-4 | | Retinoic acid receptor β2 (RARb2) | | | |
| | Denocarc mucin glycoproteins | | Gains in two or more of chromosomes 3, 7, and 17 in the same cell | Schmitz-Dräger et al (2015) | | |

| Cancer type | Biomarkers | Reference | Methylation/DNA | Reference | miRNA/mRNA | Reference |
|---|---|---|---|---|---|---|
| Germ cell cancer | Placental-like alkaline phosphatase (PLAP), OCT4 (POU5F1), NANOG, AP-2γ (TFAP2C) and LIN28 | Rajpert-De Meyts et al (2015) | Hypermethylation | Pedrazzoli et al (2021), Dieckmann et al (2019) | mi-R371a-3p | Pedrazzoli et al (2021) |
| | LDH | | | | miR-372-3p | |
| | Terato-related antigen monoclonal antibody (TRA-1-60) | Syring et al (2014) | Combination of human chorionic gonadotropin (HCG) and alfa-fetoprotein (AFP) | | miR-373-3p | |
| | Neuron-specific enolase (NSE) | | | | miR-302a-d/367-3p clusters | |
| | CD30 (TNFRSF8) | | | | | |
| Gynecological cancer | CA125 | Dochez et al (2019) | Aberrant methylation COL23A1, C2CD4D, and WNT6 | Matsas et al (2023) | miR-22, miR-93 and miR-451 (up-regulation) | Montagnana et al (2017), Ji et al (2014) |
| | Human epididymis protein 4 (HE4) | | Methylated opioid binding protein/cell adhesion molecule-like gene (OPCML) | Rein et al (2011) | miR-106b (down-regulation) | |
| | CA 15-3 | Matsas et al (2023) | Hypomethylation metastasis-related gene synuclein gamma (SNCG), satellite 2 DNA (SAT2) | | E6 and E7 mRNA | Sharma et al (2022) |
| | CA 19-9 | | | | | |
| | Inhibin | | | | | |
| | CYFRA 21-1 (serum fragments of cytokeratin 19) | | | | | |
| | Immunosuppressive acidic protein (IAP) | Ueda et al (2010) | | | | |
| | CA 72-4 | | | | | |
| | Lysophosphatidic acid (LPA) | | | | | |
| | Haptoglobin, osteopontine | | | | | |

(Continued)

**Table 4.1.** (*Continued*)

| Cancer type | Protein | References | DNA | References | miRNA/circulating cells/mRNA | References |
|---|---|---|---|---|---|---|
| Head and neck cancer | P16 | Johnson *et al* (2020) | *P16* gene inactivated (deletion/methylation) | Basheeth and Patil (2019) | E6 and E7 mRNA | Ndiaye *et al* (2014) |
| | *EGFR, HER2, FGFR1* overexpressed | | *TP53* with point mutations and loss of heterozygosity of 17p | | | |
| | *IL1RN, MAL* and *MMP1* | Basheeth and Patil (2019), Economo poulou *et al* (2019) | Hypermethylation of *CDH1* *GLT8D1* hypomethylated | | | |
| | Heat stable alkaline phosphatase, galectin, serum ferritin | | | | | |
| | Proto-oncogene eIF4E | | *C6orf136* hypermethylated | | | |
| | Tissue polypeptide antigen (TPA) | Rosati *et al* (2000), Barak *et al* (2015) | | | | |
| | *EBV* | Filippini *et al* (2023), Basheeth and Patil (2019) | | | | |
| | *VEGF* low expression | | | | | |
| | Cytokeratin-7 (CK7) and GATA binding protein 3 (GATA3) positive | | | | | |
| | Loss of TRAF3 and amplification of E2F1 | Johnson *et al* (2020) | | | | |
| Blood cancer (leukemia) | CBC (total and differential blood count) | Yilmaz *et al* (2021) | CpG methylation | Jiang *et al* (2020) | | |
| | CD200+ | Jalal (2021) | | | | |
| | CDC20 and ESM1 | | | | | |

| Cancer type | Biomarkers | Reference |
| --- | --- | --- |
| Blood cancer (lymphoma) | BCL-2/6 | Sun et al (2016) |
| | Mutated genes mID3, GNA13, RET, PIK3R1, ARID1A, and SMARCA4 as well as MYC | Sun et al (2016) |
| | PIM1, CECR1 and MYD88 | |
| | TP-53 | Sun et al (2016) |
| | vMYC | |
| | MYD88 | |
| | Overexpression of Bcl-2 and cyclin D-1 | Cho (2022) |
| | CD3, 20, 30, 56 | |
| | Beta-2 microglobulin | Morra (1999) |
| | CA 125 | |
| Musculoskeletal cancer | N-terminal propeptide of type 1 procollagen (PINP), carboxyterminal cross-linked telopeptide of type I collagen (ICTP) and bone sialoprotein (BSP) | Evola et al (2017) |
| | Serum bone-specific alkaline phosphatise (BSAP), PINP and osteoprotegerin (OPG) | |
| | EWS/FL1 fusion protein | |
| | Bax, caspase-8 and cytochrome c | |
| | Serum amyloid A (SAA) | |
| | Ezrin (EZR); α crystallin β chain (CRYAB) | |
| | Cytochrome C1 (CYC-1) | |
| | Protein NDRG1 | |
| | Gelsolin | |
| | Deletions of loci at the level of CDKN2A, EXT1, and EXT2 genes | Evola et al (2017) |

*(Continued)*

4-9

**Table 4.1.** (*Continued*)

| Cancer type | Protein | References | DNA | References | miRNA/circulating cells/mRNA | References |
|---|---|---|---|---|---|---|
| Neurologic cancer | Glial fibrillary acidic protein (GFAP) | Jelski and Mroczko (2021) | Promoter methylation of *MGMT*, overexpression of *EGFRvIII*, mutations in isocitrate dehydrogenase (*IDH1*), point mutations in the promoter of telomerase (*pTERT*), loss of heterozygosity (LOH) 10q (*PTEN* mutations or loss), LOH on chromosome 22 (loss of the tumor suppressor gene *TIMP-3*), LOH, namely 1p, 9p, 17p, and 19q | Jelski and Mroczko (2021) | Circulating tumor cells (CTCs) | Jelski and Mroczko (2021) |
| | VEGF | | *TP53* point mutations (medulloblastoma) | | Circulating tumor DNA (ctDNA) long DNA fragments (> 500 bp) | |
| | IGF2 expression | Hedborg *et al* (2010) | *ATRX* mutations (1p/19q loss and *ATRX* mutation are mutually exclusive) | Scheie *et al* (2019) | miR-21 up-regulation | |
| | Chromogranin A | | Gains at chromosome 7 and losses of chromosome 10 (+7/−10) | | mir-125b, miR-128, miR-485-3p, and miR-342-3p down-regulated | |
| | MYCN, chromosome 1p, DNA index, VMA:HVA ratio, CD44, Trk-A, NSE, | Riley *et al* (2004), Wiles *et al* (2017) | *K27M* mutation in either *H3F3A* or *HIST1H3B/C* | | | |
| | | | Fusion between *KIAA1549* exon 16 and *BRAF* exon 9 | | | |

| Cancer | Biomarkers | References | Genetic markers | References |
|---|---|---|---|---|
| | Lactate dehydrogenase, ferritin, and multidrug resistance (neuroblastoma) | | | |
| | Neuroblastoma, apoptotic index, inhibitory cell cycle proteins, matrix metalloproteinases (MMPs) (1), p53 and p21, and markers of angiogenesis, namely vascular endothelial growth factor (VEGF) (2, 3–6) and proliferative markers, e.g. Ki-67, and topoisomerases (pituitary tumors) | Sav *et al* (2012) | *MYB-QKI* fusions (glioma) *MYB, MYBL1*, and *FGFR1* *NF2* loss and monosomy of chromosome 22q (ependymomas) *CTNNB1* mutations and accumulation of beta-catenin in the tumor cell nuclei (medulloblastoma) | |
| | Higher BCL2/BAX | | Loss of *SMARCA4* expression (rahbdoid) | |
| | Induction of hypoxia-inducible factor 1α | Gossing *et al* (2020), Scheie *et al* (2019), Wiles *et al* (2017) | Focal amplification of a micro-RNA cluster on 19q13.42 (*C19MC*) (embryonal tumor) | |
| | Overexpression of vascular endothelial growth factor A | | *ALK* amplification | Wiles *et al* (2017) |
| | Overexpressed pituitary tumor transforming gene (PTTG1) | | | |
| | Overexpressed matrix metalloproteinases (MMPs) | | | |
| Respiratory cancer | CEA, hormonal peptides, and some neurogenic enzymes in small cell carcinoma | Hansen and Pedersen (1986) | | |
| | Calcitonin, ACTH, ADH, CEA, neurophysin, oxytocin, β-endorphin, neuron-specific | | | |

(Continued)

**Table 4.1.** (*Continued*)

| Cancer type | Protein | References | DNA | References | miRNA/circulating cells/mRNA | References |
|---|---|---|---|---|---|---|
| | enolase (NSE), and CK BB (small cell carcinoma) | | | | | |
| | CYFRA 21-1, NSE, ProGRP, SCC, CEA, tumor M2-PK | Schneider (2006), Wang et al (2014) | | | | |
| | CRP, LDH, tumor-suppressor genes and oncogenes, CA125, CgA, NCAM, and TPA. | | | | | |
| | High LDH | Harmsma et al (2013) | | | | |
| | Keratinization or intercellular bridges are classified as squamous cell carcinoma (SQC) | Šutić et al (2021) | | | | |
| | Tumors with mucin production or glandular architecture are classified as denocarcinoma (ADCs) | | | | | |
| | Thyroid transcription factor 1 (TTF-1) (for ADC) | | | | | |
| | p40 (for SQC) | | | | | |
| | Cytokeratin 19 fragment (CYFRA 21-1), carcinoembryonic antigen (CEA), squamous cell carcinoma antigen (SCCA), and carbohydrate antigen 125 (CA125) | | | | | |

| Skin cancer | Pmel/Pmel17/SILV/gp100 | Weinstein et al (2014) | *NRAS, BRAFnon-V600E*, or *NF1* mutations | Teixido et al (2021) | |
| | Melan-A | | *BRAFV600* mutation | | |
| | Tyrosinase | | | | |
| | MITF | | | | |
| | S100 protein family | | | | |
| | SM5-1 | | | | |
| | CSPG4/HMW-MAA | Gogas et al (2009) | | | |
| | HER2, epidermal growth factor receptor and KIT | | | | |
| Eye cancer | | | Chromosomal aberrations (chromosome 3,6,1 8) | Chattopadhyay et al (2016) | miR-16, miR-145, miR-146a, miR-204, miR-211, and miR-363-3p | Stark et al (2019), Jin and Burnier (2021) |
| | | | Mutations in guanine nucleotide-binding protein G (q) subunit alpha (*GNAQ*) | Lamas et al (2021) | | |
| | | | Mutation in guanine nucleotide-binding protein subunit alpha-11 (*GNA11*) | | | |
| | | | Mutations in the *RB1* gene | Eagle (2013) | | |

Tsai *et al* 2016, Hung *et al* 2017, Huang *et al* 2017, Wang *et al* 2017a, Ranjbar *et al* 2018, Wang *et al* 2018, Ruggieri *et al* 2019, Nik *et al* 2020). The dysregulation of the cyclo-oxygenase 2 (*COX2*) gene, driven by alterations in the methylation of its promoter, holds significant implications in gastric carcinogenesis. Elevated *COX2* levels are closely linked to reduced apoptosis and increased proliferation, particularly in gastrointestinal epithelial cells. Further understanding of these cancer mechanisms requires advancements in methylation quantification and high-throughput technologies (Akhtar *et al* 2001). Colorectal cancer serves as an informative model for exploring cancer's genetic basis, progressing with distinct genetic alterations at each stage. Epigenetic studies, particularly in DNA methylation, enhance our understanding of disease progression. Colorectal tumors exhibit varied genetic pathways, including the CpG island methylator phenotype, affecting diagnosis, prognosis, and treatment. Unanswered questions persist, requiring integrated studies to elucidate the clinical implications of molecular instability and therapeutic responses. The intricate interplay between genetic and epigenetic events provides a comprehensive understanding of colorectal cancer, influencing potential interventions and patient outcomes (Boland *et al* 1995, Markowitz *et al* 1995, Yeager *et al* 1998, Zheng *et al* 1999, Issa 2000). Prostate cancer's complex etiology involves environmental, genetic, and epigenetic factors influencing gene expression. *GSTP1*, a marker for prostate cancer detection, undergoes hypermethylation in the promoter, prevalent in potential precursor lesions, linked to GST loss. Somatic *GSTP1* inactivation, not genotype, primarily impacts prostate cancer progression, with hypermethylation correlating strongly with GST loss in adenocarcinomas but not in prostatic intraepithelial neoplasia or benign prostatic hyperplasia lesions (Jerónimo *et al* 2001, Jerónimo *et al* 2002). Ulcerative colitis, an inflammatory condition affecting the large intestine, carries the risk of colorectal carcinoma development. Investigation into hypermethylation of the *p14ARF* gene at various histological stages in ulcerative colitis patients revealed that such hypermethylation is a common and early occurrence in ulcerative-colitis-associated carcinogenesis, indicating its potential significance (Sato *et al* 2002). Barrett's esophagus, a precursor to esophageal adenocarcinoma, sees increased incidence in developed countries. The *p16INK4a* gene's frequent lesions in adenocarcinomas suggest a role in neoplastic progression, involving hypermethylation of the *CDKN2A/p16* promoter and *CDKN2A* gene loss. Methylation studies indicate early and prevalent *CDKN2A* hypermethylation in adenocarcinomas, premalignant lesions, and metaplasia. Epigenomic fingerprints reveal distinct methylation patterns at different disease stages, offering potential markers for disease progression (Eads *et al* 2001). The disorder known as Barrett's esophagus arises from the impairment of the esophageal lining due to acid reflux, resulting in a transition of the tissue from stratified squamous epithelium to simple columnar epithelium. Bladder cancer development involves frequent methylation of genes such as *CDH1*, *RASSF1A*, *APC*, and *CDH13*. Methylation of these genes is linked to various prognostic and survival indicators. Specifically, a positive status for *CDH1* methylation is associated with poor survival outcomes in individuals with bladder cancer (Kim and Kim 2016). Lung cancer is one of the leading causes of cancer-related deaths. Progress in the last two decades has focused on understanding molecular and cellular aspects, including proto-oncogene abnormalities, genetic and epigenetic changes in tumor suppressor genes, angiogenesis, and molecular abnormalities in preinvasive lesions. A marker panel, including *RAR*, *DAPK*, *GSTP1*, *FHIT*, *RASSF1*, *MGMT*, E-cad, *APC*, and *p16* detects lung cancer in early stages, with specific focus on genes such as *RAR*, *RASSF1*, and *APC* (Larsen and Minna 2011). In lymphoma and leukemia, hypermethylation of promoters in viral and cellular genes, such as the Epstein–Barr virus (EBV) latency gene *Wp* and latent membrane protein 1 (*LMP1*), can lead to transcriptional inactivation. Methylation patterns in *LMP1* regulatory sequences indicate an indirect mechanism involving methylcytosine-binding proteins in silencing the *LMP1* promoter (Verma *et al* 2001). Kaposi's sarcoma-associated herpesvirus (KSHV) is strongly linked to Kaposi's sarcoma, primary effusion lymphomas, and Castleman's disease. The mechanism of KSHV latency and reactivation involves the heavily methylated Lyta promoter region. Demethylation, crucial for Lyta expression and KSHV reactivation, is demonstrated by reversing methylation with tetradecanoylphorbol acetate. Epigenetic regulation in cancer-associated viruses, such as hepatitis B and papillomavirus, suggests potential molecular targets for intervention (Chen *et al* 2001, Laman and Boshoff 2001). Human serum and other bodily fluids are rich sources of novel biomarkers for routine clinical diagnosis. MicroRNAs, small non-coding RNA molecules, play a crucial role in regulating RNA stability and gene expression, with their dysregulation linked to cancer development and progression. Recent reports indicate stable microRNA signatures in serum and other fluids, leading to exploration of circulating microRNA profiles for identifying non-invasive biomarkers in various studies (Brase *et al* 2010). Piwi-interacting RNAs (piRNAs) are emerging as potential non-invasive diagnostic biomarkers in colorectal carcinoma (Ray and Mukherjee 2023). Large number of new and more reliable cancer biomarkers are being discovered at an unprecedented rate. All above discussion is just a primer to present an overview of biomarkers and their use in early cancer detection and prognosis.

### 4.2.2 Prognostic biomarkers

Many of the biomarkers given in table 4.1 are also prognostic markers. A prognostic biomarker provides information regarding the probable prognosis of cancer, such as disease recurrence, disease progression, or mortality, independent of the treatment administered. It is different to a predictive biomarker. A biomarker can be considered predictive when there is a significant difference in the treatment effect between patients who test positive for the biomarker and those who test negative for it, as observed in an experimental comparison with a control group (Ballman 2015). So, prognostic markers are important in the detection of cancer especially with respect to recurrence of the disease once cancer has been treated successfully. Early detection post-treatment may prevent recurrence of the disease. Table 4.2 provides a list of important prognostic markers compiled from different literature sources.

**Table 4.2.** Important prognostic markers to inform likely cancer outcome, based on a literature survey.

| Cancer type | Prognostic marker | References |
| --- | --- | --- |
| Breast cancer | N-cadherin mRNA levels | Costantini and Budillon (2020) |
| | Low expression of coiled-coil domain-containing proteins (CCDC69) | Yi et al (2022) |
| | Percentage of cells positive for Ki67 (nuclear non-histone protein) | Taneja et al (2010) |
| | Overexpression of ERα | |
| | Promoter hypermethylation of p16INK4a and p14$^{ARF}$ (tumor suppressor proteins) | |
| | TBX2 is amplified | |
| | Ki67 in more than 50% of the cells are at high risk of developing cancer | Esteva and Hortobagyi (2004) |
| Gastrointestinal cancer | High CD8+/low stroma fraction | Kerr and Yang (2021) |
| | Higher LINE-1 type transposase domain containing 1 (L1TD1) predicted longer disease-free survival | Chakraborty et al (2019) |
| | Mutations in DZIP1 were correlated with a good prognosis | Liu et al (2021) |
| | Up-regulation of BCAT1 indicated poor survival | Xu et al (2018) |
| | High c-Met expression indicated worse overall survival | Yu et al (2013) |
| Endocrine cancer | Mutations in the MEN1, ATRX and DAXX genes | Ciobanu et al (2021) |
| | INSM1 expression | |
| | Higher miR-103 and miR-107 expression | |
| | Low miR-155 expression | |
| | Loss of MGMT (O-6-methylguanine-DNA methyltransferase) | |
| | AST and LDH levels predict survival | Freis et al (2017) |

| Cancer type | Biomarker/characteristic | Reference |
|---|---|---|
| Eye cancer | Chromosomal abnormalities, especially M3, 8q gain, 6q loss and 1p loss | Zheng et al (2020) |
| | Loss of nuclear *BAP1* expression/*BAP1* mutation | Lamas et al (2021) |
| | Preferentially expressed antigen in melanoma (*PRAME*) expression | |
| | Genes involved in tumor suppressing pathways (*ABTB1*, *ADPRHL1* and *SLC17A7*) | |
| | *BRCA1*-associated protein 1 (BAP1) | Zheng et al (2020) |
| | microRNA-144 (miR-144) | Gajdzis et al (2021) |
| | Tumor-infiltrating macrophages and lymphocytes | |
| | Extravascular matrix loops and networks | |
| | Extraocular extension | |
| | Mitotic count+ | |
| Genitourinary cancer | High CD73 expression | Ku et al (2016) |
| | High apurinic/apyrimidine endonuclease 1/redox factor-1 (APE1/Ref-1) levels | |
| | Elevated neutrophil-to-lymphocyte ratio | |
| | High expression of CD45RO+, CD3+, and CD8+ lymphocytes | Ariafar et al (2022) |
| | miR-125b, -145, -183, and -221 in combination with voided urine cytology | Erdmann et al (2020) |
| Germ cell cancer | Programmed-death receptor and its ligand (PD-1 and PD-L1) | Chovanec et al (2018), Pedraza and Stephenson (2018) |
| | Level of hCG and AFP | Fosså et al (1999) |
| Gynecological cancer | Interleukin-8 (proangiogenic factor) | Huang et al (2011) |
| | MMPs (MMP-2, MMP-7, MMP-8, MMP-9, and MT1-MMP) | |
| | Overexpression of Claudin-3 and -4 | Szabo et al (2009) |
| | CA 125 | Huang et al (2011) |
| | miR-214, miR-199*, and miR-200a | |

*(Continued)*

**Table 4.2.** (*Continued*)

| Cancer type | Prognostic marker | References |
|---|---|---|
| Head and neck cancer | State of immunosuppression increases the risk of metastasis, as well as decreasing overall survival | Lubov *et al* (2021) |
| | Inflammation-associated PD-L1 expression in immune cells is associated with a good prognosis | Budach and Tinhofer (2019) |
| | E-cadherin and metalloproteinases | van den Brekel *et al* (2002) |
| Blood cancer (leukemia) | Absence of monosomy | Gbadamosi *et al* (2018) |
| | S-β2M level and s-TK level | Yun *et al* (2020) |
| | Increased expressions of CD38 and ZAP70 | |
| | miR-15a and miR-16-1, located on 13q14 | |
| | miR-155 | |
| | miR-29a and miR-29b overexpression leads to aggressive CLL, as well as miR-155 | |
| | The down regulation of miR-34a and miR-125a up regulation | |
| | miR-129-2 methylation is associated with poor survival | |
| | Gene mutations in *KIT*, Fms-like tyrosine kinase 3 (*FLT3*), nucleophosmin 1 (*NPM1*), and CCAAT enhancer-binding protein-α (*CEBPA*) | Foran (2010) |
| | Mutations of nucleophosmin gene 1 (*NPM1*), Fms-like tyrosine kinase 3 gene (*FLT3*), CCAT/enhancer binding protein alpha gene (*CEBPα*) | Gregory *et al* (2009) |
| | High levels of expression of *MN1* | |
| | Over-expression of the the ETS-related gene (*ERG*) | |

| Cancer type | Biomarker | Reference |
|---|---|---|
| Blood cancer (acute myeloid leukemia (AML)) | Inversions in chromosome 16 | Chakroborty et al (2019) |
| | Translocations between Chromosome 15 and 17 | |
| | Chromosomes 15 and 17, and | Pezo and Bedard (2015) |
| | Tumor size, nodal status, grade, and presence or absence of lymphovascular invasion | |
| Blood cancer (lymphoma) | MYC (a proto-oncogene transcription factor) overexpression | Chan and Dogan (2019) |
| | BCL2 overexpression | |
| | CD5 positive | |
| | p53 | |
| | Epigenetic modifiers such as EZH2, CREBBP/EB300, KMT2D/MLL2, as well as BCL2 alterations | |
| | CREBBP and KMT2D mutations | |
| | IL-10 | Broeckelmann et al (2016) |
| | In situ hybridization with aberrations involving the MYC and/or BCL2 and BCL6 genes | Vaidya and Witzig (2014) |
| Musculoskeltal cancer | Hematological markers such as neutrophil to lymphocyte ratio (NLR), platelet to lymphocyte ratio (PLR), and lymphocyte to macrophage ratio (LMR) can reflect the individual's tumor microenvironment to some extent and can be used to predict the prognosis of cancer patients. | Li et al (2022) |
| | Matrix metallopeptidase 9 (MMP-9), hypoxia-inducible transcription factor 1 (HIF-1), apurinic/apyrimidinic endonuclease 1 (APE1) | Zamborsky et al (2019) |
| | miR15 and miR16 were either deleted or down-regulated | |
| | Up-regulation of miR-195, miR-99, miR-181, and miR-148a | |
| | Downregulation of miR-539, miR-145, and miR-335 | |
| | TGF-$\beta$ | |
| | Abnormal TIM3 expression | |
| | Tumor-specific antibodies (IgM) can be detected in the very early stages | |
| | Expression of the Ezrin gene in circulating tumor cells | |
| | LDH level | Bacci et al (2000) |

(Continued)

**Table 4.2.** (*Continued*)

| Cancer type | Prognostic marker | References |
| --- | --- | --- |
| Neurologic cancer | Isocitrate dehydrogenase 1,2 (IDH) mutations | Śledzińska *et al* (2021), Dahlrot *et al* (2021), Aquilanti *et al* (2018), Kan *et al* (2020) |
| | *CDKN2A* deletion | |
| | *TERT* promoter mutations, *EGFR* alterations, or a combination of chromosome 7 gain and 10 loss | |
| | *MGMT* promoter methylation | |
| | *H3F3A* mutations | |
| | Up-regulation of miRNA-221, 155, 21, 222, 15b, 148a, 196, 210 | |
| | 1p/19q is a key mutation | |
| | *MYB* and *MYBL1* mutations | |
| | *MN1* | |
| | *MMP-9* | Dobra *et al* (2023) |
| Respiratory cancer | Cyclin D1 overexpression | Zhu and Tsao (2014) |
| | EGFR mutation, *ALK* and *ROS1* rearrangements | |
| | c-*SRC*, cyclin E, transcription termination factor 1 (*TTF1*), p65, checkpoint kinase 1 (*CHK1*), mitogen-activated protein kinase 8 (JNK1 also known as Mapk1) | Puderecki *et al* (2020) |
| | Epidermal growth factor receptor (EGFR), Sry-Box 2 (SOX2), E-cadherin, Akt serine/threonine kinase 1 (*AKT1*), mitogen-activated protein kinase 14 | |
| | Girdin and STAT-3 | |
| | Pten induced kinase 1 (*PINK1*) | |
| | miR-590, 155, 340, 125, 494, 148a | |
| | Long coding RNA LINC00857, RP11-284F21.7, TMPOAS1, RP11-284F21.9, LINC01137 and RP11-253E3.3 | |
| | Immunoglobulin superfamily member 10 (*IGSF10*) | Ling *et al* (2020) |
| | Ribonucleotide reductase regulatory subunit M2 | |
| | The programmed death-ligand 1 (PD-L1) protein | Šutić *et al* (2021) |
| | High excision repair cross-complementation group (ERCC1) protein | Zhu and Tsao (2014) |

| | | |
|---|---|---|
| Oral squamous cell carcinoma | Musashi 2 (*MSI2*) | Costantini and Budillon (2020) |
| Skin cancer | *CAP2*, *HER4*, CIP2A, CD73, *MCR1*, S100B, ALDH1, *MIA* | Ding *et al* (2022) |
| | miR-16, -15b, -425, -10b, -206, -4633-5p, -330-5p, -150, -199a-5p | |
| | *BAP1* (piris too) | |
| | BiP, GRP78 | |
| | *MCAM*/MUC18 | |
| | Metallothionein I and II | Weinstein *et al* (2014) |
| | *MCAM* | |
| | Ki-67 | |
| | SPRY4-IT1, a long non-coding RNA | |
| | Circulating tumor DNA (ctDNA), cell-free DNA (cfDNA), and circulating mRNA | Ding *et al* (2022) |
| | *BRAF* or *NRAS* ctDNA | |
| | mRNA expression of seven genes (*DCD, ECRG2, HES6, KBTBD, COL6A6, SCGB2A2,* and *KRT9*) | |

## 4.3 Methods used in biomarker detection

Many non-invasive methods have been developed based on the above mentioned diagnostic and prognostic biomarkers. Apart from blood testing, methods involving the analysis of stool, urine, and saliva have been developed (Heyn 2015). The detection of volatile organic compounds is being explored as an alternative non-invasive target (Liu *et al* 2023a, 2023b). Artificial intelligence based methods are also being developed for early detection of various cancers (Zhang *et al* 2023). Regarding the techniques used for the detection of cancer biomarkers, many conventional and advanced methods are being employed depending upon the type of cancer and the biomarker. The choice of method being employed also depends on the chemical nature of the biomarker. Commonly used methods in biomarker detection include polymerase chain reaction (PCR), gene expression profiling methods such as RT-PCR, microarray and RNA sequencing, flow cytometry for the detection of free cells, immunoassays, enzyme linked immunosorbant assay (ELISA), protein micro-arrays, mass spectroscopy, western blotting, immunofluorescence and immunodif-fusion for peptide-based biomarkers, and biomarkers being detected using antibodies (Wu and Qu 2015, Nimse *et al* 2016, Asci Erkocyigit *et al* 2023). Most biosensors include the above mentioned methods or a set-up to detect the by-product of these processes through electrochemical, chemiluminescent, colorimetric, and fluorescent methods through miniaturized microfluidics system (Asci Erkocyigit *et al* 2023). Nanotechnology based biosensors are emerging as great choice in the development of next-generation biosensors. The following section deals with an overview of some of the important nanotechnology-based cancer detection methods.

### 4.3.1 Cancer nanodiagnostics

Nanotechnology is being explored as a potential option for the development of more specific and sensitive detection methods. The current section provides an overview of such methods along with the basic principles involved in the function of some of these methods. Most of the nanotechnology-based cancer detection methods employ nanoparticles (NPs). NPs encompass a broad range of materials consisting of particulate compounds with at least one dimension measuring less than 100 nm (Laurent *et al* 2008). The physicochemical properties of nanoparticles differ from those of bulk materials due to their small size, which results in much greater surface to volume ratios (Moeinzadeh and Jabbari 2017). Nanoparticles often display characteristic size-dependent properties, mostly attributable to their diminutive dimensions and extensive surface area (Altammar 2023). These materials can be categorized into 0D, 1D, 2D, or 3D. This categorization is contingent upon their overall shape (Tiwari *et al* 2012). The significance of these materials became apparent when researchers discovered that the size of a substance might impact its physicochemical properties (Khan *et al* 2019).

There are different kinds of nanoparticles such as carbon-based nanoparticles, metal nanoparticles, ceramics nanoparticles, lipid-based nanoparticles, semiconductor nanoparticles, polymeric nanoparticles, etc (Altammar 2023). Metal nano-particles are of special significance with respect to the development of biosensors.

There are various kinds of metal nanoparticles. Silver nanoparticles, zinc nanoparticles, copper nanoparticles, gold nanoparticles, aluminum nanoparticles and iron nanoparticles are some important examples of metal nanoparticles. Semiconductor based nanoparticles such as quantum dots are also equally important and widely used in early cancer diagnosis. Nanoparticles offer a compelling platform for a wide range of biological applications. The surface and core characteristics of these systems can be deliberately manipulated to cater to specific applications, such as biomolecular identification, medicinal delivery, biosensing, and bioimaging (Madkour 2019) (figure 4.1).

Nanoparticle synthesis can be broadly categorized into two main approaches: top-down and bottom-up methodologies (figure 4.2). The top-down strategy involves the synthesis of NPs from bulk materials by the utilization of conventional solid-state processes such as milling, machining, or lithographic methods. The bottom-up strategy involves the synthesis of nanoparticles using various processes such as chemical interactions, self-assembly, aggregation, or chemical vapor deposition, starting from individual molecules (Moeinzadeh and Jabbari 2017).

Nanodiagnostics refers to the application of nanotechnology in the field of diagnostics. This encompasses many techniques such as single molecule manipulation and assessment, as well as the miniaturization of systems and platforms to exploit nanoscale features arising from interactions between surfaces and biomolecules, among other possibilities (Baptista 2014). Nanodiagnostic tools are designed to detect and even quantitate biomolecules such as antigens, antibodies, DNA, RNA, different proteins, metabolites, etc. These molecules may be used as biomarkers for the detection of various diseases (Alharbi and Al-Sheikh 2014,

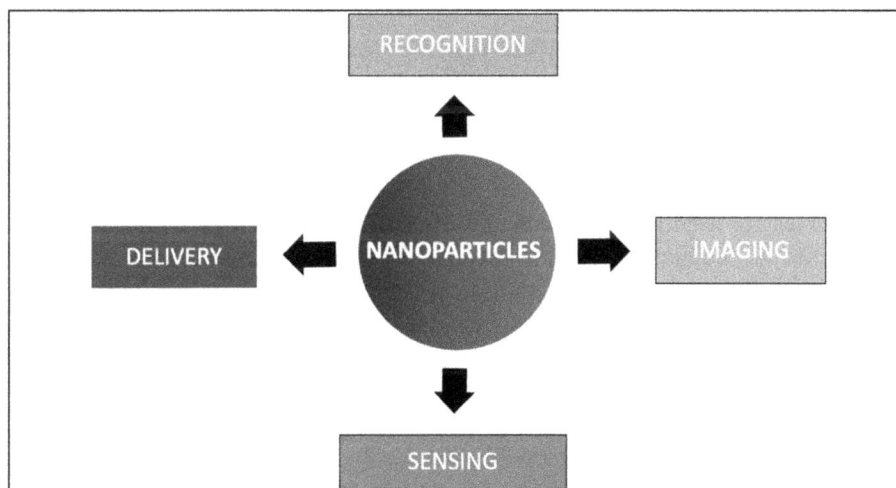

**Figure 4.1.** Applications of nanoparticles. All applications of nanoparticles fall into four broad categories. These are biomolecular identification, medicinal delivery, biosensing, and bioimaging. Biosensing and bioimaging fall under the realm of nanodiagnostics.

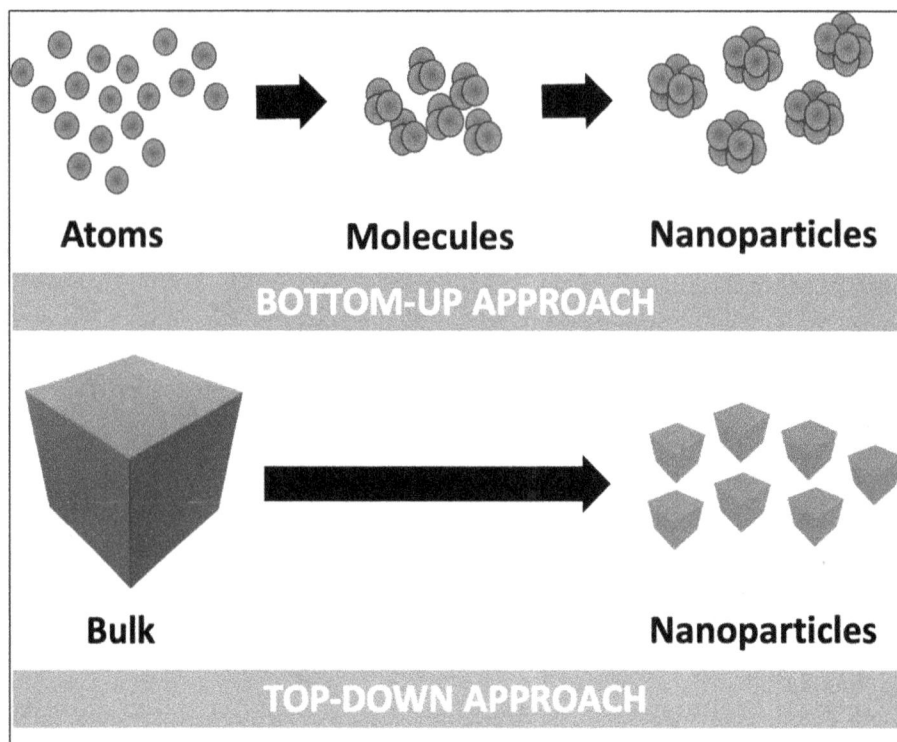

**Figure 4.2.** Different approaches of nanoparticle synthesis. The bottom-up approach involves the formation of nanoparticles by aggregation of smaller components such as atoms and molecules. The top-down approach involves the breaking down of bulk matter to nanoscale material.

Wang *et al* 2017b, Park *et al* 2017). Table 4.3 presents some examples of nano-diagnostic tools developed for detection of different types of cancer.

**4.3.2 Nanodiagnostic strategies**

Nanoparticles are used for early cancer detection in various ways. They are used in the detection of molecular biomarkers, the detection of cancer cells, and *in vivo* tumor imaging (figure 4.3). *In vivo* imaging involves either passive targeting or active targeting of nanoparticle labeled probes. Passive targeting involves the selective accumulation of macromolecules, such as nanoparticles, within neoplastic tissues due to the phenomenon of enhanced permeability and retention (EPR) (Bazak *et al* 2014, Dilliard and Siegwart 2023). Active targeting refers to a strategy wherein the surface of nanoparticles is modified biochemically to enhance its affinity towards receptors or other cell surface molecules within an organ (Dilliard and Siegwart 2023, Shi *et al* 2023). Nanoparticles offer specific targeting even if biomarker concentration is low and therefore help in developing improved, more robust next-generation biosensors (Hull *et al* 2014, Sharifi *et al* 2019). Among the different kinds of nanoparticles, gold nanoparticles (GNPs) and quantum dots (QDs) occupy a

**Table 4.3.** Some examples of recent nanodiagnostic tools for early cancer detection.

| Sl. No. | Nanoparticle | Use | Biomarker target | Sample type | Cancer type | References |
|---|---|---|---|---|---|---|
| 1 | Magnetic nanowire | Detection of circulating tumor cells (CTCs) from nonmetastatic early breast cancer cells | EpCAM | Blood (250 $\mu$l to 1 ml) | Breast cancer | Hong et al (2016) |
| 2 | ZnO nanodisks (NDs)@g-$C_3N_4$ quantum dots | CCRF-CEM cells (T lymphoblasts) | PTK7 | Cell line | Acute lymphoblastic leukemia (ALL) | Pang et al (2018) |
| 3 | Polymer dot conjugates (Pdot-IgG and Pdot-streptavidin probes) | Detection of CTCs | EpCAM | Cell line MCF-7 | Breast cancer | Wu et al (2010) |
| 4 | Hydrazine-gold nanoparticle (GNP)-aptamer bioconjugate | Detection of HER2 overexpressing breast cancer cells | HER2 | Cell lines SK-BR-3 and MCF 7 | Breast cancer | Zhu et al (2013) |
| 5 | Multi-walled carbon nanotubes (MWCNTs) | Detection of liver cancer cells in blood circulation | EpCAM | Blood | Hepatocellular carcinoma | Liu et al (2014) |
| 6 | Multifunctional nanoparticles | Detection of HER2 overexpressing breast cancer cells | HER2 | Cell line (BT474) | Breast cancer | Shen et al (2014) |
| 7 | Gelatin nanoparticle-coated silicon beads | Detection of CTCs by density-based cell isolation | EpCAM/CD146 | Blood (2 ml) | Breast cancer, colorectal cancer | Huang et al (2018) |
| 8 | Electrospun nanofiber-deposited nickel (Ni) micropillar-based cytosensor | Electrochemical detection of CTCs | EpCAM | Cell line (MCF-7) | Breast cancer | Wu et al (2018) |
| 9 | fDNA-templated magnetic nanoparticle-quantum dot (QD)-aptamer copolymers (MQAPs) | Detection of CTCs | PTK7 | Blood | Leukemia | Li et al (2018) |

(Continued)

**Table 4.3.** (*Continued*)

| Sl. No. | Nanoparticle | Use | Biomarker target | Sample type | Cancer type | References |
|---|---|---|---|---|---|---|
| 10 | Tannic acid functionalized magnetic nanoparticles (MNPs-TA) | Detection of CTCs independent of EpCAM | Glycocalyx on cancer cells | Blood (1 ml) | Breast cancer Renal cancer Prostate cancer Bronchial cancer Ovarian cancer Lung cancer Esophageal carcinoma Colon cancer | Ding *et al* (2021) |
| 11 | Label-free nanosensor coupled silicon nanoribbon detector | Detection of cancer antigens | PSA and carbohydrate antigen 15.3 (CA 15.3) | Blood | Prostate cancer and breast cancer | Stern *et al* (2010) |
| 12 | Nanosensors (nanoparticles coated with protease peptide substrates conjugated to mass-spectrometry-encoded reporters) | Detection of lung cancer (mouse model) | Tumor-associated proteases | Urine | Lung cancer | Dart (2020) |
| 13 | Nano-nose | Detection of lung cancer through exhaled breath | Volatile organic compounds (VOCs) | Exhaled breath | Lung cancer | Fernandes *et al* (2015), Baldini *et al* (2020), Peng *et al* (2009) |
| 14 | Photodiode array biochip (silver enhancement by the gold nanoparticles) | Detection of high risk HPV DNA | High risk HPV DNA | Tissue | Cervical cancer | Baek *et al* (2008) |
| 15 | NanoVelcro platform | Capture of circulating tumor cells | Cell surface carbonic anhydrase 9 and CD147 antigens | Blood | Clear cell renal cell carcinoma | Liu *et al* (2016) |

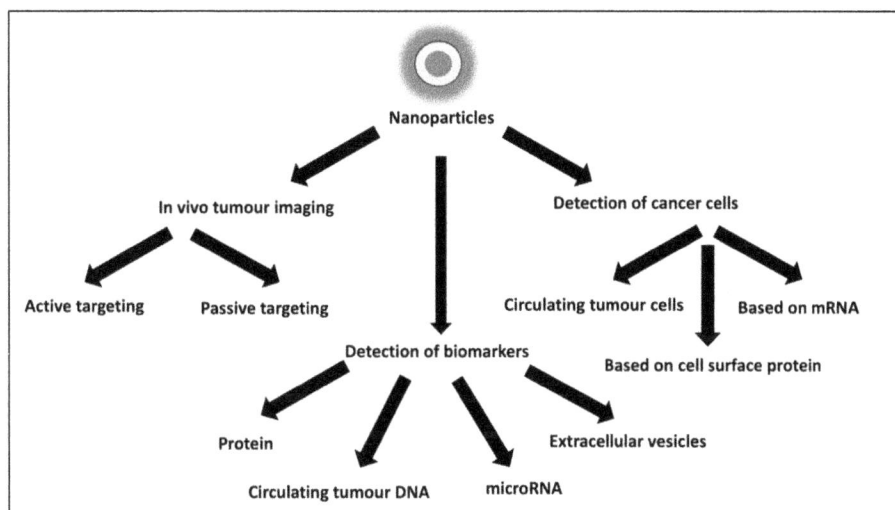

**Figure 4.3.** The application of nanoparticles in cancer detection. Nanoparticles can be used in cancer nanodiagnostics in three ways: *in vivo* tumor imaging, the detection of biomarkers and the detection of cancer cells. *In vivo* imaging is based on either active targeting or passive targeting of the probe.

central position with respect to their widespread usage in the field of nanodiagnostics. Other nanoparticles such as magnetic nanoparticles (MNPs), silver nanoparticles (AgNPs), nanowires, carbon nanotubes, dendrimers, graphene oxide, nanopillars and other polymer based nanomaterials are also being used (Huang and Lovell 2017, Zhang *et al* 2019). The following sections deal with the basic principles behind the designing and operation of three popular non-invasive nanodiagnostic approaches used in early cancer detection.

*4.3.2.1 Gold nanoparticle based biomarker detection*
Gold nanoparticles (GNPs) exhibit unique optical, electrochemical and spectral properties which make them suitable for nanodiagnostic applications. GNPs can easily be synthesized in the laboratory and can be conjugated with a variety of biomolecules such as antibodies and other peptides, oligonucleotides, aptamers, etc (Franco *et al* 2015). One of the simplest and most popular approaches in GNPs based nanodiagnostics is to conjugate oligonucleotides with GNPs to detect target DNA *in vitro*. Figure 4.4 shows the basic principle behind the generation and operation of GNP–oligonucleotide conjugate. This method is based on a simple change in color which can be detected visually. The color change is based on aggregation of GNPs under high salt concentrations. Gold nanoparticles due to their plasmon resonance properties reflect different parts of the electromagnetic spectrum depending upon its size. In figure 4.4 red colored gold nanoparticles aggregate to produce blue color under high salt concentrations. First a small oligonucleotide (usually small thiolated single stranded DNA) molecule designed to pair with the target DNA is conjugated with GNPs. This probe mixture is then

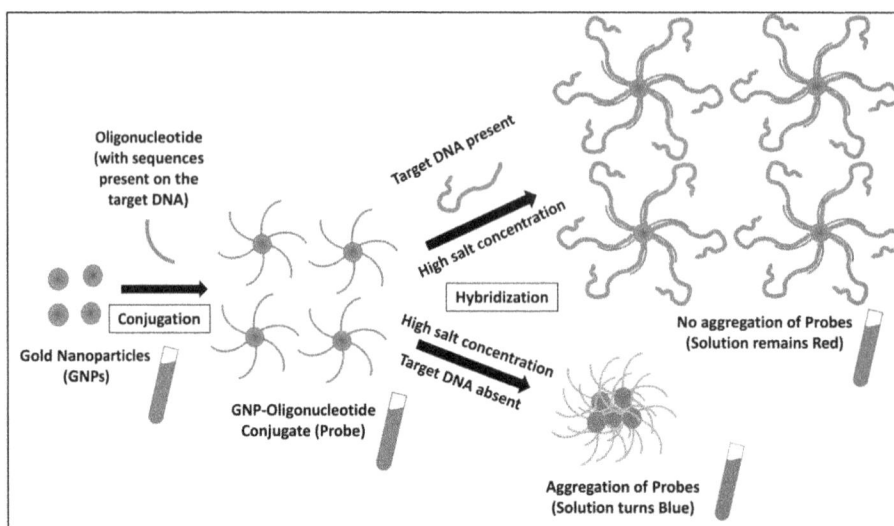

**Figure 4.4.** Gold nanoparticle (GNP) based method to detect DNA biomarkers. It is one of the most basic methods of nanotechnology-based detection of cancer biomarkers. Here GNPs are conjugated with a thiolated oligonucleotide, which is a single stranded DNA molecule which carries a thiol group at one end with sequences which can bind with the target DNA specifically. Red GNPs aggregate to produce blue color under a high salt concentration. Binding of the GNP–oligonucleotide conjugate (probe) with target prevents the GNPs from coming closer and hence a change in color is not observed when the result is positive. A change in color shows a negative result.

incubated with isolated DNA from the clinical sample for hybridization followed by the addition of salt (such as sodium chloride or magnesium sulfate). If the target is present the solution remains red as the interactions between the GNP bound oligonucleotide and target DNA prevent the GNPs from forming aggregate. Whereas if the target is absent, GNPs cluster without hindrance and the solution turns blue (from red) (Kumar and Sharma 2022). Many biosensors and diagnostic kits have been developed based on this basic and fundamental principle. One notable benefit of this approach is its minimal likelihood of producing false positive results (Iglesias and Grzelczak 2020).

Apart from this approach, many other methods have also been developed employing GNPs to detect a variety of targets with different chemical compositions. GNPs have been used to detect single nucleotide polymorphisms (SNPs) and the fusion of genes which is very common in cancers (Franco *et al* 2015). For example, *BCR-ABL* fusion gene mRNA, a hallmark of chronic myeloid leukemia, has been shown to be accurately detected using a GNP based method (Conde *et al* 2012). Table 4.3 shows some of the recently developed GNP based methods which are used in early cancer detection along with methods based on other nanoparticles. GNPs can be custom modified to detect a variety of biomarkers such ase DNA methylation, extracellular vesicles, specific proteins, CTCs, mRNAs and circulating tumor DNA (ctDNA) (Zhang *et al* 2019).

### 4.3.2.2 Quantum dot based biomarker detection

The unique optical and electrical features of quantum dots (QDs) have led to extensive research on their potential as novel probes for biomedical imaging, both *in vitro* and *in vivo*. The utilization of QD-based probes, when conjugated with biomolecules such as antibodies, peptides, or other small molecules, enables the precise targeting of cancer biomarkers with high sensitivity and specificity (Fang *et al* 2012). QDs are nanocrystals made of semiconductor materials that emit fluorescence when excited by a light source (Zhang *et al* 2008). Figure 4.5(B) shows one of the basic methods where QDs are used in biomarker detection *in vivo*. Antibodies raised against a particular antigen can be labeled with QDs. QDs such as CdSe based QDs fluoresce in the presence of UV light to produce different colors depending upon the particle size (figure 4.5(A)). When the patient cells are treated with these QD labeled antibodies, fluorescence is detected on illumination with UV light if the target antigen (biomarker) is present. No fluorescence means the absence of the target. This simple strategy has been variously modified by different scientists. Table 4.3 shows some examples of QDs based nanodiagnostic methods along with other methods. QDs can be used efficiently to detect CTCs, cell surface proteins, microRNA, and many other kinds of biomarkers (Zhang *et al* 2019).

### 4.3.2.3 Integrative approach

To achieve more sensitivity and specificity, nanodiagnostic methods have been developed using more than one kind of nanoparticles. Such an approach helps in signal enhancement when the amount of patient sample is limited or the concentration of biomarker is very low. Detecting biomarkers even at low concentrations aids in early detection of cancer as well as prognosis so that therapeutic measures can be taken at the right time. One such approach is integrating QDs and magnetic nanoparticles (MNPs) in one diagnostic system. Here, two different antibodies are raised against different epitopes (say epitope-1 and epitope-2) of the same antigen (say antigen-A). One of these two antibodies is labeled with quantum dots while the other is labeled with MNPs. Treating patient samples in a solution with MNP labeled antibodies is followed by treatment with QD labeled antibodies. If the target antigen (biomarker) is present in the solution, both antibodies bind to it. The MNP labeled antibodies aggregate together and form a clump under a magnetic field. This aggregate produces a greater fluorescence signal under UV light due to the aggregation of QD labeled antibodies as these are bound to the same antigen with which MNP labeled antibodies are associated (figure 4.6). Human papilloma virus (HPV) is known to be the causative agent of cervical cancers. A similar QD-MNP based strategy has been employed to develop a method to detect patient's susceptibility to cervical cancer by confirming the presence or absence of HPV protein in a solution containing pap smear samples (Raman *et al* 2021). A similar strategy has been used in the development of multiplexed nanobiosensors. Multiplexing facilitates a biosensor to run different samples in parallel and take multiple readings simultaneously (Jarockyte *et al* 2020).

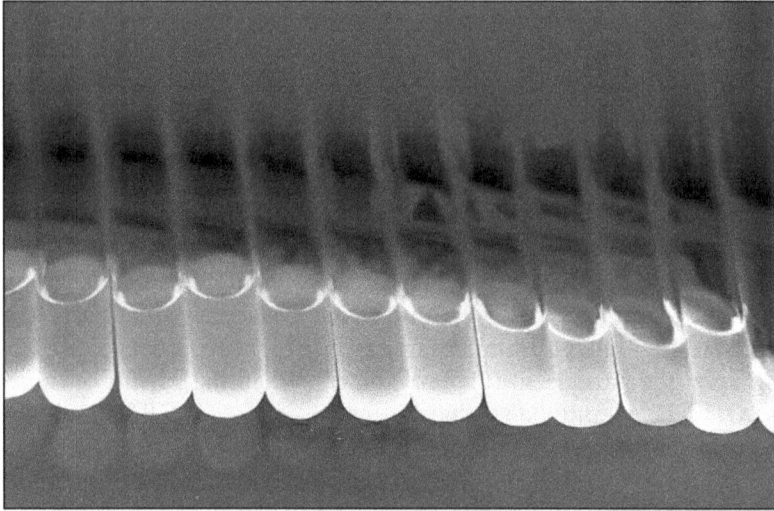

A

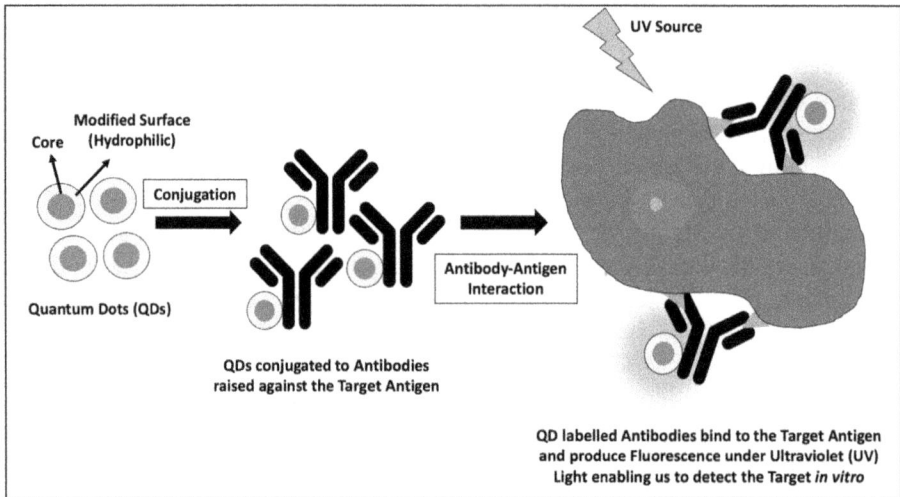

B

**Figure 4.5.** Quantum dots (QDs). (A) CdSe QDs of different sizes producing fluorescence of different colors under UV light. The smallest QDs are blue-green in color whereas the largest are red. These quantum dots were synthesized at Nanotechnology Lab, Electron Microscopy Facility, All India Institute of Medical Sciences, New Delhi, India (unpublished). (B) Schematic representation of the basic principle behind the detection of a biomarker using QD labeled antibodies.

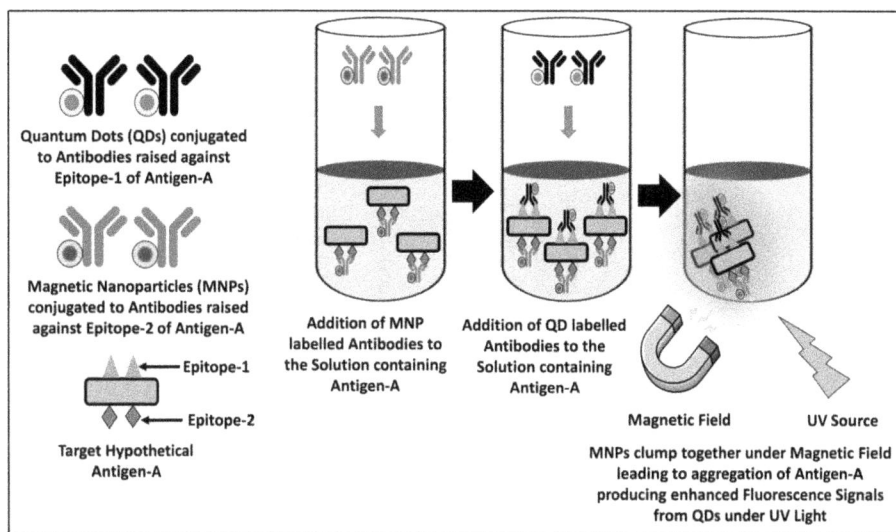

**Figure 4.6.** A hybrid nanodiagnostic system involving two different nanoparticles. Two different antibodies are against different epitopes of the same antigen. These antibodies bind to the same antigen and produce enhanced fluorescence signals under a magnetic field and UV light.

The account of different nanodiagnostic methods used for the early detection of cancer given in the present chapter is not exhaustive. The number of currently available methods are much higher. Only a few important and popular methods have been discussed for the sake of simplicity and ease of understanding. Several of these approaches are currently in various phases of clinical trials (table 4.4), many are still in the process of being developed and some of these procedures are being utilized by pathologists and physicians worldwide for diagnostic purposes. The days are not far away when nanotechnology based diagnostics will dominate the biomedical industry.

## 4.4 Conclusion

Nanotechnology has the potential to fulfill increasing demands of fast, easy to use, cheap and reliable diagnostic tools for early cancer detection. Today it is possible to develop an effective diagnostic tool against any kind of biomarker for any type of cancer. More robust next-generation biosensors are being developed with enhanced sensitivity and high specificity with almost zero probability of measurement errors. Biosensors have achieved detection capabilities at ultralow concentrations of biomarkers. Nanotechnology has made this possible. Nanotechnology is revolutionizing biosensor research and development globally and has the potential to thousands upon thousands of human lives from succumbing to cancer worldwide by providing cheap and reliable early cancer detection platforms.

**Table 4.4.** Examples of clinical trials of some nanotechnology-based cancer detection methods (sources: Zhang *et al* 2019, Kemp and Kwon 2021).

| Sl. No. | Trial no. | Intervention | Cancer type | Clinical trial status | Study type |
|---|---|---|---|---|---|
| 1 | NCT04482803 | Carbon nanoparticles | Breast cancer | Completed | Interventional |
| 2 | NCT04696744 | Biological: CTC detection | Oropharyngeal squamous cell carcinoma | Recruiting | Observational |
| 3 | NCT04825002 | Diagnostic test: urinary multimarker sensor (*ANXA3*, PSMA, *ERG*, ENG) | Prostate cancer | Recruiting | Interventional |
| 4 | NCT04661176 | Diagnostic test: miR Sentinel™ PCC4 Assay | Prostate cancer | Active, not recruiting | Observational |
| 5 | NCT04300673 | Procedure: radio guided surgery (RGS) using indium-labeled PSMA | Prostate cancer | Active, not recruiting | Phase 1 and 2 |
| 6 | NCT04261777 | Drug: Ferrotran® (Ferumoxtran-10) | Prostate cancer | Recruiting | Phase 3 |
| 7 | NCT04290923 | NA | Leukemia | Completed | Observational |
| 8 | NCT04239105 | Device: microfluidic and Raman spectrum | Breast cancer | Unknown | Observational |
| 9 | NCT04167969 | Drug: (64Cu)-labeled PSMA-targeting particle tracer, or 64Cu-NOTA-PSMAi-PEG-Cy5.5-C' dots | Prostate cancer | Recruiting | Phase 1 |
| 10 | NCT03817307 | Diagnostic test: ultrasmall superparamagnetic iron oxide (USPIO)-enhanced MRI | Head and neck squamous cell carcinoma | Recruiting | Interventional |
| 11 | NCT03550001 | Procedure: injection CNP before NAT | Rectal cancer | Unknown | Interventional |
| 12 | NCT04167722 | Procedure: robotic radical prostatectomy | Prostate cancer | Recruiting | Observational |
| 13 | NCT03134846 | Drug: Cetuximab-IRDye800CW | Head and neck squamous cell carcinoma | Unknown | Phase 1 and 2 |
| 14 | NCT02751606 | Drug: ferumoxtran-10; Device: 7 Tesla MRI; Device: 3 Tesla MRI | Breast neoplasms rectal neoplasms | Unknown | Phase 3 |
| 15 | NCT02106598 | Drug: fluorescent cRGDY-PEG-Cy5.5-C dots | Head and neck melanoma | Active, not recruiting | Phase 1 and 2 |
| 16 | NCT01359436 | Device: electrosensing antibody probing system (e-Ab sensing) | Non-small cell lung cancer | Unknown | Interventional |
| 17 | NCT03656835 | Procedure: molecular nanotechnology | Diffuse large B-cell lymphoma | Recruiting | Interventional |
| 18 | NCT03350945 | Procedure: device: tumor localization | Colorectal cancer | Unknown | Interventional |
| 19 | NCT03778268 | Procedure: sentinel lymph node biopsy | Cervical cancer | Unknown | Interventional |

# References

Afzal S, Hassan M, Ullah S, Abbas H, Tawakkal F and Khan M A 2022. Breast cancer; discovery of novel diagnostic biomarkers, drug resistance, and therapeutic implications *Front. Mol. Biosci.* **9** 783450

Akhtar M, Cheng Y, Magno R M, Ashktorab H, Smoot D T, Meltzer S J and Wilson K T 2001 Promoter methylation regulates *Helicobacter pylori*-stimulated cyclooxygenase-2 expression in gastric epithelial cells *Cancer Res.* **61** 2399–403

Alharbi K K and Al-Sheikh Y A 2014 Role and implications of nanodiagnostics in the changing trends of clinical diagnosis *Saudi J. Biol. Sci.* **21** 109–17

Altammar K A 2023 A review on nanoparticles: characteristics, synthesis, applications, and challenges *Front. Microbiol.* **14** 1155622

Ananth R 2000 Downstaging of cervical cancer *J. Indian Med. Assoc.* **98** 41–4

Aquilanti E, Miller J, Santagata S, Cahill D P and Brastianos P K 2018 Updates in prognostic markers for gliomas *Neuro-Oncology* **20** vii17–26

Ariafar A, Sanati A, Ahmadvand S, Shekarkhar G, Safaei A, Shayan Z and Faghih Z 2022 Prognostic significance of immunoscore related markers in bladder cancer *BMC Urol.* **22** 133

Arroyo J D, Chevillet J R, Kroh E M, Ruf I K, Pritchard C C, Gibson D F and Tewari M 2011 Argonaute2 complexes carry a population of circulating microRNAs independent of vesicles in human plasma *Proc. Natl Acad. Sci.* **108** 5003–8

Asci Erkocyigit B, Ozufuklar O, Yardim A, Guler Celik E and Timur S 2023 Biomarker detection in early diagnosis of cancer: recent achievements in point-of-care devices based on paper microfluidics *Biosensors* **13** 387

Bacci G, Ferrari S, Bertoni F, Rimondini S, Longhi A, Bacchini P and Picci P 2000 Prognostic factors in nonmetastatic Ewing's sarcoma of bone treated with adjuvant chemotherapy: analysis of 359 patients at the Istituto Ortopedico Rizzoli *J. Clin. Oncol.* **18** 4-4

Baek T J, Park P Y, Han K N, Kwon H T and Seong G H 2008 Development of a photodiode array biochip using a bipolar semiconductor and its application to detection of human papilloma virus *Anal. Bioanal. Chem.* **390** 1373–8

Baldini C, Billeci L, Sansone F, Conte R, Domenici C and Tonacci A 2020 Electronic nose as a novel method for diagnosing cancer: a systematic review *Biosensors* **10** 84

Ballman K V 2015 Biomarker: predictive or prognostic? *J. Clin. Oncol.* **33** 3968–71

Baptista P V 2014 Nanodiagnostics: leaving the research lab to enter the clinics? *Diagnosis* **1** 305–309

Barak V, Meirovitz A, Leibovici V, Rachmut J, Peretz T, Eliashar R and Gross M 2015 The diagnostic and prognostic value of tumor markers (CEA, SCC, CYFRA 21-1, TPS) in head and neck cancer patients *Anticancer Res.* **35** 5519–24

Basheeth N and Patil N 2019 Biomarkers in head and neck cancer an update *Indian J. Otolaryngol. Head Neck Surg.* **71** 1002–11

Bazak R, Houri M, El Achy S, Hussein W and Refaat T 2014 Passive targeting of nanoparticles to cancer: a comprehensive review of the literature *Mol. Clin. Oncol.* **2** 904–8

Boland C R, Sato J, Appelman H D, Bresalier R S and Feinberg A P 1995 Microallelotyping defines the sequence and tempo of alleiic losses at tumour suppressor gene loci during colorectal cancer progression *Nat. Med.* **1** 902

Brase J C, Wuttig D, Kuner R and Sültmann H 2010 Serum microRNAs as non-invasive biomarkers for cancer *Mol. Cancer* **9** 1–9

Bratu O, Marcu D, Anghel R, Spinu D, Iorga L, Balescu I and Cherciu A 2021 Tumoral markers in bladder cancer *Exp. Ther. Med.* **22** 1–8

Broeckelmann P J, Angelopoulou M K and Vassilakopoulos T P 2016 Prognostic factors in Hodgkin lymphoma *Semin. Hematol.* **53** 155–64

Budach V and Tinhofer I 2019 Novel prognostic clinical factors and biomarkers for outcome prediction in head and neck cancer: a systematic review *Lancet Oncol.* **20** e313–26

Căinap C, Nagy V, Gherman A, Cetean S, Laszlo I, Constantin A M and Căinap S 2015 Classic tumor markers in gastric cancer. Current standards and limitations *Clujul Med.* **88** 111

Chakroborty D, Emani M R, Klén R, Böckelman C, Hagström J, Haglund C and Elo L L 2019 L1TD1-a prognostic marker for colon cancer *BMC Cancer* **19** 1–9

Chan A and Dogan A 2019 Prognostic and predictive biomarkers in diffuse large B-cell lymphoma *Surg. Pathol. Clin.* **12** 699–707

Chattopadhyay C, Kim D W, Gombos D S, Oba J, Qin Y, Williams M D and Patel S P 2016 Uveal melanoma: from diagnosis to treatment and the science in between *Cancer* **122** 2299–312

Chen J, Ueda K, Sakakibara S, Okuno T, Parravicini C, Corbellino M and Yamanishi K 2001 Activation of latent Kaposi's sarcoma-associated herpesvirus by demethylation of the promoter of the lytic transactivator *Proc. Natl Acad. Sci.* **98** 4119–24

Chen X, Gole J, Gore A, He Q, Lu M, Min J and Jin L 2020 Non-invasive early detection of cancer four years before conventional diagnosis using a blood test *Nat. Commun.* **11** 1–10

Cho J 2022 Basic immunohistochemistry for lymphoma diagnosis *Blood Res.* **57** 55

Chovanec M, Albany C, Mego M, Montironi R, Cimadamore A and Cheng L 2018 Emerging prognostic biomarkers in testicular germ cell tumors: looking beyond established practice *Front. Oncol.* **8** 571

Ciobanu O A, Martin S and Fica S 2021 Perspectives on the diagnostic, predictive and prognostic markers of neuroendocrine neoplasms *Exp. Ther. Med.* **22** 1–14

Conde J, Doria G, de la Fuente J M and Baptista P V 2012 RNA quantification using noble metal nanoprobes: simultaneous identification of several different mRNA targets using color multiplexing and application to cancer diagnostics *Nanoparticles in Biology and Medicine: Methods and Protocols* (Berlin: Springer) pp 71–87

Costantini S and Budillon A 2020 New prognostic and predictive markers in cancer progression *Int. J. Mol. Sci.* **21** 8667

Dahlrot R H, Bangsø J A, Petersen J K, Rosager A M, Sørensen M D, Reifenberger G and Kristensen B W 2021 Prognostic role of Ki-67 in glioblastomas excluding contribution from non-neoplastic cells *Sci. Rep.* **11** 17918

Dart A 2020 Catching cancer *Nat. Rev. Cancer* **20** 299

Dieckmann K P, Simonsen-Richter H, Kulejewski M, Anheuser P, Zecha H, Isbarn H and Pichlmeier U 2019 Serum tumour markers in testicular germ cell tumours: frequencies of elevated levels and extents of marker elevation are significantly associated with clinical parameters and with response to treatment *BioMed Res. Int.* **2019** 5030349

Dilliard S A and Siegwart D J 2023 Passive, active and endogenous organ-targeted lipid and polymer nanoparticles for delivery of genetic drugs *Nat. Rev. Mat.* **8** 282–300

Ding L, Gosh A, Lee D J, Emri G, Huss W J, Bogner P N and Paragh G 2022 Prognostic biomarkers of cutaneous melanoma *Photodermatol. Photoimmunol. Photomed.* **38** 418–34

Ding P, Wang Z, Wu Z, Hu M, Zhu W, Sun N and Pei R 2021 Tannic acid (TA)-functionalized magnetic nanoparticles for EpCAM-independent circulating tumor cell (CTC) isolation from patients with different cancers *ACS Appl. Mater. Interfaces* **13** 3694–700

Dobra G, Gyukity-Sebestyén E, Bukva M, Harmati M, Nagy V, Szabó Z and Buzás K 2023 MMP-9 as prognostic marker for brain tumours: a comparative study on serum-derived small extracellular vesicles *Cancers* **15** 712

Dochez V, Caillon H, Vaucel E, Dimet J, Winer N and Ducarme G 2019. Biomarkers and algorithms for diagnosis of ovarian cancer: CA125, HE4, RMI and ROMA, a review *J. Ovarian Res.* **12** 28

Eads C A, Lord R V, Wickramasinghe K, Long T I, Kurumboor S K, Bernstein L and Laird P W 2001 Epigenetic patterns in the progression of esophageal adenocarcinoma *Cancer Res.* **61** 3410–8

Eagle R C 2013 The pathology of ocular cancer *Eye* **27** 128–36

Economopoulou P, De Bree R, Kotsantis I and Psyrri A 2019 Diagnostic tumor markers in head and neck squamous cell carcinoma (HNSCC) in the clinical setting *Front. Oncol.* **9** 827

Erdmann K, Salomo K, Klimova A, Heberling U, Lohse-Fischer A, Fuehrer R and Fuessel S 2020 Urinary MicroRNAs as potential markers for non-invasive diagnosis of bladder cancer *Int. J. Mol. Sci.* **21** 3814

Erickson L A and Lloyd R V 2004 Practical markers used in the diagnosis of endocrine tumors *Adv. Anat. Pathol.* **11** 175–89

Eriksson B, Öberg K and Stridsberg M 2000 Tumor markers in neuroendocrine tumors *Digestion* **62** 33–8

Esteva F J and Hortobagyi G N 2004 Prognostic molecular markers in early breast cancer *Breast Cancer Res.* **6** 1–10

Evola F R, Costarella L, Pavone V, Caff G, Cannavò L, Sessa A and Sessa G 2017 Biomarkers of osteosarcoma, chondrosarcoma, and Ewing sarcoma *Front. Pharmacol.* **8** 239591

Fang M, Peng C W, Pang D W and Li Y 2012 Quantum dots for cancer research: current status, remaining issues, and future perspectives *Cancer Biol. Med.* **9** 151

Fernandes M P, Venkatesh S and Sudarshan B G 2015 Early detection of lung cancer using nano-nose—a review *Open Biomed. Eng. J.* **9** 228–33

Filippini D M, Broseghini E, Carosi F, Molin D D, Riefolo M, Fabbri L and Ferracin M 2023 A systematic review of diagnostic and prognostic biomarkers for head and neck cancer of unknown primary: an unmet clinical need *Diagnostics* **13** 1492

Foran J M 2010 New prognostic markers in acute myeloid leukemia: perspective from the clinic *Hematology Am. Soc. Hematol. Educ. Program.* **2010** 47–55

Fosså S D, Stenning S P, Gerl A, Horwich A, Clark P I, Wilkinson P M and Cook P A 1999 Prognostic factors in patients progressing after cisplatin-based chemotherapy for malignant non-seminomatous germ cell tumours *Br. J. Cancer* **80** 1392–9

Franco R, Pedrosa P, Carlos F F, Veigas B and Baptista P V 2015 Gold nanoparticles for DNA/RNA-based diagnostics *Handbook of Nanoparticles* (Berlin: Springer) p 1339

Freis P, Graillot E, Rousset P, Hervieu V, Chardon L, Lombard-Bohas C and Walter T 2017 Prognostic factors in neuroendocrine carcinoma: biological markers are more useful than histomorphological markers *Sci. Rep.* **7** 40609

Gajdzis M, Kaczmarek R and Gajdzis P 2021 Novel prognostic immunohistochemical markers in uveal melanoma-literature review *Cancers* **13** 4031

García-Alfonso P, Muñoz Martín A J, Ortega Morán L, Soto Alsar J, Torres Perez-Solero G, Blanco Codesido M and Grasso Cicala S 2021 Oral drugs in the treatment of metastatic colorectal cancer *Ther. Adv. Med. Oncol.* **13** 17588359211009001

Gbadamosi B, Ezekwudo D, Bastola S and Jaiyesimi I 2018 Predictive and prognostic markers in adults with acute myeloid leukemia: a single-institution experience *Clin. Lymphoma Myeloma Leuk.* **18** e287–94

Geisler L, Mohr R, Lambrecht J, Knorr J, Jann H, Loosen S H and Roderburg C 2021 The role of miRNA in the pathophysiology of neuroendocrine tumors *Int. J. Mol. Sci.* **22** 8569

Gogas H, Eggermont A M M, Hauschild A, Hersey P, Mohr P, Schadendorf D and Dummer R 2009 Biomarkers in melanoma *Ann. Oncol.* **20** vi8–vi13

Gossing W, Frohme M and Radke L 2020 Biomarkers for liquid biopsies of pituitary neuro-endocrine tumors *Biomedicines* **8** 148

Green J 2012 *The Fault in Our Stars* (New York: Dutton)

Gregory T K, Wald D, Chen Y, Vermaat J M, Xiong Y and Tse W 2009 Molecular prognostic markers for adult acute myeloid leukemia with normal cytogenetics *J. Hematol. Oncol.* **2** 1–10

Hanke M, Hoefig K, Merz H, Feller A C, Kausch I, Jocham D and Sczakiel G 2010 A robust methodology to study urine microRNA as tumor marker: microRNA-126 and microRNA-182 are related to urinary bladder cancer *Urol. Oncol.* **28** 655–61

Hansen M and Pedersen A G 1986 Tumor markers in patients with lung cancer *Chest* **89** 219S–24S

Harmsma M, Schutte B and Ramaekers F C 2013 Serum markers in small cell lung cancer: opportunities for improvement *Biochim. Biophys. Acta.* **1836** 255–72

Hedborg F, Fischer-Colbrie R, Östlin N, Sandstedt B, Tran M G and Maxwell P H 2010 Differentiation in neuroblastoma: diffusion-limited hypoxia induces neuro-endocrine secretory protein 55 and other markers of a chromaffin phenotype *PLoS One* **5** e12825

Heyn H 2015 Personalized therapy—epigenetic profiling as predictors of prognosis and response *Epigenetic Cancer Therapy* (New York: Academic) pp 677–98

Hong W, Lee S, Chang H J, Lee E S and Cho Y 2016 Multifunctional magnetic nanowires: a novel breakthrough for ultrasensitive detection and isolation of rare cancer cells from non-metastatic early breast cancer patients using small volumes of blood *Biomaterials* **106** 78–86

Huang H and Lovell J F 2017 Advanced functional nanomaterials for theranostics *Adv. Funct. Mater.* **27** 1603524

Huang J, Hu W and Sood A K 2011 Prognostic biomarkers in ovarian cancer *Cancer Biomark.* **8** 231–51

Huang Q *et al* 2018 Gelatin nanoparticle-coated silicon beads for density-selective capture and release of heterogeneous circulating tumor cells with high purity *Theranostics* **8** 1624–35

Huang Z, Zhu D, Wu L, He M, Zhou X, Zhang L and Liu P 2017 Six serum-based miRNAs as potential diagnostic biomarkers for gastric cancer *Cancer Epidemiol. Biomarkers Prev.* **26** 188–96

Hull L C, Farrell D and Grodzinski P 2014 Highlights of recent developments and trends in cancer nanotechnology research—view from NCI Alliance for Nanotechnology in Cancer *Biotechnol. Adv.* **32** 666–78

Hung P S, Chen C Y, Chen W T, Kuo C Y, Fang W L, Huang K H and Lo S S 2017 miR-376c promotes carcinogenesis and serves as a plasma marker for gastric carcinoma *PLoS One* **12** e0177346

Iglesias M S and Grzelczak M 2020 Using gold nanoparticles to detect single-nucleotide polymorphisms: toward liquid biopsy *Beilstein J. Nanotechnol.* **11** 263–84

Issa J P 2000 The epigenetics of colorectal cancer *Ann. N.Y. Acad. Sci.* **910** 140–55

Jalal S D 2021 The contribution of CD200 to the diagnostic accuracy of Matutes score in the diagnosis of chronic lymphocytic leukemia in limited resources laboratories *PLoS One* **16** e0247491

Jarockyte G, Karabanovas V, Rotomskis R and Mobasheri A 2020 Multiplexed nanobiosensors: current trends in early diagnostics *Sensors* **20** 6890

Jelski W and Mroczko B 2021 Molecular and circulating biomarkers of brain tumors *Int. J. Mol. Sci.* **22** 7039

Jeong S H and Ku J H 2022 Urinary markers for bladder cancer diagnosis and monitoring *Front. Cell Dev. Biol.* **10** 892067

Jerónimo C, Usadel H, Henrique R, Oliveira J, Lopes C, Nelson W G and Sidransky D 2001 Quantitation of *GSTP1* methylation in non-neoplastic prostatic tissue and organ-confined prostate adenocarcinoma *J. Natl Cancer Inst.* **93** 1747–52

Jerónimo C, Varzim G, Henrique R, Oliveira J, Bento M J, Silva C and Sidransky D 2002 I105V polymorphism and promoter methylation of the *GSTP1* gene in prostate adenocarcinoma *Cancer Epidemiol. Biomarkers Prev.* **11** 445–50

Ji T, Zheng Z G, Wang F M, Xu L J, Li L F, Cheng Q H and Ding X F 2014 Differential microRNA expression by Solexa sequencing in the sera of ovarian cancer patients *Asian Pac. J. Cancer Prev.* **15** 1739–43

Jiang H, Ou Z, He Y, Yu M, Wu S, Li G and Zhang K 2020 DNA methylation markers in the diagnosis and prognosis of common leukemias *Signal Trans. Target. Ther.* **5** 3

Jin E and Burnier J V 2021 Liquid biopsy in uveal melanoma: are we there yet? *Ocul. Oncol. Pathol.* **7** 1–16

Johnson D E, Burtness B, Leemans C R, Lui V W Y, Bauman J E and Grandis J R 2020 Head and neck squamous cell carcinoma *Nat. Rev. Dis. Primers* **6** 92

Kabel A M 2017 Tumor markers of breast cancer: new prospectives *J. Oncol. Sci.* **3** 5–11

Kan L K, Drummond K, Hunn M, Williams D, O'Brien T J and Monif M 2020 Potential biomarkers and challenges in glioma diagnosis, therapy and prognosis *BMJ Neurol. Open* **2** e000069

Kemp J A and Kwon Y J 2021 Cancer nanotechnology: current status and perspectives *Nano Converg.* **8** 34

Kerr D J and Yang L 2021 Personalising cancer medicine with prognostic markers *EBioMedicine* **72** 103577

Khan I, Saeed K and Khan I 2019 Nanoparticles: properties, applications and toxicities *Arabian J. Chem.* **12** 908–31

Kim Y J and Kim W J 2016 Can we use methylation markers as diagnostic and prognostic indicators for bladder cancer ? *Invest. Clin. Urol.* **57** S77

Korotaeva A, Mansorunov D, Apanovich N, Kuzevanova A and Karpukhin A 2021 MiRNA expression in neuroendocrine neoplasms of frequent localizations *Non-coding RNA* **7** 38

Ku J H, Kim W J, Lerner S P, Chun F and Kluth L A 2016 Diagnostic and prognostic markers in bladder cancer *Dis. Markers* **2016**

Kumar R and Sharma A K 2022 Conferring midas touch on integrative taxonomy: a nanogold-oligonucletide conjugate-based quick species detection tool *Int. J. Ecol.* **2022** 1009066

Laman H and Boshoff C 2001 Is KSHV lytic growth induced by a methylation-sensitive switch? *Trends Microbiol.* **9** 464–6

Lamas N J, Martel A, Nahon-Estève S, Goffinet S, Macocco A, Bertolotto C and Hofman P 2021 Prognostic biomarkers in uveal melanoma: the status quo, recent advances and future directions *Cancers* **14** 96

Larsen J E and Minna J D 2011 Molecular biology of lung cancer: clinical implications *Clin. Chest Med.* **32** 703–40

Laurent S, Forge D, Port M, Roch A, Robic C, Vander Elst L and Muller R N 2008 Magnetic iron oxide nanoparticles: synthesis, stabilization, vectorization, physicochemical characterizations, and biological applications *Chem. Rev.* **108** 2064–110

Law C C, Wong C H, Chong P S, Mang O W, Lam A W, Chak M M and Ho R K 2022 Effectiveness of population-based colorectal cancer screening programme in down-staging *Cancer Epidemiol.* **79** 102184

Lawrence R, Watters M, Davies C R, Pantel K and Lu Y J 2023 Circulating tumour cells for early detection of clinically relevant cancer *Nat. Rev. Clin. Oncol.* **20** 487–500

Li L, Wang Y, He X and Min L 2022 Hematological prognostic scoring system can predict overall survival and can indicate response to immunotherapy in patients with osteosarcoma *Front. Immunol.* **13** 879560

Li Z, Wang G, Shen Y, Guo N and Ma N 2018 DNA-templated magnetic nanoparticle-quantum dot polymers for ultrasensitive capture and detection of circulating tumor cells *Adv. Funct. Mater.* **28** 1707152

Ling B, Liao X, Huang Y, Liang L, Jiang Y, Pang Y and Qi G 2020 Identification of prognostic markers of lung cancer through bioinformatics analysis and *in vitro* experiments *Int. J. Oncol.* **56** 193–205

Liu J, Chen H, Li Y, Fang Y, Guo Y, Li S and Wang X 2023a A novel non-invasive exhaled breath biopsy for the diagnosis and screening of breast cancer *J. Hematol. Oncol.* **16** 63

Liu Q *et al* 2023b Identification of urinary volatile organic compounds as a potential non-invasive biomarker for esophageal cancer *Sci. Rep.* **13** 18587

Liu S *et al* 2016 Combined cell surface carbonic anhydrase 9 and CD147 antigens enable high-efficiency capture of circulating tumor cells in clear cell renal cell carcinoma patients *Oncotarget* **7** 59877–91

Liu Y J, Li J P, Zeng S H, Han M, Liu S L and Zou X 2021 DZIP1 expression as a prognostic marker in gastric cancer: a bioinformatics-based analysis *Pharmacogenomics Pers. Med.* **14** 1151–68

Liu Y, Zhu F, Dan W, Fu Y and Liu S 2014 Construction of carbon nanotube based nanoarchitectures for selective impedimetric detection of cancer cells in whole blood *Analyst* **139** 5086–92

Lorio M V, Ferracin M, Liu C G, Veronese A, Spizzo R, Sabbioni S and Croce C M 2005 MicroRNA gene expression deregulation in human breast cancer *Cancer Res.* **65** 7065–70

Lubov J, Labbé M, Sioufi K, Morand G B, Hier M P, Khanna M and Mlynarek A M 2021 Prognostic factors of head and neck cutaneous squamous cell carcinoma: a systematic review *J. Otolaryngol. Head Neck Surg.* **50** 54

Luo J, Xiao J, Yang Y, Chen G, Hu D and Zeng J 2023. Strategies for five tumour markers in the screening and diagnosis of female breast cancer *Front. Oncol.* **12** 1055855

Madkour L H 2019 Examples of nanomaterials with various morphologies *Nanoelectronic Materials* (Advanced Structured Materials vol 116) (Cham: Springer)

Magnes T, Wagner S, Kiem D, Weiss L, Rinnerthaler G, Greil R and Melchardt T 2021 Prognostic and predictive factors in advanced head and neck squamous cell carcinoma *Int. J. Mol. Sci.* **22** 4981

Markowitz S, Wang J, Myeroff L, Parsons R, Sun L, Lutterbaugh J and Willson J K 1995 Inactivation of the type II TGF-$\beta$ receptor in colon cancer cells with microsatellite instability *Science* **268** 1336–8

Matsas A, Stefanoudakis D, Troupis T, Kontzoglou K, Eleftheriades M, Christopoulos P and Iliopoulos D C 2023 Tumor markers and their diagnostic significance in ovarian cancer *Life* **13** 1689

Matsuoka T and Yashiro M 2018 Biomarkers of gastric cancer: current topics and future perspective *World J. Gastroenterol.* **24** 2818

Mayo Clinic 2022 Cancer: diagnosis and treatment https://mayoclinic.org/diseases-conditions/cancer/diagnosis-treatment/drc-20370594 (Accessed: 17 November 2023)

Moeinzadeh S and Jabbari E 2017 Nanoparticles and their applications *Springer Handbook of Nanotechnology* (Berlin: Springer) pp 335–61

Montagnana M, Benati M and Danese E 2017 Circulating biomarkers in epithelial ovarian cancer diagnosis: from present to future perspective *Ann. Transl. Med.* **5**

Morra E 1999 The biological market of non-Hodgkin's lymphomas their role in diagnosis, prognostic assessment and therapeutic strategy *Int. J. Biol. Markers* **14** 149–53

NCCN 2024 NCCN guidelines https://nccn.org/guidelines/category_1 (Accessed: 17 November 2023)

Ndiaye C, Mena M, Alemany L, Arbyn M, Castellsagué X, Laporte L and Trottier H 2014 HPV DNA, E6/E7 mRNA, and p16INK4a detection in head and neck cancers: a systematic review and meta-analysis *Lancet Oncol.* **15** 1319–31

Nik M, Kamal N N S B and Shahidan W N S 2020 Non-exosomal and exosomal circulatory microRNAs: which are more valid as biomarkers? *Front. Pharmacol.* **10** 487717

Nimse S B, Sonawane M D, Song K S and Kim T 2016 Biomarker detection technologies and future directions *Analyst* **141** 740–55

Pang X, Cui C, Su M, Wang Y, Wei Q and Tan W 2018 Construction of self-powered cytosensing device based on ZnO nanodisks@g-$C_3N_4$ quantum dots and application in the detection of CCRF-CEM cells *Nano Energy* **46** 101–9

Park S M, Aalipour A, Vermesh O, Yu J H and Gambhir S S 2017 Towards clinically translatable *in vivo* nanodiagnostics *Nat. Rev. Mater.* **2** 1–20

Pedraza A M and Stephenson A J 2018 Prognostic markers in clinical stage I seminoma and nonseminomatous germ cell tumours *Curr. Opin. Urol.* **28** 448–53

Pedrazzoli P, Rosti G, Soresini E, Ciani S and Secondino S 2021 Serum tumour markers in germ cell tumours: from diagnosis to cure *Crit. Rev. Oncol. Hematol.* **159** 103224

Peng G, Tisch U, Adams O, Hakim M, Shehada N, Broza Y Y, Billan S, Abdah-Bortnyak R, Kuten A and Haick H 2009 Diagnosing lung cancer in exhaled breath using gold nanoparticles *Nat. Nanotechnol.* **4** 669–73

Pezo R C and Bedard P L 2015 Definition: translational and personalised medicine, biomarkers, pharmacodynamics *ESMO Handbook of Translational Research* (Lugano: ESMO)

Puderecki M, Szumiło J and Marzec Kotarska B 2020 Novel prognostic molecular markers in lung cancer *Oncol. Lett.* **20** 9–18

Qu Y, Dang S and Hou P 2013 Gene methylation in gastric cancer *Clin. Chim. Acta* **424** 53–65

Rajpert-De Meyts E, Nielsen J E, Skakkebaek N E and Almstrup K 2015 Diagnostic markers for germ cell neoplasms: from placental-like alkaline phosphatase to micro-RNAs *Folia Histochem. Cytobiol.* **53** 177–88

Raman S, Tanwar P, Bhatla N and Yadav S C 2021 An immuno-nano-fluorescence assay, antibodies and a kit thereof for detection of human papillomavirus (HPV) infection associated cervical cancer *Patent* India 202111035011 (filed 3 August 2021)

Ranjbar R, Hesari A, Ghasemi F and Sahebkar A 2018 Expression of microRNAs and IRAK1 pathway genes are altered in gastric cancer patients with *Helicobacter pylori* infection *J. Cell. Biochem.* **119** 7570–6

Ray S K and Mukherjee S 2023 Piwi-interacting RNAs (piRNAs) and colorectal carcinoma: emerging non-invasive diagnostic biomarkers with potential therapeutic target based clinical implications *Curr. Mol. Med.* **23** 300–11

Rein B J, Gupta S, Dada R, Safi J, Michener C and Agarwal A 2011 Potential markers for detection and monitoring of ovarian cancer *J. Oncol.* **2011**

Riley R D, Heney D, Jones D R, Sutton A J, Lambert P C, Abrams K R and Burchill S A 2004 A systematic review of molecular and biological tumor markers in neuroblastoma *Clin. Cancer Res.* **10** 4–12

Rosati G, Riccardi F and Tucci A 2000 Use of tumor markers in the management of head and neck cancer *Int. J. Biol. Markers* **15** 179–83

Ruggieri V, Russi S, Zoppoli P, La Rocca F, Angrisano T, Falco G and Laurino S 2019 The role of microRNAs in the regulation of gastric cancer stem cells: a meta-analysis of the current status *J. Clin. Med.* **8** 639

Santoni G, Morelli M B, Amantini C and Battelli N 2018 Urinary markers in bladder cancer: an update *Front. Oncol.* **8** 362

Sarhadi V K and Armengol G 2022 Molecular biomarkers in cancer *Biomolecules* **12** 1021

Sato F, Harpaz N, Shibata D, Xu Y, Yin J, Mori Y and Meltzer S J 2002 Hypermethylation of the p14 ARF gene in ulcerative colitis-associated colorectal carcinogenesis *Cancer Res.* **62** 1148–51

Sav A, Rotondo F, Syro L V, Scheithauer B W and Kovacs K 2012 Biomarkers of pituitary neoplasms *Anticancer Res.* **32** 4639–54

Scheie D, Kufaishi H H A, Broholm H, Lund E L, de Stricker K, Melchior L C and Grauslund M 2019 Biomarkers in tumors of the central nervous system—a review *Apmis* **127** 265–87

Schmitz-Dräger B J, Droller M, Lokeshwar V B, Lotan Y, Hudson M L A, Van Rhijn B W and Shariat S F 2015 Molecular markers for bladder cancer screening, early diagnosis, and surveillance: the WHO/ICUD consensus *Urol. Int.* **94** 1–24

Schneider J 2006 Tumor markers in detection of lung cancer *Adv. Clin. Chem.* **42** 1–41

Sharifi M, Avadi M R, Attar F, Dashtestani F, Ghorchian H, Rezayat S M and Falahati M 2019 Cancer diagnosis using nanomaterials based electrochemical nanobiosensors *Biosens. Bioelectron.* **126** 773–84

Sharma B, Lakhanpal V, Singh K, Oberoi L, Bedi P K and Devi P 2022 Evaluation of HPV E6/E7 mRNA detection in clinically suspected cases of cervical cancer with abnormal cytology: time to upgrade the screening protocols *J. Lab. Physicians* **14** 336–42

Shen J, Li K, Cheng L, Liu Z, Lee S T and Liu J 2014 Specific detection and simultaneously localized photothermal treatment of cancer cells using layer-by-layer assembled multifunctional nanoparticles *ACS Appl. Mater. Interfaces* **6** 6443–52

Shi P, Cheng Z, Zhao K, Chen Y, Zhang A, Gan W and Zhang Y 2023 Active targeting schemes for nano-drug delivery systems in osteosarcoma therapeutics *J. Nanobiotechnol.* **21** 103

Śledzińska P, Bebyn M G, Furtak J, Kowalewski J and Lewandowska M A 2021 Prognostic and predictive biomarkers in gliomas *Int. J. Mol. Sci.* **22** 10373

Stark M S *et al* 2019. A panel of circulating microRNAs detects uveal melanoma with high precision *Transl. Vis. Sci. Technol.* **8** 12

Stern E, Vacic A, Rajan N K, Criscione J M, Park J, Ilic B R, Mooney D J, Reed M A and Fahmy T M 2010 Label-free biomarker detection from whole blood *Nat. Nanotechnol.* **5** 138–42

Sun R, Medeiros L J and Young K H 2016 Diagnostic and predictive biomarkers for lymphoma diagnosis and treatment in the era of precision medicine *Mod. Pathol.* **29** 1118–42

Šutić M, Vukić A, Baranašić J, Försti A, Džubur F, Samaržija M and Knežević J 2021 Diagnostic, predictive, and prognostic biomarkers in non-small cell lung cancer (NSCLC) management *J. Pers. Med.* **11** 1102

Syring I, Müller S C and Ellinger J 2014 Novel tumor markers in the serum of testicular germ cell cancer patients: a review *Curr. Biomark. Find.* **4** 133–7

Szabo I, Kiss A, Schaff Z and Sobel G 2009 Claudins as diagnostic and prognostic markers in gynecological cancer *Histol. Histopathol.* **24** 1607–15

Taneja P, Maglic D, Kai F, Zhu S, Kendig R D, Elizabeth A F and Inoue K 2010 Classical and novel prognostic markers for breast cancer and their clinical significance *Clin. Med. Insights Oncol.* **4** CMO-S4773

Teixido C, Castillo P, Martinez-Vila C, Arance A and Alos L 2021 Molecular markers and targets in melanoma *Cells* **10** 2320

Tiwari J N, Tiwari R N and Kim K S 2012 Zero-dimensional, one-dimensional, two-dimensional and three-dimensional nanostructured materials for advanced electrochemical energy devices *Prog. Mater Sci.* **57** 724–803

Tsai M M, Wang C S, Tsai C Y, Huang C G, Lee K F, Huang H W and Lin K H 2016 Circulating microRNA-196a/b are novel biomarkers associated with metastatic gastric cancer *Eur. J. Cancer* **64** 137–48

Ueda Y, Enomoto T, Kimura T, Miyatake T, Yoshino K, Fujita M and Kimura T 2010 Serum biomarkers for early detection of gynecologic cancers *Cancers* **2** 1312–27

Vaidya R and Witzig T E 2014 Prognostic factors for diffuse large B-cell lymphoma in the R (*X*) CHOP era *Ann. Oncol.* **25** 2124–33

van den Brekel M W M, Bindels E M J and Balm A J M 2002 Prognostic factors in head and neck cancer *Eur. J. Cancer* **38** 1041–3

Verma M, Lambert P F and Srivastava S K 2001 Meeting highlights: National Cancer Institute workshop on molecular signatures of infectious agents *Dis. Markers* **17** 191–201

Wang J, Zhang H, Zhou X, Wang T, Zhang J, Zhu W and Cheng W 2018 Five serum-based miRNAs were identified as potential diagnostic biomarkers in gastric cardia adenocarcinoma *Cancer Biomark.* **23** 193–203

Wang L, Zhan C, Zhang Y, Ma J, Xi J, Jiang W and Wang Q 2014 Quantifying the expression of tumor marker genes in lung squamous cell cancer with RNA sequencing *J. Thorac. Dis.* **6** 1380

Wang N, Wang L, Yang Y, Gong L, Xiao B and Liu X 2017a A serum exosomal microRNA panel as a potential biomarker test for gastric cancer *Biochem. Biophys. Res. Commun.* **493** 1322–8

Wang Y, Yu L, Kong X and Sun L 2017b Application of nanodiagnostics in point-of-care tests for infectious diseases *Int. J. Nanomed.* **12** 4789–803

Weinstein D, Leininger J, Hamby C and Safai B 2014 Diagnostic and prognostic biomarkers in melanoma *J. Clin. Aesthet. Dermatol.* **7** 13

Wiles A B, Karrs J X, Pitt S, Almenara J, Powers C N and Smith S C 2017 GATA3 is a reliable marker for neuroblastoma in limited samples, including FNA cell blocks, core biopsies, and touch imprints *Cancer Cytopathol.* **125** 940–6

World Health Organization 2022 Cancer https://who.int/news-room/fact-sheets/detail/cancer (Accessed: 17 November 2023)

Wu C, Schneider T, Zeigler M, Yu J, Schiro P G, Burnham D R, McNeill J D and Chiu D T 2010 Bioconjugation of ultrabright semiconducting polymer dots for specific cellular targeting *JACS* **132** 15410–7

Wu L and Qu X 2015 Cancer biomarker detection: recent achievements and challenges *Chemical Society Reviews* **44** 2963–97

Wu X, Xiao T, Luo Z, He R, Cao Y, Guo Z, Zhang W and Chen Y 2018 A micro-/nano-chip and quantum dots-based 3D cytosensor for quantitative analysis of circulating tumor cells *J. Nanobiotechnol.* **16** 65

Xu Y, Yu W, Yang T, Zhang M, Liang C, Cai X and Shao Q 2018 Overexpression of BCAT1 is a prognostic marker in gastric cancer *Human Pathol.* **75** 41–6

Yeager T R, DeVries S, Jarrard D F, Kao C, Nakada S Y, Moon T D and Reznikoff C A 1998 Overcoming cellular senescence in human cancer pathogenesis *Genes Dev.* **12** 163–74

Yi Y, Xu T, Tan Y, Lv W, Zhao C, Wu M and Zhang Q 2022 *CCDC69* is a prognostic marker of breast cancer and correlates with tumor immune cell infiltration *Front. Surg.* **9** 879921

Yılmaz H, Toy H I, Marquardt S, Karakülah G, Küçük C, Kontou P I and Pavlopoulou A 2021 *In silico* methods for the identification of diagnostic and favorable prognostic markers in acute myeloid leukemia *Int. J. Mol. Sci.* **22** 9601

Yin Y, Li J, Chen S, Zhou T and Si J 2012 MicroRNAs as diagnostic biomarkers in gastric cancer *Int. J. Mol. Sci.* **13** 12544–55

Yip C H 2019 Downstaging is more important than screening for asymptomatic breast cancer *Lancet Glob. Health* **7** e690–1

Yu S, Yu Y, Zhao N, Cui J, Li W and Liu T 2013 C-Met as a prognostic marker in gastric cancer: a systematic review and meta-analysis *PLoS One* **8** e79137

Yun X, Zhang Y and Wang X 2020 Recent progress of prognostic biomarkers and risk scoring systems in chronic lymphocytic leukemia *Biomark. Res.* **8** 1–11

Zamborsky R, Kokavec M, Harsanyi S and Danisovic L 2019 Identification of prognostic and predictive osteosarcoma biomarkers *Med. Sci.* **7** 28

Zhang H, Yee D and Wang C 2008 Quantum dots for cancer diagnosis and therapy: biological and clinical perspectives *Nanomedicine* **3** 83–91

Zhang Y, Li M, Gao X, Chen Y and Liu T 2019 Nanotechnology in cancer diagnosis: progress, challenges and opportunities *J. Hematol. Oncol.* **12** 137

Zhang B, Shi H and Wang H 2023 Machine learning and AI in cancer prognosis, prediction, and treatment selection: a critical approach *J. Multidisc. Healthc.* **2023** 1779–91

Zheng M, Wang H, Zhang H, Ou Q, Shen B, Li N and Yu B 1999 The influence of the p53 gene on the *in vitro* chemosensitivity of colorectal cancer cells *J. Cancer Res. Clin. Oncol.* **125** 357–60

Zheng Q, Zhu Q, Li C, Hao S, Li J, Yu X and Pan Y 2020 microRNA-144 functions as a diagnostic and prognostic marker for retinoblastoma *Clinics* **75** e1804

Zhou J, Gong G, Tan H, Dai F, Zhu X, Chen Y and Wen J 2015 Urinary microRNA-30a-5p is a potential biomarker for ovarian serous adenocarcinoma *Oncol. Rep.* **33** 2915–23

Zhu C Q and Tsao M S 2014 Prognostic markers in lung cancer: is it ready for prime time? *Transl. Lung Cancer Res.* **3** 149

Zhu C, Ren C, Han J, Ding Y, Du J, Dai N and Jin G 2014 A five-microRNA panel in plasma was identified as potential biomarker for early detection of gastric cancer *Br. J. Cancer* **110** 2291–9

Zhu Y, Chandra P and Shim Y B 2013 Ultrasensitive and selective electrochemical diagnosis of breast cancer based on a hydrazine-Au nanoparticle-aptamer bioconjugate *Anal. Chem.* **85** 1058–64

# Chapter 5

# Detection of circulatory cancerous cells for early diagnosis of breast cancer

**Priyanka Sonkar and Amit Kumar Sonkar**

Over recent decades, extensive scientific research has focused on various critical elements in the early detection and management of breast cancer, significantly transforming how this condition is addressed in clinical practice. This transformation encompasses several key areas of advancements in detection technologies such as digital mammography, computer-assisted readings, and tomosynthesis, the establishment of standardized systems for interpreting imaging results, the adoption of less invasive surgical approaches, enhancements in systemic therapies, and breakthroughs in genomics. Simultaneously, there has been a notable increase in social awareness and acceptance of breast cancer, prompting governments in many countries to allocate resources toward implementing early detection strategies due to the high rates of incidence and mortality.

Despite these strides, breast cancer remains the primary cause of cancer-related deaths among women. Moreover, alongside the apparent progress, there have been emerging risks and adverse events, the precise impact of which is challenging to gauge accurately. These factors cast doubt on the genuine benefits derived from mammography screenings, prompting a critical re-evaluation of their efficacy and overall impact on breast cancer management. This chapter explores the significance of detecting circulating cancerous cells in the bloodstream for the early diagnosis of breast cancer. Various techniques and methodologies are discussed, including liquid biopsy, immunocytochemistry, microfluidic devices, and next-generation sequencing. The chapter emphasizes the importance of early detection in improving patient outcomes and highlights the potential of these innovative approaches in breast cancer management.

doi:10.1088/978-0-7503-6234-4ch5

## Abbreviations

| | |
|---|---|
| BC | breast cancer |
| cfDNA | cell-free DNA |
| CTCs | circulatory tumor cells |
| ctDNA | circulating tutor DNA |
| EMT | epithelial–mesenchymal transition |
| EpCAM | epithelial cell adhesion molecule |
| EV | extracellular vesicles |
| ICC | immunocytochemistry |
| NGS | next-generation sequencing |

## 5.1 Introduction

Breast cancer is the most common malignancy affecting women worldwide and is characterized by the abnormal growth of cells in the breast tissue. Epidemiologically, it is estimated that one in eight women will develop breast cancer during their lifetime. Breast cancer (BC) stands as one of the most prevalent forms of cancer globally, impacting millions of women each year (Addanki *et al* 2022). In 2020 alone, approximately 2.3 million new cases were diagnosed, constituting a quarter of all new cancer diagnoses. Tragically, it also remains a leading cause of cancer-related deaths among females, claiming the lives of an estimated 685 000 individuals, representing one in six cancer-related deaths (Sedeta *et al* 2023, Bray *et al* 2018). While the exact causes of breast cancer remain elusive, several risk factors have been identified, including genetic predisposition (*BRCA* mutations), hormonal factors (estrogen exposure), lifestyle choices (obesity, alcohol consumption), and environmental factors (exposure to ionizing radiation).

Breast cancer typically originates in the milk ducts (ductal carcinoma) or lobules (lobular carcinoma) of the breast tissue (Creighton 2012). Mechanistically, genetic mutations, such as alterations in tumor suppressor genes (e.g. *BRCA1*, *BRCA2*) or oncogenes (e.g. *HER2*/neu), contribute to the uncontrolled proliferation of cells (Panesar *et al* 2016, Qiu *et al* 2023). This dysregulated cell growth leads to the formation of tumors, which may eventually invade surrounding tissues and metastasize to distant organs. Early detection through screening programs and advancements in treatment modalities, including surgery, chemotherapy, radiation therapy, and targeted therapies, have significantly improved the prognosis for breast cancer patients.

The early detection of breast cancer is of paramount importance due to its significant impact on patient outcomes, treatment options, and overall healthcare efficacy. Prompt identification of breast cancer at an early stage offers patients a wider array of treatment choices, including less invasive procedures such as lumpectomy or hormone therapy. This not only enhances the quality of life for patients but also contributes to improved long-term prognosis (Merino Bonilla *et al* 2017, Li *et al* 2020). Liquid biopsies, capturing circulating tumor cells (CTCs) from blood, offer a non-invasive, frequent monitoring method (Kilgour *et al* 2020, Lin *et al* 2018). Unlike tissue biopsies, they reflect tumor heterogeneity and facilitate real-time tracking of cancer evolution and treatment response, potentially revolutionizing cancer diagnosis and personalized therapy (Descamps *et al* 2022). Studies consistently demonstrate that early detection leads to higher survival rates among breast cancer patients, highlighting its critical role in mitigating the impact of this disease (Mehlen and Puisieux 2006). Moreover, early diagnosis can help reduce morbidity by minimizing the need for aggressive treatments such as chemotherapy or extensive surgeries, thereby alleviating treatment-related adverse effects and expediting recovery (Galizia *et al* 2018). Economically, early detection proves cost-effective, as it averts the necessity for expensive advanced-stage interventions and reduces the burden on healthcare systems. Beyond its tangible benefits, early detection empowers individuals through routine screening programs, offering them the opportunity to detect cancer before symptoms emerge, thereby facilitating timely diagnostic evaluations and interventions. The integration of liquid biopsy techniques, such as the analysis of CTCs, circulating tumor DNA (ctDNA), cell-free RNA, tumor-educated platelets, and exosomes, addresses the limitations of traditional methods such as tissue biopsy in breast cancer management (Bardelli and Pantel 2017). These methods offer a comprehensive view of the genomic landscape, facilitating early diagnosis, prognosis prediction, relapse detection, and longitudinal monitoring of treatment response. This approach enhances the efficiency of breast cancer management by enabling early interventions and personalized treatment strategies tailored to the dynamic nature of the disease (Alimirzaie *et al* 2019). Ultimately, early detection not only extends survival but also enhances the overall quality of life for breast cancer survivors by preserving physical function, emotional well-being, and social connections. Hence, efforts to promote early detection strategies, such as public awareness campaigns and accessible screening programs, are crucial in mitigating the impact of breast cancer and improving patient outcomes on a global scale.

## 5.2 Role of circulating tumor cells in cancer metastasis

The discovery of CTCs in 1869 marked a significant milestone in cancer research, offering insights into metastatic processes (Addanki *et al* 2022). Subsequently, in 1948, circulating nucleic acids were identified, broadening our understanding of cancer biomarkers (Mandel and Metais 1948). Building upon these discoveries, the revelation of circulating cell-free DNA (cfDNA) further advanced diagnostic capabilities by enabling the detection of specific mutations associated with various cancers. This progression underscores the continuous evolution in our ability to detect and characterize cancer through blood-based markers. CTCs comprise a diverse population, including highly differentiated cells and those with stem cell-like properties (Bidard *et al* 2018, Micalizzi *et al* 2017, Gkountela *et al* 2019). They can adapt and survive in different tissues, promoting metastasis through interactions with blood components and immune cells. CTC detection has shown promise in evaluating treatment efficacy, early diagnosis, and prognosis, particularly in metastatic breast cancer. Studies have demonstrated its prognostic relevance and potential for guiding therapy decisions. CTCs play a pivotal role in cancer metastasis, the spread of cancer from its original site to distant organs (Qiu *et al* 2023). As cancer cells detach from the primary tumor and enter the bloodstream, CTCs can travel to other parts of the body, initiating the formation of secondary tumors. Their presence in the bloodstream serves as a key indicator of metastatic potential and disease progression (Jahr *et al* 2001). Additionally, CTCs can undergo epithelial–mesenchymal transition (EMT), enhancing their ability to invade surrounding tissues and evade the immune system (Yu *et al* 2013). Understanding the biology of CTCs is critical for developing targeted therapies to prevent metastasis and improve patient outcomes.

While more research is needed for validation, CTCs offer a promising avenue for real-time monitoring of treatment response and detecting relapses. Recent investigations have also explored CTC enumeration in cerebrospinal fluid for diagnosing leptomeningeal metastases, further highlighting its clinical value in prognosis and treatment monitoring.

### 5.2.1 Liquid biopsy: a promising approach

Liquid biopsy is a ground-breaking diagnostic technique revolutionizing cancer diagnosis and monitoring (figure 5.1). Liquid biopsy samples, derived from body fluids, encompass diverse tumor-related materials such as tumor DNA, RNA, intact CTCs, tumor-educated platelets, and extracellular vesicles (DiNicolantonio *et al* 2013; Nagrath *et al* 2007). Despite similar acquisition methods, such as blood draw or urine collection, isolating distinct tumor-derived components, such as CTCs and ctDNA, necessitates varied technologies (Tay and Tan 2021). It involves the analysis of biomarkers present in these bodily fluids, offering a minimally invasive alternative to traditional tissue biopsies. The principle of liquid biopsy lies in detecting various biomarkers, including CTCs (Freitas *et al* 2022), cfDNA, and extracellular vesicles (EVs), shed by tumors into the bloodstream or other bodily fluids (Jahr *et al* 2001, Nikanjam *et al* 2022, Palmirotta *et al* 2018).

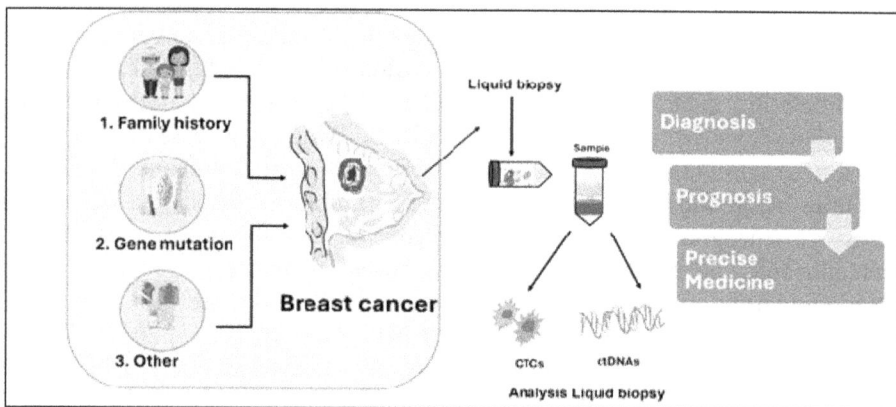

**Figure 5.1.** Overview of the liquid biopsy method for breast cancer diagnosis: body fluids from BC patients enable liquid biopsy analysis of circulating tumor cells, DNA and extracellular vesicles, offering advantages such as real-time monitoring, reduced pain and easier sample collection compared to tissue biopsy.

Several studies explore the potential of tumor-derived materials in blood for early breast cancer detection. Kruspe *et al* demonstrated the discriminatory ability of probes activated by nucleases from CTCs, isolating CTCs via ScreenCell technology (Kruspe *et al* 2017). While promising for detecting metastatic breast cancer, its efficacy in early detection remains uncertain due to lower CTC levels in early-stage disease. Additionally, elevated cfDNA levels in breast cancer patients, although higher than in healthy controls, pose challenges in distinguishing from benign conditions. Agostini *et al* proposed the ALU247 integrity index, showing its accuracy in discriminating cancer patients from non-cancer subjects, with potential for lymph node metastasis detection (Agostini *et al* 2012). Moreover, PCR-based fluorescence microsatellite analyses of cfDNA reveal significant correlations with lymph node status, suggesting further diagnostic potential in breast cancer detection.

In breast cancer diagnosis and monitoring, liquid biopsy has emerged as a promising tool with various clinical applications (Alimirzaie *et al* 2019). Liquid biopsy can aid in the early detection of breast cancer by identifying circulating tumor cells or cell-free DNA carrying breast cancer-specific mutations. Moreover, liquid biopsy enables the monitoring of treatment response and disease progression by tracking changes in biomarker levels over time (Palmirotta *et al* 2018). This dynamic approach facilitates the identification of resistance mutations or the emergence of metastatic disease, guiding treatment adjustments accordingly. Liquid biopsies provide numerous benefits over traditional tissue biopsies, as listed in table 5.1.

However, liquid biopsy also presents challenges and limitations (Wang *et al* 2017). One major challenge is the sensitivity and specificity of detection methods, as circulating biomarkers may be present in low concentrations and can be obscured by background noise. Standardization of procedures and validation of biomarker assays are crucial for ensuring reliable and reproducible results across different laboratories and platforms. Interpretation of liquid biopsy results requires expertise in molecular biology and oncology, as well as consideration of factors such as tumor type, stage, and treatment history (Banys-Paluchowski *et al* 2022). Moreover, cost and accessibility may limit the widespread adoption of liquid biopsy in certain healthcare settings (figure 5.2).

**Table 5.1.** Advantages of liquid biopsy over traditional biopsy for breast cancer diagnosis and monitoring.

1. *Non-invasive*: Liquid biopsies require only a simple blood draw or urine sample, eliminating the need for invasive surgical procedures associated with traditional tissue biopsies.
2. *Real-time monitoring*: They enable repeated sampling over time, allowing for dynamic monitoring of disease progression and treatment response.
3. *Early detection*: Liquid biopsies can detect cancer at earlier stages by identifying circulating tumor cells or cell-free DNA even before symptoms manifest.
4. *Tumor heterogeneity*: They capture the genetic diversity of tumors across different sites, providing a more comprehensive understanding compared to single-site tissue biopsies.

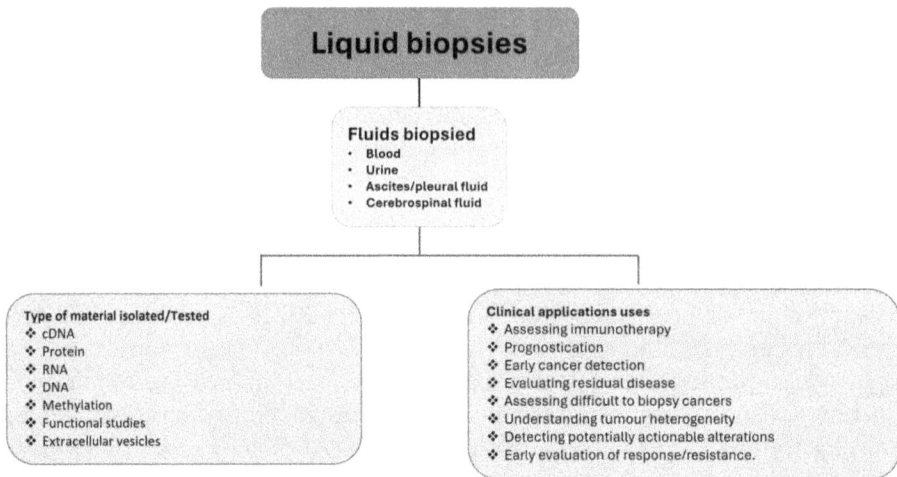

**Figure 5.2.** Liquid biopsy, primarily acquired through blood sampling, but also from various other body fluids, yields valuable materials such as cfDNA/ctDNA and CTCs. These materials enable the assessment of protein expression, methylation patterns, and RNA, driving diverse clinical applications in cancer diagnosis and monitoring.

In conclusion, liquid biopsy holds immense promise in the field of cancer diagnosis and monitoring, offering numerous advantages over traditional tissue biopsies (Poulet *et al* 2019).

### 5.2.2 Detection techniques for liquid biopsy

Isolating CTCs from blood involves distinguishing them from other blood cells, often by exploiting differences in size or identifying surface molecules unique to cancer cells (Alimirzaie *et al* 2019). While methods such as CellSearch target epithelial cell adhesion molecule (EpCAM) to isolate CTCs, it is noted that not all CTCs express EpCAM due to EMT. Alternative markers such as lysine-specific demethylase 1 (LSD1) or programmed cell death ligand 1 (PD-L1) are explored for EMT-induced CTC isolation. Novel techniques such as multi-orifice flow fractionation (MOFF) enhance CTC isolation by size, while analysis of CTC contents, including protein markers such as cancer antigen 15-3 (CA15-3), reveals potential discrepancies between CTCs and primary tumors, impacting treatment decisions. Moreover, CTC profiling, especially regarding hormone receptors and HER2, highlights tumor heterogeneity and dynamic functional states, crucial for understanding and treating metastatic breast cancer effectively. These recent developments in detection are provided in the comprehensive table 5.2 (Wu *et al* 2022).

### 5.2.3 Immunocytochemistry in CTC detection

Immunocytochemistry (ICC) plays a crucial role in the detection and characterization of CTCs, offering insights into cancer progression, treatment response, and metastasis (Hillig *et al* 2014). This technique involves the use of specific antibodies to

**Table 5.2.** Recent detection methods for circulating tumor markers among breast cancer.

| Detection techniques | Target | Advantages | References |
|---|---|---|---|
| CellSearch® | CTCs isolation by targeting epithelial cell adhesion molecule (EpCAM) | High specificity, FDA-approved | Sparano *et al* (2018) |
| Adnatest (QIAGEN®) | A combination of antibodies conjugated with magnetic beads for selecting tumor and epithelial markers and an RT-PCR for detecting breast cancer mRNA biomarkers. | Isolate CTCs in the breast cancer neoadjuvant setting | Kasimir *et al* (2016) |
| CTC-iChip | CTC-iChip a digital RNA signature | For CTC isolation and detection in early and metastatic breast cancer patients | Kwan *et al* (2018) |
| AFMchip | EpCAM, CK19, CD45, and DAPI | Highly efficient at rapidly capturing CTCs from cancer patients' whole blood, without requiring extra equipment | Abdulla *et al* (2022) |

target proteins or antigens expressed on the surface of CTCs, allowing for their identification and analysis within peripheral blood samples.

The process of ICC begins with the isolation of CTCs from blood samples using various enrichment methods, such as density gradient centrifugation or microfluidic devices. Once isolated, CTCs are fixed onto a slide or a membrane and treated with fluorescently labeled antibodies targeting epithelial markers such as cytokeratins (e.g. CK8, CK18, CK19) or tumor-associated antigens (e.g. EpCAM, HER2). These markers distinguish CTCs from surrounding blood cells based on their epithelial origin and cancer-specific characteristics.

Following antibody labeling, the samples are examined under a fluorescence microscope, where CTCs appear as distinct fluorescently labeled cells against a background of non-fluorescent blood cells. The presence of CTCs can be quantified and further characterized based on their morphological features, protein expression profiles, and molecular alterations. Additionally, multiplexing techniques allow for the simultaneous detection of multiple biomarkers, enhancing the sensitivity and specificity of CTC detection. The complete process is demonstrated by the stepwise process in figure 5.3.

ICC-based CTC detection offers several advantages over traditional methods, including its non-invasive nature, ability to capture heterogeneous CTC populations,

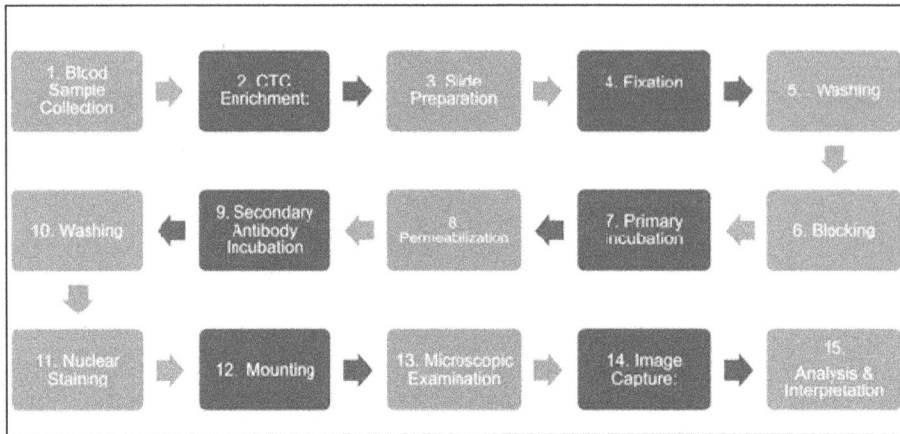

**Figure 5.3.** Stepwise process demonstrating CTC detection for breast cancer using immunocytochemistry.

and real-time monitoring capabilities (Zaha 2014). By providing a snapshot of tumor biology, ICC enables clinicians to assess disease progression, monitor treatment response, and predict patient outcomes. Furthermore, the molecular characterization of CTCs holds promise for guiding personalized cancer therapy and identifying therapeutic targets or drug resistance mechanisms (Lowes and Allan 2014).

However, ICC-based CTC detection also faces challenges, including the rarity of CTCs in circulation, low sensitivity of detection methods, and technical variability between assays. Ongoing research efforts focus on improving the efficiency and accuracy of ICC techniques, standardizing protocols, and validating CTC biomarkers for clinical use. Overall, ICC remains a valuable tool in the study of CTCs, offering valuable insights into cancer biology and clinical management.

### 5.2.4 Microfluidic devices for CTC isolation

Microfluidic technology has emerged as a powerful tool in biomedical research, offering innovative solutions for various applications, including the capture and analysis of CTCs for breast cancer detection (Hou *et al* 2009, Descamps *et al* 2022, Ohnaga *et al* 2016). These devices manipulate small volumes of fluids in microscale channels, enabling precise control over fluid flow and reaction conditions.

Microfluidic devices typically consist of a network of interconnected channels, chambers, and valves fabricated on a small chip. They can be designed using various materials such as glass, silicon, or polymers, and fabrication techniques such as soft lithography or microfabrication processes (Ohnaga *et al* 2016, Nora Dickson *et al* 2011). The design of microfluidic devices is tailored to specific applications, allowing for efficient and high-throughput processing of biological samples (Saadi *et al* 2006).

In the context of CTC capture and analysis, microfluidic devices employ various strategies to isolate and characterize CTCs from blood samples. Common methods include immunoaffinity capture, where antibodies targeting CTC-specific biomarkers are immobilized onto the device's surface, and physical properties-based sorting, which separates CTCs from blood cells based on differences in size, deformability, or electrical properties (Kwon *et al* 2007).

Microfluidic technology offers several advantages over conventional methods for CTC capture and analysis (Panesar *et al* 2016). First, microfluidic devices enable the processing of small sample volumes, minimizing sample requirements and reducing reagent consumption. Second, they provide precise control over fluid flow and reaction conditions, leading to enhanced sensitivity and specificity in CTC detection. Additionally, microfluidic devices offer integration capabilities, allowing for multiplexed assays and streamlined workflows within a single platform (Bhagat and Lim 2012).

The clinical implications of microfluidic-based CTC capture and analysis are significant. These devices have the potential to revolutionize cancer diagnosis, prognosis, and treatment monitoring by providing real-time insights into disease progression and treatment response. They enable the detection of rare CTCs present in peripheral blood, which can serve as biomarkers for early cancer detection, minimal residual disease monitoring, and prediction of patient outcomes.

However, microfluidic-based CTC capture and analysis also face challenges. Standardization of device fabrication and assay protocols is essential to ensure reproducibility and reliability across different laboratories and platforms. Moreover, the translation of microfluidic technology from research settings to clinical practice requires addressing regulatory and commercialization hurdles (Wülfing *et al* 2006).

In summary, microfluidic technology offers innovative solutions for CTC capture and analysis, with significant potential for improving cancer diagnosis and management. Despite challenges, ongoing advancements in device design, integration, and validation hold promise for the widespread adoption of microfluidic-based approaches in clinical oncology.

### 5.2.5 Next-generation sequencing in CTC analysis

Next-generation sequencing (NGS) is a high-throughput DNA sequencing technology that has revolutionized genomic research and clinical diagnostics. It enables the rapid and cost-effective analysis of entire genomes, transcriptomes, or targeted gene panels, providing comprehensive insights into the genetic variations, gene expression profiles, and molecular pathways underlying various diseases, including cancer (Cristall *et al* 2021).

In cancer genomics, NGS plays a pivotal role in elucidating the genetic landscape of tumors, identifying driver mutations, and uncovering mechanisms of tumor progression and therapeutic resistance. By sequencing the entire tumor genome or specific gene regions, NGS enables the identification of somatic mutations, copy number alterations, and structural variants associated with cancer development (De Luca *et al* 2016). Additionally, NGS facilitates the characterization of tumor heterogeneity and clonal evolution, providing valuable information for personalized treatment strategies (Zhu *et al* 2022).

The workflow for NGS-based analysis of CTCs involves several steps that are described in figure 5.4. Initially, CTCs are isolated from blood samples using microfluidic devices or immunomagnetic separation techniques. Subsequently,

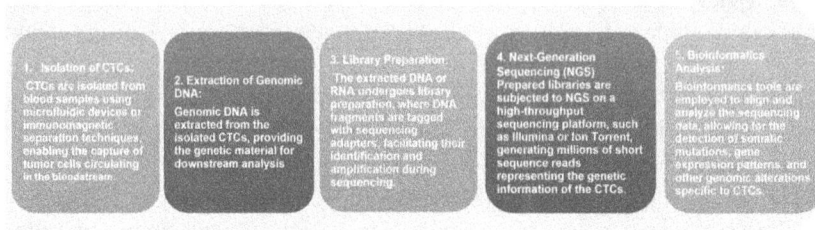

**Figure 5.4.** Diagram illustrating the workflow for NGS-based analysis of CTCs, focusing on breast cancer, showcasing the process from isolation to genomic profiling, crucial for elucidating tumor heterogeneity and guiding personalized treatment strategies.

genomic DNA or RNA is extracted from isolated CTCs, followed by library preparation, where DNA fragments are tagged with sequencing adapters. The prepared libraries are then subjected to NGS on a sequencing platform, such as Illumina or Ion Torrent, generating millions of short sequence reads. Bioinformatics tools are employed to align and analyse the sequencing data, allowing for the detection of somatic mutations, gene expression patterns, and other genomic alterations specific to CTCs (Moorcraft *et al* 2015).

In breast cancer, NGS has provided molecular insights into tumor heterogeneity, metastasis, and treatment response (Rossi *et al* 2020). By profiling the genomic landscape of breast tumors, NGS has identified recurrent mutations in key driver genes, such as *BRCA1*, *BRCA2*, and *PIK3CA*, as well as novel therapeutic targets (Falcone *et al* 2023, Liang *et al* 2018, Teirno *et al* 2023). Furthermore, NGS-based gene expression profiling has enabled the classification of breast cancer subtypes and the prediction of patient outcomes, guiding treatment decisions in clinical practice (Madic *et al* 2015).

NGS is integral to precision medicine approaches in oncology, where genomic data are utilized to tailor therapy based on individual patient characteristics (Gremke *et al* 2024). By integrating NGS data with clinical and pathological information, clinicians can identify actionable genetic alterations and match patients with targeted therapies or clinical trials. Additionally, NGS-based liquid biopsies, including CTC analysis, offer non-invasive methods for monitoring treatment response and disease progression in real time.

In conclusion, NGS has transformed cancer genomics research and clinical practice, providing molecular insights into tumor biology and guiding personalized treatment approaches. Its application in CTC analysis offers new opportunities for understanding cancer progression and improving patient outcomes, particularly in breast cancer and other malignancies.

## 5.2.6 Comparative analysis of techniques

Various techniques for the early detection of breast cancer via liquid biopsy, particularly focusing on CTCs (Tay and Tan 2021), offer distinct advantages and limitations, as listed in table 5.3, contributing to the ongoing quest for improved diagnostic precision and patient outcomes. ICC stands as established method within liquid biopsy approaches, utilizing specific antibodies to identify and characterize CTCs in blood samples. Its high sensitivity and specificity enable the detection of rare CTCs, crucial for early diagnosis and monitoring of disease progression. However, ICC's reliance on protein markers may limit its ability to capture the full heterogeneity of CTC populations and detect cells undergoing EMT, potentially missing aggressive tumor subtypes.

In contrast, NGS represents a cutting-edge approach within liquid biopsy, offering unparalleled genomic insights into CTCs. By analysing the entire genome or specific gene panels, NGS can identify genetic alterations indicative of breast cancer, including mutations, amplifications, and chromosomal rearrangements. This technique holds promise for personalized medicine by guiding treatment selection based on the unique molecular profile of each patient's tumor. Nonetheless, NGS's high cost, complexity, and reliance on intact DNA may pose challenges for routine clinical implementation, particularly in resource-limited settings.

Microfluidic-based technologies present an innovative paradigm for CTC detection within liquid biopsy, capitalizing on miniaturized devices to isolate and analyse CTCs with enhanced efficiency and sensitivity. These platforms enable label-free isolation or capture based on physical properties, such as size or deformability, circumventing the need for specific biomarkers and preserving CTC integrity for downstream analyses. Despite their promise, microfluidic devices may encounter technical hurdles, including clogging and sample contamination, requiring further optimization for robust clinical utility.

Overall, a multifaceted approach integrating complementary techniques, such as ICC, NGS, and microfluidics, within liquid biopsy holds the potential to overcome

**Table 5.3.** Advantages and limitations of techniques for the early detection of breast cancer.

| Technique | Advantages | Limitations |
| --- | --- | --- |
| ICC | High sensitivity and specificity for CTC detection | Reliance on protein markers may limit the detection of CTC heterogeneity and EMT |
| NGS | Comprehensive genomic insights into CTCs | High cost, complexity, and reliance on intact DNA may limit routine clinical use |
| Microfluidic-based technologies | Enhanced efficiency and sensitivity for CTC isolation | Technical hurdles such as clogging and sample contamination may occur |

**Table 5.4.** Comparison of techniques utilized in the early detection of breast cancer.

| Technique | Sensitivity | Specificity | Scalability | Clinical utility | References |
|---|---|---|---|---|---|
| Immunocytochemistry (ICC) | Moderate | High | Limited | Diagnosis, prognosis | Zaha (2014), Zhang et al (2013) |
| Microfluidic devices | High | Moderate | Limited | Early detection, prognosis | Adams et al (2008) |
| Next-generation sequencing (NGS) | High | High | Moderate | Early detection, prognosis, treatment | De Luca et al (2016), Heitzer et al (2013), Magbanua et al (2015) |

individual limitations and maximize the efficacy of CTC-based early detection strategies for breast cancer. By leveraging the strengths of each method, clinicians can enhance diagnostic accuracy, tailor treatment regimens, and ultimately improve patient outcomes in the fight against this prevalent and heterogeneous disease.

Table 5.4 compares the three techniques utilized in liquid biopsy for breast cancer detection: ICC, NGS, and microfluidic-based technologies. It compares their sensitivity, specificity, scalability and clinical utility. This comparison aids in understanding the diverse approaches available for early breast cancer diagnosis through liquid biopsy.

### 5.2.7 Clinical significance and translation into practice

The clinical significance of techniques such as liquid biopsy (Eigeliene et al 2019), ICC, microfluidic devices, and NGS lies in their potential to improve patient outcomes and survival rates in breast cancer.

These techniques offer non-invasive and comprehensive approaches to diagnose and monitor breast cancer, allowing for early detection of disease progression, assessment of treatment response, and identification of therapeutic targets. By providing real-time insights into tumor biology and treatment efficacy, they enable clinicians to tailor therapy to individual patients, ultimately improving outcomes and survival rates.

Incorporation of these techniques into clinical guidelines and practice guidelines is crucial for their widespread adoption and impact on patient care. While some techniques, such as NGS, have already been integrated into clinical practice guidelines for breast cancer management, others such as liquid biopsy and microfluidic devices are still in the process of validation and standardization.

### 5.2.8 Future perspectives and conclusions

Future perspectives in the field of breast cancer diagnosis and management are promising, with continued advancements in techniques such as liquid biopsy, ICC, microfluidic devices, and NGS expected to drive personalized and precise approaches to patient care.

## Conflict of interest

The authors declare no conflict of interest.

## References

Abdulla A, Zhang Z, Ahmad K Z, Warden A R, Li H and Ding X 2022 Rapid and efficient capturing of circulating tumor cells from breast cancer patient's whole blood via the antibody functionalized microfluidic (AFM) chip *Biosens. Bioelectron.* **201** 113965

Adams A A *et al* 2008 Highly efficient circulating tumor cell isolation from whole blood and label-free enumeration using polymer-based microfluidics with an integrated conductivity sensor *J. Am. Chem. Soc.* **130** 8633–41

Addanki S, Meas S, Sarli V N, Singh B and Lucci A 2022 Applications of circulating tumor cells and circulating tumor DNA in precision oncology for breast cancers *Int. J. Mol. Sci.* **23** 7843

Agostini M *et al* 2012 Circulating cell-free DNA: a promising marker of regional lymphonode metastasis in breast cancer patients *Cancer Biomark.* **11** 89–98

Alimirzaie S, Bagherzadeh M and Akbari M R 2019 Liquid biopsy in breast cancer: a comprehensive review *Clin. Genet.* **95** 643–60

Banys-Paluchowski M, Fehm T N, Grimm-Glang D, Rody A and Krawczyk N 2022 Liquid biopsy in metastatic breast cancer: current role of circulating tumor cells and circulating tumor DNA *Oncol. Res. Treat.* **45** 4–11

Bardelli A and Pantel K 2017 Liquid biopsies, what we do not know (yet) *Cancer Cell* **31** 172–9

Bhagat A A and Lim C T 2012 Microfluidic technologies *Recent Results Cancer Res.* **195** 59–67

Bidard F C *et al* 2018 Circulating tumor cells in breast cancer patients treated by neoadjuvant chemotherapy: a meta-analysis *J. Nat. Cancer Inst.* **110** 560–7

Bray F, Ferlay J, Soerjomataram I, Siegel R L, Torre L and Jemel A 2018 GLOBOCAN estimates of incidence and mortality worldwide for 36 cancers in 185 countries *CA Cancer J. Clin.* **68** 394–424

Creighton C J 2012 The molecular profile of luminal B breast cancer *Biologics* **6** 289–97

Cristall K, Bidard F C, Pierga J Y, Rauh M J, Popova T, Sebbag C, Lantz O, Stern M H and Mueller C R 2021 A DNA methylation-based liquid biopsy for triple-negative breast cancer *NPJ Precis. Oncol.* **5** 53

De Luca F *et al* 2016 Mutational analysis of single circulating tumor cells by next generation sequencing in metastatic breast cancer *Oncotarget* **7** 26107–19

Descamps L, Le Roy D and Deman A L 2022 Microfluidic-based technologies for CTC isolation: a review of 10 years of intense efforts towards liquid biopsy *Int. J. Mol. Sci.* **23** 1981

DiNicolantonio F, Newell-Price J and Tan D S 2013 Liquid biopsy: a potential and promising diagnostic tool for advanced stage non-small cell lung cancer *Expert Rev. Mol. Diagn.* **13** 649–51

Eigeliene N, Saarenheimo J and Jekunen A 2019 Potential of liquid biopsies for breast cancer screening, diagnosis, and response to treatment *Oncology* **96** 115–24

Falcone R, Lombardi P, Filetti M, Fabi A, Altamura V, Scambia G and Daniele G 2023 Molecular profile and matched targeted therapy for advanced breast cancer patients *Curr. Oncol* **30** 2501–9

Freitas A J A, Causin R L, Varuzza M B, Calfa S, Hidalgo Filho C M T, Komoto T T, Souza C P and Marques M M C 2022 Liquid biopsy as a tool for the diagnosis, treatment, and monitoring of breast cancer *Int. J. Mol. Sci.* **23** 9952

Galizia D *et al* 2018 Self-evaluation of duration of adjuvant chemotherapy side effects in breast cancer patients: a prospective study *Cancer Med.* **7** 4339–44

Gkountela S *et al* 2019 Circulating tumor cell clustering shapes DNA methylation to enable metastasis seeding *Cell* **176** 98–112.e14

Gremke N *et al* 2024 NGS-guided precision oncology in breast cancer and gynecological tumors-a retrospective molecular tumor board analysis *Cancers* **16** 1561

Heitzer E *et al* 2013 Tumor-associated copy number changes in the circulation of patients with prostate cancer identified through whole-genome sequencing *Genome Med.* **5** 30

Hillig T, Nygaard A B, Nekiunaite L, Klingelhöfer J and Sölétormos G 2014 *In vitro* validation of an ultra-sensitive scanning fluorescence microscope for analysis of circulating tumor cells *APMIS* **122** 545–51

Hou H W, Li Q, Lee G, Kumar A, Ong C and Lim C T 2009 Deformability study of breast cancer cells using microfluidics *Biomed. Microdevices* **11** 557–64

Jahr S, Hentze H, Englisch S, Hardt D, Fackelmayer F O, Hesch R D and Knippers R 2001 DNA fragments in the blood plasma of cancer patients: quantitations and evidence for their origin from apoptotic and necrotic cells *Cancer Res.* **61** 1659–65

Kasimir-Bauer S, Reiter K, Aktas B, Bittner A K, Weber S, Keller T, Kimmig R and Hoffmann O 2016 Different prognostic value of circulating and disseminated tumor cells in primary breast cancer: Influence of bisphosphonate intake? *Sci. Rep.* **6** 26355

Kilgour E, Rothwell D G, Brady G and Dive C 2020 Liquid biopsy-based biomarkers of treatment response and resistance *Cancer Cell* **37** 485–95

Kruspe S *et al* 2017 Rapid and sensitive detection of breast cancer cells in patient blood with nuclease-activated probe technology *Mol. Ther. Nucleic Acids* **8** 542–57

Kwan T T *et al* 2018 A digital RNA signature of circulating tumor cells predicting early therapeutic response in localized and metastatic breast cancer *Cancer Discov.* **8** 1286–99

Kwon K W, Choi S S, Lee S H, Kim B, Lee S N, Park M C, Kim P, Hwang S Y and Suh K Y 2007 Label-free, microfluidic separation and enrichment of human breast cancer cells by adhesion difference *Lab Chip* **7** 1461–8

Li J, Guan X, Fan Z, Ching L M, Li Y, Wang X, Cao W M and Liu D X 2020 Non-invasive biomarkers for early detection of breast cancer *Cancers* **12** 2767

Liang X, Vacher S, Boulai A, Bernard V, Baulande S, Bohec M, Bièche I, Lerebours F and Callens C 2018 Targeted next-generation sequencing identifies clinically relevant somatic mutations in a large cohort of inflammatory breast cancer *Breast Cancer Res.* **20** 88

Lin E, Cao T, Nagrath S and King M R 2018 Circulating tumor cells: diagnostic and therapeutic applications *Annu. Rev. Biomed. Eng.* **20** 329–52

Lowes L E and Allan A L 2014 Recent advances in the molecular characterization of circulating tumor cells *Cancers* **6** 595–624

Madic J *et al* 2015 Circulating tumor DNA and circulating tumor cells in metastatic triple negative breast cancer patients *Int. J. Cancer* **136** 2158–65

Magbanua M J M *et al* 2015 Circulating tumor cell analysis in metastatic triple-negative breast cancers *Clin. Cancer Res.* **21** 1098–105

Mandel P and Metais P 1948 Nuclear acids in human blood plasma *C. R. Seances Soc. Biol. Fil.* **142** 241–3

Mehlen P and Puisieux A 2006 Metastasis: a question of life or death *Nat. Rev. Cancer* **6** 449–58

Merino Bonilla J A, Torres Tabanera M and Ros Mendoza L H 2017 Breast cancer in the 21st century: from early detection to new therapies. El cáncer de mama en el siglo XXI: de la detección precoz a los nuevos tratamientos *Radiologia* **59** 368–79

Micalizzi D S, Maheswaran S and Haber D A 2017 A conduit to metastasis: circulating tumor cell biology *Genes Dev.* **31** 1827–40

Moorcraft S Y, Gonzalez D and Walker B A 2015 Understanding next generation sequencing in oncology: a guide for oncologists *Crit. Rev. Oncol. Hematol.* **96** 463–74

Nagrath S *et al* 2007 Isolation of rare circulating tumour cells in cancer patients by microchip technology *Nature* **450** 1235–9

Nikanjam M, Kato S and Kurzrock R 2022 Liquid biopsy: current technology and clinical applications *J. Hematol. Oncol.* **15** 131

Nora Dickson M, Tsinberg P, Tang Z, Bischoff F Z, Wilson T and Leonard E F 2011 Efficient capture of circulating tumor cells with a novel immunocytochemical microfluidic device *Biomicrofluidics* **5** 34119–3411915

Ohnaga T, Shimada Y, Takata K, Obata T, Okumura T, Nagata T, Kishi H, Muraguchi A and Tsukada K 2016 Capture of esophageal and breast cancer cells with polymeric microfluidic devices for CTC isolation *Mol. Clin. Oncol.* **4** 599–602

Palmirotta R, Lovero D, Cafforio P, Felici C, Mannavola F, Pellè E, Quaresmini D, Tucci M and Silvestris F 2018 Liquid biopsy of cancer: a multimodal diagnostic tool in clinical oncology *Ther. Adv. Med. Oncol.* **10** 1758835918794630

Panesar S and Neethirajan S 2016 Microfluidics: rapid diagnosis for breast cancer *Nanomicro Lett.* **8** 204–20

Poulet G, Massias J and Taly V 2019 Liquid biopsy: general concepts *Acta Cytol.* **63** 449–55

Qiu J, Qian D, Jiang Y, Meng L and Huang L 2023 Circulating tumor biomarkers in early-stage breast cancer: characteristics, detection, and clinical developments *Front. Oncol.* **13** 1288077

Rossi T *et al* 2020 Single-cell NGS-based analysis of copy number alterations reveals new insights in circulating tumor cells persistence in early-stage breast cancer *Cancers* **12** 2490

Saadi W, Wang S-J, Lin F and Jeon N L 2006 A parallel-gradient microfluidic chamber for quantitative analysis of breast cancer cell chemotaxis *Biomed. Microdevices* **8** 109–18

Sedeta E T *et al* 2023 Breast cancer: global patterns of incidence, mortality, and trends *J. Clin. Oncol.* **41** 10528

Sparano J, O'Neill A, Alpaugh K, Wolff A C, Northfelt D W, Dang C T, Sledge G W and Miller K D 2018 Association of circulating tumor cells with late recurrence of estrogen receptor-positive breast cancer: a secondary analysis of a randomized clinical trial *JAMA Oncol.* **4** 1700–6

Tay T K Y and Tan P H 2021 Liquid biopsy in breast cancer: a focused review *Arch. Pathol. Lab Med.* **145** 678–86

Tierno D, Grassi G, Scomersi S, Bortul M, Generali D, Zanconati F and Scaggiante B 2023 Next-generation sequencing and triple-negative breast cancer: insights and applications *Int. J. Mol. Sci.* **24** 9688

Wang J, Chang S, Li G and Sun Y 2017 Application of liquid biopsy in precision medicine: opportunities and challenges *Front. Med.* **11** 522–7

Wu Q *et al* 2022 Detection of folate receptor-positive circulating tumor cells as a biomarker for diagnosis, prognostication, and therapeutic monitoring in breast cancer *J. Clin. Lab. Anal.* **36** e241801

Wülfing P, Borchard J, Buerger H, Heidl S, Zänker K S, Kiesel L and Brandt B 2006 HER2-positive circulating tumor cells indicate poor clinical outcome in stage I to III breast cancer patients *Clin. Cancer Res.* **12** 1715–20

Yu M *et al* 2013 Circulating breast tumor cells exhibit dynamic changes in epithelial and mesenchymal composition *Science* **339** 580–4

Yu M *et al* 2019 Erratum for the report "Circulating breast tumor cells exhibit dynamic changes in epithelial and mesenchymal composition" *Science* **363** 6425 (erratum)

Zaha D C 2014 Significance of immunohistochemistry in breast cancer *World J. Clin. Oncol.* **5** 382–92

Zhang L, Ridgway L D, Wetzel M D, Ngo J, Yin W, Kumar D, Goodman J C, Groves M D and Marchetti D 2013 The identification and characterization of breast cancer CTCs competent for brain metastasis *Sci. Transl. Med.* **5** 180ra48

Zhang L *et al* 2013 A correction to the research article titled: "The identification and characterization of breast cancer CTCs competent for brain metastasis" *Sci. Transl. Med.* **5** 189er5

Zhu C *et al* 2022 Circulating tumor cells and breast cancer metastasis: from enumeration to somatic mutational profile *J. Clin. Med.* **11** 6067

# Chapter 6

## Insight into the role of non-coding RNA as a potential biomarker for the early detection of breast cancer

**Alibha Rawat, N Ganesh, Gresh Chander and Shiv Kumar Yadav**

The key to better cancer prognosis and management is its early detection. All the established techniques available for cancer diagnosis are mostly invasive and thus present some obvious challenges, the foremost of which is the apprehension and reluctance of people to undergo screening investigations in the first place. There is an urgent need for more effective, sensitive, and improved screening tests than are available clinically. Unfortunately, many cancers still lack effective screening methods. Biopsies remain the cornerstone of cancer diagnosis but are invasive and painful leading to dread among the individuals undergoing investigations. In this regard, liquid biopsies, in the form of circulating DNA or RNA in the blood, have generated tremendous interest and advantages in the diagnostic screening scenario. Lately, long non-coding RNAs (lncRNAs) that are secreted by tumor cells and are stable components that do not become degraded easily, have gained much attention in the research community as one of the potential liquid biopsy biomarkers for cancer detection and are being studied extensively for cancer screening. The current chapter reviews the relevance of ncRNA as a potential biomarker for cancer detection with special reference to breast cancer.

## 6.1 Introduction

Cancer is one of the leading causes of death worldwide and has been increasing alarmingly during the last decade or so. Several advanced technologies are now available in the clinical world and provide tremendous data that can be explored by biomedical research for even more effective management of cancer, both in diagnosis and as a therapeutic target. Early cancer detection is the most important part of cancer management and cure. All the diagnostic techniques and markers are being explored for their potential to detect cancer effectively with high specificity and sensitivity. In this regard, the existing diagnostic methods, although effective, are mostly invasive and thus pose pressure on the patient. Therefore, more non-invasive techniques, such as liquid biopsy, are being explored now. One of the explored biomarkers with the most potential is non-coding RNA obtained from this so-called 'liquid biopsy'.

Across the world, breast cancer is the most frequently diagnosed malignant tumor in women and the leading cause of cancer-related deaths. Around the world, the prevalence of breast cancer is steadily rising (Smolarz *et al* 2022). Breast cancer commonly presents as a lump in the breast and is typically painless. The size of the tumor and whether it has spread to other regions determine the stage of cancer. Additionally, it depends on the kind of tumor cells. Breast cancer can occur in five stages, denoted by 0, I, II, III, and IV.

A favorable prognosis for all cancer types depends on early detection and efficient treatment. Individuals diagnosed with tumors at an early stage have a far better chance of surviving. To effectively manage breast cancer, numerous innovative technologies are being developed for the early diagnosis of original tumors as well as distant metastases and recurrent diseases (Bhushan *et al* 2021). Imaging techniques including x-ray, magnetic-field, and nuclear imaging techniques are commonly used for breast cancer detection, however, mammography is utilized for both screening and diagnosis of breast cancer and is known as the gold standard screening technique. Breast cancer screening and diagnosis are of three types, clinical examination, imaging modalities, and biopsy, as shown in figure 6.1.

Imaging techniques are invasive, require sophisticated instruments, and are also painful for patients. Therefore, researchers are more and more focused on developing non-invasive assays for the detection of biomarkers present in biological fluids (whole blood, plasma, serum, urine, lymph, etc). Different kinds of biomarkers are found in biological fluids, such as circulatory cancer cells, cancerous proteins, DNA, RNA, non-coding RNA (ncRNA), exosomes, and other metabolites. Cancerous protein, DNA, and RNA are major biomarkers, and their characteristics are shown in table 6.1. Recently, non-coding RNAs have attracted researcher's attention as diagnostic and therapeutic targets for cancer. ncRNAs have a range of regulatory activities and are dysregulated in numerous malignancies, including breast cancer; therefore, they have received a lot of interest in cancer research. Several ncRNAs are being studied for specific cancer types, in particular lung cancer, breast cancer, gastric cancer, liver cancer, prostate cancer, etc. lncRNA, namely MALAT1 (Weber *et al* 2013), SPRY4-IT1, ANRIL, NEAT1 (Hu *et al* 2016), and GAS5 (Liang *et al* 2016), are some markers that have shown high sensitivity and specificity in non-small cell lung cancer (NSCLC).

Research has demonstrated that ncRNAs have regulatory role in response of immune cells as well as anti-inflammatory factors. Recent studies have revealed its potential role in regulating the tumor microenvironment that affects tumor immune response in different types of cancer, including breast cancer. Studies have identified

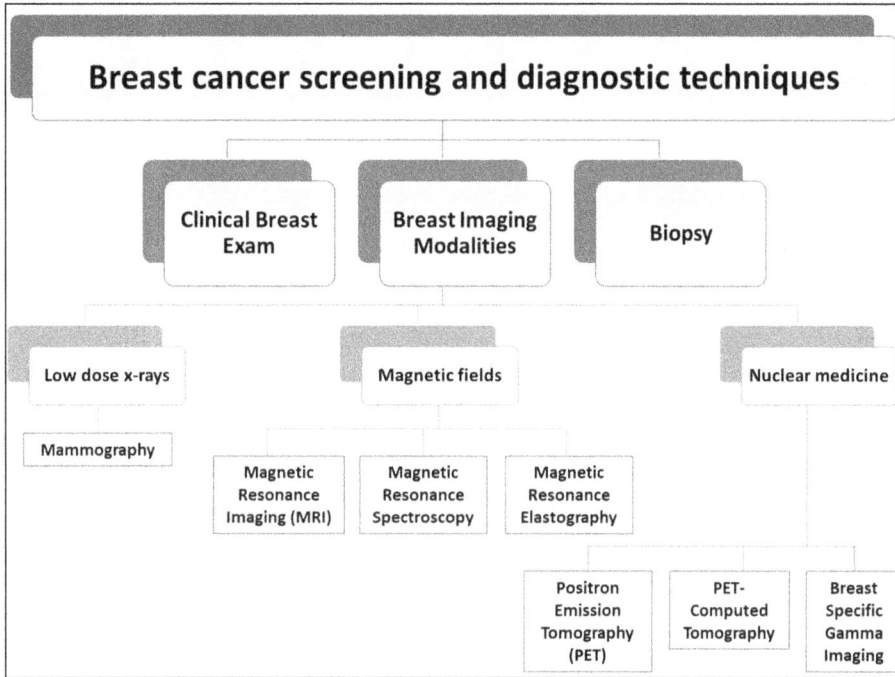

**Figure 6.1.** A basic representation of breast cancer screening and diagnostic techniques. Reproduced with permission from Huan *et al* 2021.

diverse genes associated with the development and progression of breast carcinoma including *TP53, BRCA1, GATA3, ERBB2, PIK3CA, MYC, PTEN, CDH1*, etc (Harbeck *et al* 2019). Similarly, dysregulation in signaling pathways (such as PI2K/AKT/Mtor, MAPK/ERK, TGF-$\beta$, NF$\kappa$B, WNT/Catenin, Notch, Hippo, and SHH), are also associated with cell survival, proliferation, and epithelial–mesenchymal transition. Merlano *et al* (2019) studied the role of ncRNAs in the context of cancer immune-biology in several types of cancer and found them to be a critical regulator of anti-tumoral immune response. The study demonstrated that ncRNAs play a key role in regulating the tumor microenvironment and tumor cell immune escape. As a result, lncRNA is a good candidate for targeted cancer immunotherapy and, with further advancements in molecular techniques, lncRNA can be used as a novel cancer therapeutic target. More research needs to be done to understand more such pathways and gain a deeper understanding of the role of ncRNAs in cancer immune-biology that can be utilized for targeted therapy for better management of cancer progression.

The functional role of ncRNAs in cancer and their potential clinical applications as diagnostic biomarkers and therapeutic targets for cancer are being explored and utilized in recent times.

**Table 6.1.** Correlation of genomic biomarkers.

| Characteristics | DNA | RNA | Protein |
| --- | --- | --- | --- |
| Biological activity | Carrier of genomic data catalyst or regulating factor | Transmitter of the genetic makeup regulating factor | The structural element |
| Biological resilience | Stable in alkaline conditions; less reactive than RNAs | Not stable in alkaline conditions; reactive | Usually more stable than nucleic acids |
| Developing phase as a form of biomarker | During advanced research; used in therapeutic counseling | During advanced research; used in therapeutic counseling | Commonly used for regular assessment |
| Biomarker characteristics | Mutation, epigenetic variation | Expressive profiles | Proteomics profile |
| Techniques for identification | qPCR, DNA-seq microarray | RT-qPCR, RNA-seq, microarray | Electrophoresis, immunoassay mass spectrometry |
| Efficiency and applicability | Comparatively higher | Moderately higher | Comparatively lower (mostly rely on good antibodies being found) |
| Quantity per human cell | –6 pg (Russo and Russo 2014) | 10–30 pg (Russo and Russo 2014) | 130–150 pg (Finka and Goloubinoff 2013) |
| Quantity in 1 ml of plasma | 1–1000 ng (Fleischhacker and Schmidt 2007) | 1–1000 ng (Schwarzenbach et al 2011) | –6 × 10⁴ ng (Caby et al 2005) |
| Example | *BRCA1* mutation (breast cancer) | PAM50 (breast cancer) | AFP (liver cancer) |

## 6.2 Noncoding RNAs and their characteristics

The sequencing of the human genome led to the discovery of a lot of hidden information regarding DNA, one of the most significant discoveries being the fact that not all DNA is coded into proteins and a whole lot of non-coding RNAs form a large chunk of the human genome, and these have a range of functions to perform. It has been established that a very small percentage of nucleic acids in a human genome are used for protein-encoding, and the majority of it is made up of more than 98% nucleic acids that do not encode proteins (Quinn and Chang 2016). Next-generation sequencing has opened a gate for information on the mechanism of eukaryotic genomes and has demonstrated that most of the complex eukaryotic genomes are transcribed into ncRNAs. ncRNAs have several functions in gene regulation, such as housekeeping functions and even specialized functions such as dosage compensation and regulatory roles in mRNA degradation (Heather and Chain 2016). They also regulate protein-coding genes and interact with RNAs, proteins, and chromatin structures (Statello *et al* 2021). Therefore, in the last decade the scientific community worldwide has been exploring these lncRNAs to understand their role in cancer development.

Thus, an ncRNA is a functional RNA molecule not translated into a protein. The DNA sequence from which a functional ncRNA is transcribed is often called an RNA gene. Various kinds of ncRNAs are found in nature and have different functions. The most well-known ncRNAs are transfer RNAs (tRNAs) and ribosomal RNAs (rRNAs) and in addition to these two there are small RNAs such as microRNAs, snRNAs, siRNAs, piRNAs, and snoRNAs, and the long ncRNAs, as shown in figure 6.2. Several studies have revealed their role in tumorogenesis over the years and several regulatory pathways are under study to understand ncRNA more clearly.

The ncRNAs have been associated with various types of cancers as regulators of gene expression (Loh *et al* 2019, Yuan *et al* 2019) as shown in figure 6.3 (miRNAs and lncRNAs). Thus the ncRNA with no protein-coding potential has gained much attention during the last decade with its large diverse family comprising various RNAs with regulatory functions such as lncRNA, miRNA, and a recently discovered circular RNA (circRNA) that is found to be more stable and formed by back-splicing (Loh *et al* 2019). In transcription and the processing of lncRNA compared to mRNAs, a higher proportion of lncRNAs are localized in the nucleus, posing the key issue of what drives their differential localization (Derrien *et al* 2012, Guo *et al* 2020). A comparison of the global characteristics of lncRNAs and mRNAs indicates that lncRNA genes are less evolutionarily conserved, have fewer exons, and are less abundantly expressed (Hezroni *et al* 2015).

lncRNAs are non-protein-coding RNAs of around 200 nucleotides. Depending upon their position relative to protein-encoding genes, these lncRNAs are classified

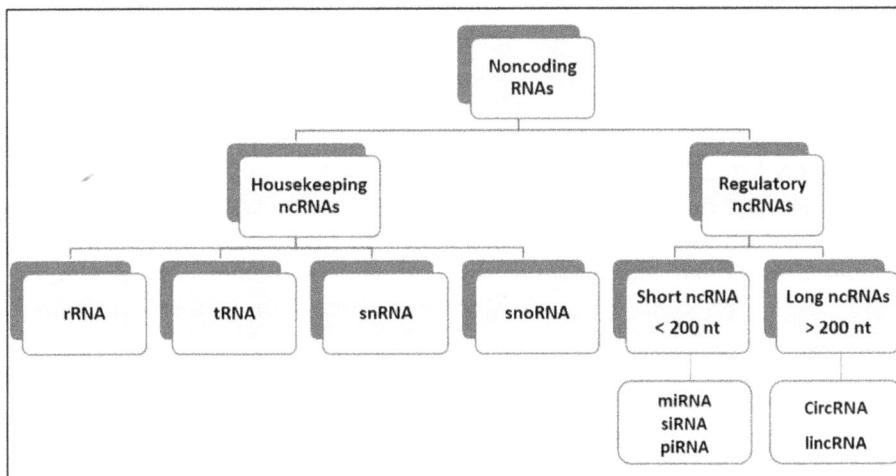

**Figure 6.2.** Noncoding RNA classification. On the basis of function, ncRNAs are divided into two main types, housekeeping ncRNAs and regulatory ncRNAs that are further divided on the basis of nucleotide size, structure and functions.

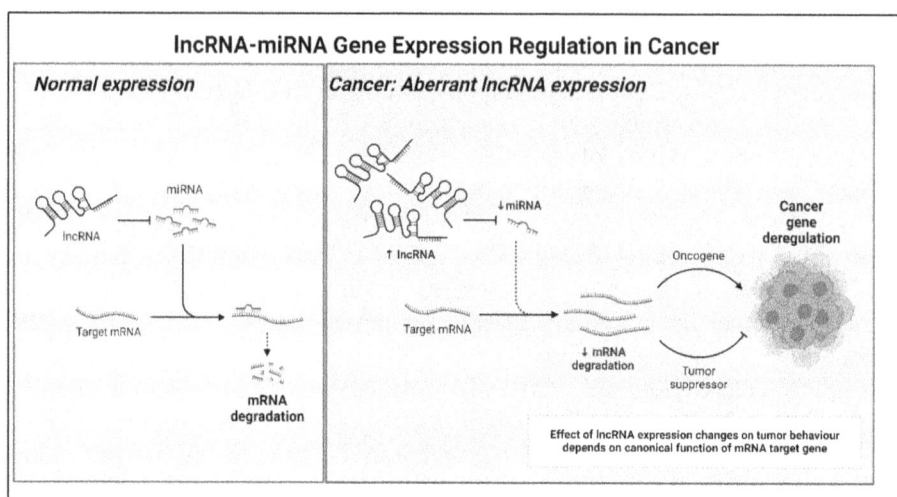

**Figure 6.3.** lncRNA and miRNA gene expression regulation in cancer. In normal conditions (healthy cells), miRNA degrade the target mRNA. However in tumor cells, lncRNA is up-regulated and miRNA is down-regulated which decreases the target mRNA degradation and increase in oncogene expression that leads to tumor development and progression.

as sense lncRNAs, antisense lncRNAs, bidirectional lncRNAs, intron lncRNAs, intergenic lncRNAs (lincRNAs), and enhancer intergenic lncRNAs (Wang and Chang 2011, Bhatti *et al* 2021). Recent transcriptomic and bio-informatics studies have made it possible to explore these molecules in detail and it has been revealed that there are thousands of non-coding transcripts or ncRNAs present in the genome (Cheng *et al* 2005, Birney *et al* 2007). Until recently, these ncRNAs were thought to be non-functional and considered 'junk RNA' (Brosius 2005, Palazzo and Lee 2015), however, many recent studies have argued for their functional role, especially in regulation, and this needs to be studied in more detail (Lee *et al* 2019, Mattick and Amaral 2022).

The lncRNA mechanisms of action include as signal molecule, guide molecule, scaffold molecule, etc. miRNAs are a small (around –20 nt) species of ncRNA that have been found to have a regulatory role in gene expression and they are also found to be more stable than mRNAs and resistant to degradation. A huge number of miRNAs have been identified lately that have been found to have implications across hundreds of diseases including cancer, heart disease, renal diseases, dysfunction of the nervous system, obesity, and even infectious diseases. miRNA is also found in other body fluids, including saliva, tears, cerebrospinal fluid, and urine.

lncRNA acts as a signal molecule that can modify transcription in the downstream genes by combining with some protein molecules which are transcription factors. lncRNAs can also act as guide molecules that carry functional proteins and locate them in the target area to perform functions. lncRNA can act as a scaffold molecule to guide different protein assemblies in the target area to perform their function.

Studies have reported circulating miRNA as a biomarker for liver, breast, and prostate cancers, however, extracellular miRNA tends to degrade rapidly, making them less useful as biomarkers. In some cases, these circulating miRNAs can form complexes with other bio-molecules such as proteins and persist longer in the blood, but still, a very high degree of variability makes them less specific and therefore not a very good candidate for diagnosing with precision.

## 6.3 Non-coding RNA as biomarker for breast cancer

Breast cancer has been one of the most common cancers in females worldwide and has recently increased at an alarming rate. Although mammography and sono-mammography are the cornerstone diagnostic methods for the detection of breast cancer, more and more specific tumor markers that can detect cancer at an early stage, preferably non-invasive, are the need of the hour, since early detection is the key to a complete cure in cancer management. Therefore, over the last decade, studies are being devoted to the exploration of several specific tumor markers for the early detection of cancer.

The role of lncRNA in breast cancer has been studied and turns out that in breast cancer, 91H lncRNA prevents DNA methylation of the maternal allele at the H19/IGF2 locus, which leads to the aggressiveness of the breast cancer cells. In addition, lncRNA also inhibits gene transcription by recruiting histone modification or chromatin remodeling proteins. In a case-controlled study done by Xu et al (2015), circulating lncRNA, RP11-445H22.4 expressions were studied in both groups and its expressions were found to be significantly higher in the serum of breast cancer patients, indicating its potential as a good biomarker of breast cancer. The study also compared this biomarker with other common tumor serum markers such as AFP, CEA, CA125, and CA-153 as well as the imaging diagnostic method, and showed that lncRNA RP11-445H22.4 has the highest sensitivity and specificity (Xu et al 2015). Another study examined lncRNA MALAT1 from the tissue samples of breast cancer patients and found significantly higher expression of this marker, especially in lymph node metastases (Miao et al 2016). Therefore, it can be utilized in detecting the stage of breast cancer also. Similarly, Zhang et al (2016) evaluated the differentiated H19 lncRNA expression in both cancer tissues and serum samples of breast cancer patients and healthy subjects and found significantly higher expression ($P < 0.05$) in breast cancer patients, which was even higher than the clinically established markers CEA and CA-153. Several lncRNAs have been explored and studied for their role in breast cancer diagnosis and prognosis, as shown in table 6.2. The role of various lincRNAs in breast cancer progression and metastasis is summarized in table 6.3.

snRNAs and snoRNAs regulate mRNA splicing and rRNA maturation, respectively (Karijolich and Yu 2010). A study done in breast cancer patients showed that elevated snoRNA synthesis is essential for high rRNA expression and is also needed for protein synthesis (Su et al 2014). SNORD46 and SNORD42A have been detected in the mammary gland and lymphoblastoid cells. Thirteen snoRNAs have been recognized as predictive indicators of breast cancer, notably the down-regulation of SNORD46 and SNORD89 (Krishnan et al 2016).

**Table 6.2.** Some clinically relevant lncRNAs in breast cancer. Reproduced from Smolarz *et al* (2021). CC BY 4.0.

| Clinicopathological features | lncRNA |
|---|---|
| PR status | MALAT1 |
| HER status | TUSC7 |
| Histological grade | MEG3 |
| TNM stage | NEAT1, TP73-AS1 |
| **Survival** | |
| Shorter overall survival | CCAT2, MALAT1, NEAT1 |
| Longer overall survival | MEG3 |
| Overall survival (better prognosis) | FGF14-AS2, AFAP1-AS1, EPB4L4A-AS2, BC040587, EGOT, GAS6-AS1, FENDERR |
| Overall survival (worse prognosis) | BCAR4, HOTTIP, CCAT1,Z38, TUNAR, CRNDE, HULC,MVIH, TP73-AS1, linc-ITGB1, UCA1,OR3A4, DANCR, LINP1, SNHG15, SUMO1P3 |
| Metastasis-free survival | CCAT2, HOTAIR, BCAR4 |
| Disease-free survival | MALAT1, HOTTIP, MVIH, LINC00978, linc-ITGB1, GAS6-AS1, HOTAIR, LINP1 |
| Progression-free survival | MALAT1, MEG3, HOTAIR, RFS, CCAT1, MEG3, FENDRR |

The clonal development of effective cancer cells is governed by intracellular and interstitial mutations that confer positive or negative effects on cell lines. Mutations in *uL18/RPL5* ribosomal protein genes contribute to the evolution of breast cancers in around 34% of cases (Bastide and David 2018). Several snoRNAs are converted into stable miRNA-like oligomers known as 'small nucleolar RNA-derived RNAs' (sdRNAs) (Scott and Ono 2011). sdRNA-93 has been shown to play a function in MDA-MB-231 cell invasiveness and is highly expressed in luminal B/HER2+ breast tumors compared to other types of breast tumors or normal breast tissue (Patterson *et al* 2017). Other research indicates that changes in snoRNAs can encourage tumorigenesis and favor cancer stem cell characteristics (Bastide and David 2018). The role of various snoRNAs in breast cancer and their level compared to healthy controls was reviewed by Louca and Gkretsi (2022) and is presented in table 6.4.

miRNAs have acquired much attention due to their ease of detection and reproducibility, and have been reported in various research and review articles, and they may play a potential role in the development and progression of breast cancer (Jordan-Alejandre *et al* 2023), and have diagnostic potential as a biomarker. miRNAs that play a critical role in cancer development are known as oncomiRs. These oncomiRs have different roles in breast cancer development and progression, such as sustained growth and breast cell proliferation, metastasis and invasion, inhibiting apoptosis and cell death, inducing angiogenesis, avoiding immune

**Table 6.3.** Role of lincRNAs in breast cancer. Table adapted from Louca and Gkretsi (2022).

| | Levels in breast cancer compared to normal | Survival | ceRNA function | miRNA targeted | Pathway | Proliferation, migration, invasion and EMT | In vivo growth and metastasis | Chemoresistance (drug) |
|---|---|---|---|---|---|---|---|---|
| Linc00337 | ↑ | | | | ↑M2 tumor associated macrophage markers | ↑ | ↑ | ↑(Paclitaxel) |
| Linc00460 | ↑ | → | Yes | | | | ↑ | |
| Linc00518 | ↑ | | Yes | miR199 | ↑Wnt, β-catenin MRP1 | ↑ | ↑ | ↑(Doxorubicin, Paclitaxel) |
| Linc00894 | ↑ | → | Yes | miR429 | ZEB1 | ↑ | ↑ | |
| Linc00922 | ↑ | | | | Wnt, NKD2 | ↑ | ↑ | |
| Linc01119 | | | | | ↑SOCS5, ↓JAK1/2, ↓STAT1/3 | ↑ | ↑ | |
| Linc01977 | ↑ | → | Yes | miR-212-3p | ↓GOLNM1 | ↑ | | ↑(Doxorubicin) |
| Linc02163 | ↑ | → | Yes | miR-511-3p | ↑HMGA1 | ↑ | | |
| Linc00641 | → | | Yes | miR-194-5p | ↓Wnt, β-catenin | → | ↑ | |
| Linc01087 | ↓In TNBC | | | | | | → | |
| Linc02615 | → | | Yes | miR-129-5p | ↑Lamins | | | |

**Table 6.4.** Role of various snoRNAs in breast cancer. Table adapted from Louca and Gkretsi (2022).

| | Elevated levels in breast cancer compared to normal | ceRNA function | miRNA targeted and/or pathway involved | Increased proliferation, migration, invasion and EMT (in vitro) | In vivo growth and metastasis |
|---|---|---|---|---|---|
| SNHG1 | ✓ | ✓ | miR-193a-5p → HOXA1 | ✓ | ✓ |
| | | | miR-199a-3p → TFAM | | |
| | | | miR-18b-5p → TERT | | |
| | | | miR-382 | | |
| | | | miR-448 | | |
| SNHG3 | ✓ | ✓ | miR-186-5p → ZEB1 | ✓ | ✓ |
| | | | miR-154-3p → Notch | | |
| | | | miR-330-5p → PKM | | |
| | | | miR-384-5p → HDGF | | |
| SNHG5 | | ✓ | miR-154-5p → PCNA | ✓ | |
| SNHG6 | | ✓ | miR-26a-5p → VASP | ✓ | |
| SNHG7 | ✓ | ✓ | c-Myc | ✓ | |
| | | | miR-34a→Notch1 | | |
| | | | miR-186 | | |
| | | | miR-381 | | |
| | | | miR-15a | | |
| SNHG12 | ✓ | ✓ | c-Myc | ✓ | ✓ |
| SNHG14 | ✓ | ✓ | miR-15a-5p→SALL4 | ✓ | |
| | | | miR-543→KLF7 | ✓ | |
| | | | acetylation of H2K27 | | |
| | | | miR-193a-3p | | |
| SNHG15 | ✓ | ✓ | miR-411-5p | ✓ | |
| SNHG16 | | ✓ | miR-211-3p | ✓ | |
| SNHG17 | | ✓ | miR-20a | ✓ | |
| SNHG20 | | ✓ | miR-124-3p | ✓ | |
| | | | miR-495 | | |
| SNORA71A | | | | ✓ | ✓ |
| SNORA71B | ✓ | | ROCK2 | ✓ | |

destruction, and making the breast tumor cell immortal (Loh *et al* 2019). A study by Zhou *et al* revealed that miR-301b-3p and miR-301b-5p are tumor promoters in breast cancer via different signaling pathways and miR-301b-3p could be a prognostic molecule while miR-301b-5p may be utilized as a potential diagnostic marker (Zhou *et al* 2023). Breast cancer has high expression levels of miR-423 and boosted cisplatin resistance and increased proliferation in breast cancer cell lines. Additional research revealed that pre-miR-423-A expression enhanced breast cancer cell motility and invasion while inhibiting cisplatin-induced apoptosis. The study concluded by suggesting that the rs6505162-A allele increases the expression of miR-423, which in turn increases the proliferation, viability, chemoresistance, migration, and invasion of breast cancer cells while decreasing their apoptosis (Morales-Pison *et al* 2021). Farré *et al* revealed that breast cancer patient breast tissue compared to normal breast tissue has up-regulated miR-21–5p and miR-106b-5p, while miR-205–5p and miR-143–3p were found to be down-regulated. These two groups of cells share a number of target genes, including *GAB1*, *GNG12*, *HBP1*, and *SESN1*, which were down-regulated in breast primary tumors and metastases and could be promising biomarkers for breast cancer diagnosis (Farré *et al* 2021). Breast cancer tissue exhibits high expression levels of miR-21 and miR-210, which have a substantial correlation with lymph node metastases, clinical staging, and differentiation. It is possible to employ miR-210 as a prognostic indicator to determine the prognosis of breast cancer patients, as its up-regulated expression is associated with a bad prognosis for these patients (Xiaofei 2020). To date, huge numbers of miRNAs have been observed to be linked with breast cancer development and progression and are involved in the hallmarks of breast cancer, as shown in figure 6.4.

## 6.4 Detection approaches of non-coding RNAs

ncRNAs are identified using high-throughput techniques, including RNA sequencing (RNA-seq), microarrays, Northern blotting, reverse transcription-polymerase chain reaction, next-generation sequencers, and *in situ* hybridization (Sargazi *et al* 2022). Each technology has limitations and advantages (Beylerli *et al* 2022), as shown in table 6.3. These techniques evaluate ncRNA expression and its function in cell pathways. The microarray technique is most commonly used for ncRNA detection.

Microarray technology is a laboratory technique that involves binding an array of thousands to millions of known nucleic acid fragments to a solid surface, referred to as a 'chip'. The chip is then made to bind with nucleic acids (DNA or RNA) isolated from a study sample (such as cells or tissue). The principle behind microarrays is that complementary sequences will bind to each other. Therefore, in this technique probes are made and unknown DNA molecules cut into fragments by restriction endo-nucleases and attached to fluorescent markers and are then allowed to react with probes of the DNA chip.

The most advanced method of studying nucleic acids is now the microarray technique that can profile both miRNAs and lncRNAs in addition to protein-coding

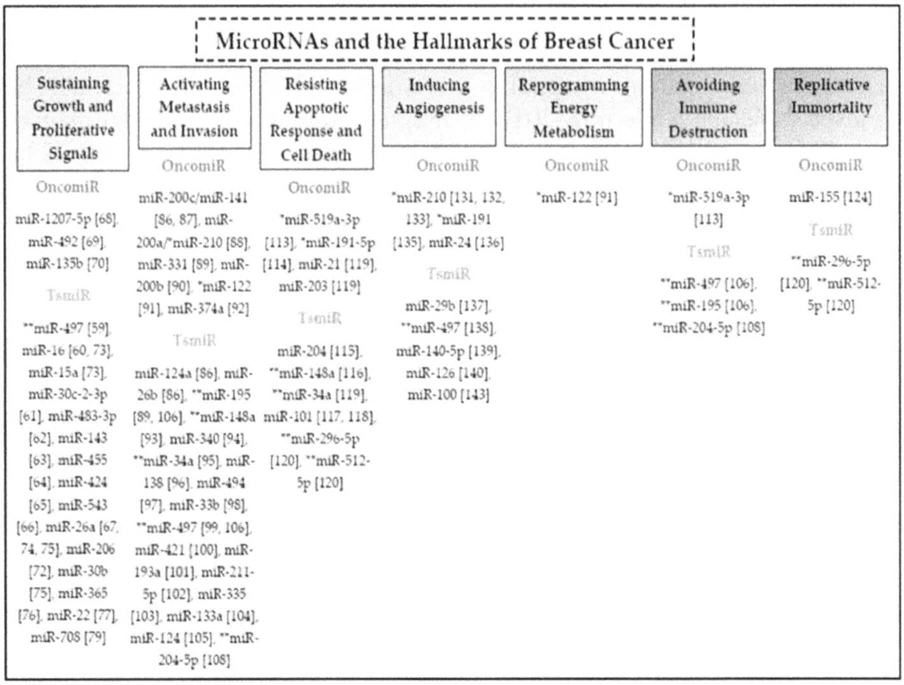

| MicroRNAs and the Hallmarks of Breast Cancer | | | | | | |
|---|---|---|---|---|---|---|
| Sustaining Growth and Proliferative Signals | Activating Metastasis and Invasion | Resisting Apoptotic Response and Cell Death | Inducing Angiogenesis | Reprogramming Energy Metabolism | Avoiding Immune Destruction | Replicative Immortality |
| OncomiR | OncomiR | OncomiR | OncomiR | OncomiR | OncomiR | OncomiR |
| miR-1207-5p [68], miR-492 [69], miR-135b [70] | miR-200c/miR-141 [86, 87], miR-200a/*miR-210 [88], miR-331 [89], miR-200b [90], *miR-122 [91], miR-374a [92] | *miR-519a-3p [113], *miR-191-5p [114], miR-21 [119], miR-203 [119] | *miR-210 [131, 132, 133], *miR-191 [135], miR-24 [136] | *miR-122 [91] | *miR-519a-3p [113] | miR-155 [124] |
| TsmiR | | | TsmiR | | TsmiR | TsmiR |
| **miR-497 [59], miR-16 [60, 73], miR-15a [73], miR-30c-2-3p [61], miR-483-3p [62], miR-143 [63], miR-455 [64], miR-424 [65], miR-543 [66], miR-26a [67, 74, 75], miR-206 [72], miR-30b [75], miR-365 [76], miR-22 [77], miR-708 [79] | TsmiR | TsmiR | miR-29b [137], **miR-497 [138], miR-140-5p [139], miR-126 [140], miR-100 [143] | | **miR-497 [106], **miR-195 [106], **miR-204-5p [108] | **miR-296-5p [120], **miR-512-5p [120] |
| | miR-124a [86], miR-26b [86], **miR-195 [89, 106], **miR-148a [93], miR-340 [94], **miR-34a [95], miR-138 [96], miR-494 [97], miR-33b [98], **miR-497 [99, 106], miR-421 [100], miR-193a [101], miR-211-5p [102], miR-335 [103], miR-133a [104], miR-124 [105], **miR-204-5p [108] | miR-204 [115], **miR-148a [116], **miR-34a [119], miR-101 [117, 118], **miR-296-5p [120], **miR-512-5p [120] | | | | |

**Figure 6.4.** Role of various miRNA in breast cancer development and progression. (Figure from Loh *et al* 2019.)

mRNAs. In this method, probes are hybridized with labeled mRNA to target and detect the lncRNA or miRNA. Advantages of microarrays include cost effectiveness, simultaneous analysis of large nucleic acids, no need for PCR steps, and the ability to detect even low levels of molecules of RNAs. Microarrays have some limitations when compared to RNA-seq, as they only evaluate known sequences (Uchida 2017, see table 6.5).

## 6.5 Challenges

Over the past decade, there have been thousands of publications that have highlighted the role of 'long non-coding RNA' in biological processes and around 2000 publications have reported its validated functions (Statello *et al* 2021). This in itself shows the increasing interest in the field. In recent years, several studies have explored the role of lncRNA as a cancer biomarker and a therapeutic target.

The ncRNA technology is a very effective technology that has found application in clinical diagnostic set-ups for the diagnosis of various diseases including cancer. There are various areas, however, that need to be improved and tackled to make use of this very effective technology. The emerging technology of the analysis of ncRNA as regulators of diverse biological functions is not without its challenges. First of all, they are not very cost-effective as of yet, particularly for a developing country such

**Table 6.5.** The main technology for the detection of circulating lncRNA and their advantages and disadvantages. (Adapted from Beylerli *et al* 2022.)

| Method | Advantages | Disadvantages |
|---|---|---|
| Microarray | High-throughput screening | High-cost, large-scale data, complicated operation, low sensitivity and specificity |
| Quantitative RT-PCR | Simple operation, low cost | Low throughput, low specificity |
| Northern blotting | Low cost, wide application | Complicated operation, low sensitivity, harmful experimental supplies |
| RNA sequencing | Time-saving, comprehensive, precision | High-cost, large-scale sequence data, not applicable for single gene |
| *In situ* hybridization | Spatial and tissue specificity | Low sensitivity, low specificity |

as India. In addition to this, the technical know-how is still very lacking in remote areas and second- and third-tier cities in India. The field also needs better model systems to interpret the functions of ncRNAs and their roles in both physiological and pathological conditions.

The field of ncRNA is still in its infancy and a lot needs to be done, in particular to improving the technologies used to analyse these components in order to utilize their full potential. Currently, techniques use the available biochemical and genetic methods to extract information about the ncRNA mechanism but these have many gaps. The main technical challenges that are faced in utilizing ncRNA as a diagnostic marker are weak expression, low sequence conservation, and capricious functions.

One of the main challenges in exploring ncRNAs is that they are present in low amounts and are expressed very little (Derrien *et al* 2012), and are known to be just 'transcriptional noise' with no valuable function. Studies in different tetrapods also showed that most (81%) lncRNAs are poorly conserved in the DNA sequence and are primate-specific. However, other studies (Necsulea *et al* 2014) revealed some ultra-conserved lncRNAs in the DNA sequence the appear to have originated more than 300 million years ago and can be found in organisms ranging from *Xenopus* to humans.

## 6.6 Future scope

Noncoding RNAs were once considered junk due to their inability to code proteins, and coding RNAs translating some or other proteins was their only known function. But in the last decade or so, several pieces of evidence have indicated that ncRNAs participate in various other biological processes that regulate gene expression, including the occurrence and development of cancers, making them potential targets for cancer management. The emerging roles of ncRNAs in the pathogenesis of cancer are diverse and complex and need to be explored in more detail. Further research needs to be done to throw some more light on the correlations between ncRNAs and cancers. The study confirmed that ncRNAs can be used as biomarkers and therapeutic targets, and also to predict the prognosis of cancer patients in the future.

## 6.7 Conclusion

Numerous studies carried out over the last decades have paid more attention to ncRNAs, in particular miRNA and lncRNA, that have been shown to play an important role in the regulation of gene expression, which in turn regulates the growth, proliferation, apoptosis, and cellular communication of cells. These RNAs have been identified as potential biomarkers of cancer as they show different levels of expression change in tumors (Ganepola *et al* 2014). Several tumor marker studies have been done in various cancer types to explore these ncRNA levels. The property that makes these circulating ncRNAs good candidates as cancer biomarkers is their stable nature in blood and other body fluids (urine, saliva, cerebrospinal fluid, etc), which makes it easy to detect them (Li *et al* 2014).

Thus, this molecular marker has paved the way for other such studies and this can certainly benefit the medical community in diagnosing cancer at an early stage with a specific and sensitive tumor marker that is non-invasive in nature, making it an ideal marker.

Therefore, understanding the role of ncRNAs and their mechanism of actions and pathways inside the cell more deeply will reveal a lot of information to understand the mystery of life and the interaction between genes and the environment, and will pave the way for the prevention of diseases including cancer, and the development of more and more specific targeted therapies for better disease management.

## References

Bastide A and David A 2018 The ribosome, (slow) beating heart of cancer (stem) cell *Oncogenesis* **7** 34

Beylerli O, Gareev I, Sufianov A, Ilyasova T and Guang Y 2022 Long noncoding RNAs as promising biomarkers in cancer *Non-coding RNA Res.* **7** 66–70

Bhatti G K, Khullar N, Sidhu I S, Navik U S, Reddy A P, Reddy P H and Bhatti J S 2021 Emerging role of non-coding RNA in health and disease *Metab. Brain Dis.* **36** 1119–34

Bhushan A, Gonsalves A and Menon J U 2021 Current state of breast cancer diagnosis, treatment, and theranostics *Pharmaceutics* **13** 723

Birney EThe ENCODE Project Consortium *et al* 2007 Identification and analysis of functional elements in 1% of the human genome by the ENCODE pilot project *Nature* **447** 799–816

Brosius J 2005 Waste not, want not—transcript excess in multicellular eukaryotes *Trends Genet.* **21** 287–8

Caby M P, Lankar D, Vincendeau-Scherrer C, Raposo G and Bonnerot C 2005 Exosomal-like vesicles are present in human blood plasma *Int. Immunol.* **17** 879–87

Cheng J *et al* 2005 Transcriptional maps of 10 human chromosomes at 5-nucleotide resolution *Science* **308** 1149–54

Derrien T *et al* 2012 The GENCODE v7 catalog of human long noncoding RNAs: analysis of their gene structure, evolution, and expression *Genome Res.* **22** 1775–89

Farré P L, Duca R B, Massillo C, Dalton G N, Graña K D, Gardner K, Lacunza E and De Siervi A 2021 MiR-106b-5p: a master regulator of potential biomarkers for breast cancer aggressiveness and prognosis *Int. J. Mol. Sci.* **22** 11135

Finka A and Goloubinoff P 2013 Proteomic data from human cell cultures refine mechanisms of chaperone-mediated protein homeostasis *Cell Stress Chaperones* **18** 591–605

Fleischhacker M and Schmidt B 2007 Circulating nucleic acids (CNAs) and cancer—a survey *Biochim. Biophys. Acta* **1775** 181–232

Ganepola G A, Nizin J, Rutledge J R and Chang D H 2014 Use of blood-based biomarkers for early diagnosis and surveillance of colorectal cancer *World J. Gastrointest Oncol.* **l6** 83–97

Guo C J *et al* 2020 Distinct processing of lncRNAs contributes to non-conserved functions in stem cells *Cell* **181** 621–636.e622

Harbeck N, Penault-Llorca F, Cortes J, Gnant M, Houssami N, Poortmans P, Ruddy K, Tsang J and Cardoso F 2019 Breast cancer *Nat. Rev. Dis. Primers* **5** 66

Heather J M and Chain B 2016 The sequence of sequencers: the history of sequencing DNA *Genomics* **107** 1–8

Hezroni H, Koppstein D, Schwartz M G, Avrutin A, Bartel D P and Ulitsky I 2015 Principles of long noncoding RNA evolution derived from direct comparison of transcriptomes in 17 species *Cell Rep.* **11** 1110–22

Hu X, Bao J, Wang Z, Zhang Z, Gu P, Tao F, Cui D and Jiang W 2016 The plasma lncRNA acting as fingerprint in non-small-cell lung cancer *Tumour Biol.* **37** 3497–504

Huan J, Wei D, Wentao H, Jiajing Y, Qing T, Yibing C and Zhengzhi Z 2021 lncRNA and breast cancer: Progress from identifying mechanisms to challenges and opportunities of clinical treatment *Mol. Ther. Nucleic Acids* **25** 613–37

Jordan-Alejandre E, Campos-Parra A D, Castro-López D L and Silva-Cázares M B 2023 Potential miRNA use as a biomarker: from breast cancer diagnosis to metastasis *Cells* **12** 525

Karijolich J and Yu Y T 2010 Spliceosomal snRNA modifications and their function *RNA Bio.* **l7** 192–204

Krishnan P, Ghosh S, Wang B, Heyns M, Graham K, Mackey J R, Kovalchuk O and Damaraju S 2016 Profiling of small nucleolar rnas by next generation sequencing: potential new players for breast cancer prognosis *PLoS One* **11** e0162622

Lee H, Zhang Z and Krause H M 2019 Long noncoding RNAs and repetitive elements: junk or intimate evolutionary partners? *Trends Genet.* **35** 892–902

Li H, Yu B, Li J, Su L, Yan M, Zhu Z and Liu B 2014 Overexpression of lncRNA H19 enhances carcinogenesis and metastasis of gastric cancer *Oncotarget* **5** 2318–29

Liang G, Zhang H, Lou D and Yu D 2016 Selection of highly efficient sgRNAs for CRISPR/Cas9-based plant genome editing *Sci. Rep.* **6** 21451

Loh H Y, Norman B P, Lai K S, Rahman N, Alitheen N B M and Osman M A 2019 The regulatory role of microRNAs in breast cancer *Int. J. Mol. Sci.* **20** 4940

Louca M and Gkretsi V 2022 LincRNAs and snoRNAs in breast cancer cell metastasis: the unknown players *Cancers* **14** 4528

Mattick J and Amaral P 2022 *RNA, the Epicenter of Genetic Information: A New Understanding of Molecular Biology* (Abingdon: CRC Press)

Merlano M C, Denaro N and Lo Nigro C 2019 Long noncoding RNAs as regulators of cancer immunity *Mol. Oncol.* **13** 61–73

Miao Y, Fan R, Chen L and Qian H 2016 Clinical significance of long non-coding RNA MALAT1 expression in tissue and serum of breast cancer *Ann. Clin. Lab Sci.* **46** 418–24

Morales-Pison S, Jara L, Carrasco V, Gutiérrez-Vera C, Reyes J M, Gonzalez-Hormazabal P, Carreño L J, Tapia J C and Contreras H R 2021 Genetic variation in microRNA-423 promotes proliferation, migration, invasion, and chemoresistance in breast cancer cells *Int. J. Mol. Sci.* **23** 380

Necsulea A, Soumillon M, Warnefors M, Liechti A, Daish T, Zeller U, Baker J C, Grützner F and Kaessmann H 2014 The evolution of lncRNA repertoires and expression patterns in tetrapods *Nature* **505** 635–40

Palazzo A F and Lee E S 2015 Non-coding RNA: what is functional and what is junk? *Front. Genet.* **6** 2

Patterson D G *et al* 2017 Human snoRNA-93 is processed into a microRNA-like RNA that promotes breast cancer cell invasion *npj Breast Cancer* **3** 25

Quinn J J and Chang H Y 2016 Unique features of long non-coding RNA biogenesis and function *Nat. Rev. Genet.* **17** 47–62

Russo J R and Russo I H 2014 *Techniques and Methodological Approaches in Breast Cancer Research* (New York: Springer)

Sargazi S, Mukhtar M, Rahdar A, Bilal M, Barani M, Díez-Pascual A M, Behzadmehr R and Pandey S 2022 Opportunities and challenges of using high-sensitivity nanobiosensors to detect long noncoding RNAs: a preliminary review *Int. J. Biol. Macromol.* **205** 304–15

Schwarzenbach H, Hoon D S and Pantel K 2011 Cell-free nucleic acids as biomarkers in cancer patients *Nat. Rev. Cancer* **11** 426–37

Scott M S and Ono M 2011 From snoRNA to miRNA: dual function regulatory non-coding RNAs *Biochimie* **93** 1987–92

Smolarz B, Nowak A Z and Romanowicz H 2022 Breast cancer—epidemiology, classification, pathogenesis and treatment (review of literature) *Cancers* **14** 2569

Smolarz B, Zadrożna-Nowak A and Romanowicz H 2021 The role of lncRNA in the development of tumors, including breast cancer *Int. J. Mol. Sci.* **22** 8427

Statello L, Guo C-J, Chen L-L and Huarte M 2021 Gene regulation by long non-coding RNAs and its biological functions *Nat. Rev. Mol. Cell Biol.* **22** 96–118

Su H, Xu T, Ganapathy S, Shadfan M, Long M, Huang T H, Thompson I and Yuan Z M 2014 Elevated snoRNA biogenesis is essential in breast cancer *Oncogene* **33** 1348–58

Uchida S 2017 High-throughput methods to detect long non-coding RNAs *High Throughput* **6** 12

Wang K C and Chang H Y 2011 Molecular mechanisms of long noncoding RNAs *Mol. Cell.* **43** 904–14

Weber D G, Johnen G, Casjens S, Bryk O, Pesch B, Jöckel K H, Kollmeier J and Brüning T 2013 Evaluation of long noncoding RNA MALAT1 as a candidate blood-based biomarker for the diagnosis of non-small cell lung cancer *BMC Res. Notes* **6** 518

Xiaofei W U 2020 Expressions of miR-21 and miR-210 in breast cancer and their predictive values for prognosis *Iran. J. Public Health* **49** 21

Xu N, Chen F, Wang F, Lu X, Wang X, Lv M and Lu C 2015 Clinical significance of high expression of circulating serum lncRNA RP11–445H22.4 in breast cancer patients: a Chinese population-based study *Tumour Biol.* **36** 7659–65

Yuan C L, Jiang X M, Yi Y, Jian-Fei E , Zhang N D, Luo X, Zou N, Wei W and Liu Y Y 2019 Identification of differentially expressed lncRNAs and mRNAs in luminal-B breast cancer by RNA-sequencing *BMC Cancer* **19** 1171

Zhang K, Luo Z, Zhang Y, Zhang L, Wu L, Liu L, Yang J, Song X and Liu J 2016 Circulating
   lncRNA H19 in plasma as a novel biomarker for breast cancer *Cancer Biomark* **24** 187–94
Zhou Q, Wang F, Sun E, Liu X and Lu C 2023 Role of miR-301b-3p/5p in breast cancer: a study
   based on the cancer GenomeAtlas program (TCGA) and bioinformatics analysis *Non-Coding
   RNA Res.* **8** 571–8

# Chapter 7

## Insight into the role of non-coding RNAs as potential biomarkers for the early detection of lung cancer

**Santosh Kumar, Alisha Behara, Bimal Prashad Jit, Rohit Kumar Singh and Ashok Sharma**

Lung cancer is the second most common malignancy with the highest mortality worldwide. There are two forms of lung cancer, non-small cell lung cancer (NSCLC), which affects over 85% of people with lung cancer, and small cell lung cancer. Liquid biopsies are less invasive and more easily implemented than standard tissue biopsies. In the past ten years, there has been a lot of interest in the use of liquid biopsies in cancer treatment. Circulating tumor cells (CTCs), extracellular vehicles (EVs), cell-free DNA (cfDNA)/circulating tumor DNA (ctDNA), and circulating non-coding RNAs (ncRNAs) are frequently used as indicators and markers for the detection of disease in blood samples. ncRNAs, which are RNAs that do not encode proteins, are still a major focus in cancer research and are essential to the onset and progression of NSCLC. Based on their structural characteristics, ncRNAs can be categorized as either linear RNAs or circular RNAs (circRNAs). Based on their lengths, linear RNAs can be classified as long non-coding RNAs (lncRNAs) or microRNAs (miRNAs). Numerous studies have revealed the involvement of ncRNAs such MALAT1, miR-21, and miR-155 in the advancement of lung cancer. Microarrays, RT-PCR, and next-generation sequencing are commonly used to develop ncRNA biomarkers. However, costs, sensitivity, and specificity remain concerns for biomarker validation in patient samples. Because they are highly sensitive and cost-effective, recently discovered methods based on CRISPR Cas, rolling circle amplification, and biosensor-based non-coding RNA detection are attracting a lot of attention from researchers. In this chapter, we will review the various methods for finding ncRNAs, along with their potential use as biomarkers for lung cancer identification.

doi:10.1088/978-0-7503-6234-4ch7

## 7.1 Introduction

Globally, lung cancer (LC) is the largest cause of cancer-related deaths and ranks second in terms of diagnosis frequency. Almost two thirds of deaths from LC are due to tobacco smoking. LC is also significantly influenced by the use of coal and other biomass fuels for cooking and heating, as well as by indoor and outdoor air pollution from PM2.5 (2.5 $\mu$m pollutants) [1]. The most prevalent type of LC, non-small cell lung cancer (NSCLC), affects 85% of individuals among all other types [2]. Large cell carcinoma, adenocarcinoma, and squamous cell carcinoma are the three most common types of NSCLC. These days, low-dose computed tomography (LDCT) is a helpful screening method for LC that is not small cell. However, in some densely populated nations, it may be difficult to screen for NSCLC and distinguish benign from malignant pulmonary micronodules [3]. Consequently, there is a need for a more potent screening method for early-stage NSCLC that can forecast prognosis and show treatment resistance to tyrosine kinase inhibitors (TKIs) and chemotherapy. Comparatively speaking, liquid biopsies are easier to perform, less invasive, and more accessible than standard tissue biopsies. Throughout the past ten years, there has been a lot of interest in the application of liquid biopsies in cancer treatment. Samples of biological fluid, including blood, urine, saliva, and even cerebrospinal fluid, can be used for liquid biopsies. Peripheral blood is easier to obtain and contains promising markers for serum and plasma [4]. In addition, circulating non-coding RNAs (ncRNAs), extracellular vesicles (EVs), and circulating tumor DNA (ctDNA) are a few of the indications that are frequently discovered in blood samples. ncRNAs are RNAs that lack the ability to encode proteins. They continue to serve as the primary focus of cancer research and have significance in the initiation and progression of NSCLC [5]. Based on the variations in their structures, ncRNAs can be categorized as linear RNA and circular RNA (circRNA). Long non-coding RNA (lncRNA) and microRNA (miRNA) are the two categories into which linear RNAs can be divided according to their length. While miRNAs are only roughly 22 nt long, lncRNAs frequently have lengths greater than 200 nt. Furthermore, polyadenylated tails and whole circular structures devoid of 5′–3′ polarity are characteristics of highly stable circRNAs.

Research has demonstrated a strong correlation between circulating ncRNAs and carcinogenesis. Abnormal expression of ncRNAs can initiate tumorigenesis and often alter their expression during tumor development, hence rendering ncRNAs promising biomarkers for tumor diagnosis as well as prognosis [6]. Furthermore, because ncRNA expression is specific to tissue and is frequently released into the extracellular space by certain tumor cells via exosomes, a particular ncRNA can be utilized as a specific tumor biomarker in determining the origin of a tumor. Additionally, saliva, urine, serum, and plasma all showed stable expression of miRNAs. Compared to mRNA with a protein-coding function, lncRNAs' half-life in serum was nevertheless comparatively lengthy, despite their instability and not being as steady as miRNAs [7]. As a result of these findings, circulating ncRNA was found to be a highly specific and sensitive biomarker for NSCLC in subsequent studies. circRNAs, lncRNAs, and miRNAs may be extracted through a few common laboratory techniques, are stable, and do not degrade easily. Moreover, they may be assessed with great sensitivity and specificity using RT-qPCR, which is widely used in clinical laboratories. Additionally, next-generation sequencing, RT-qPCR panels, or microarrays can yield global profiles in a single experiment, which emphasizes the importance of circulatory ncRNAs as disease markers for quick clinical detection and diagnosis [8]. Currently, circulating ncRNAs such as miR-21, miR-25, and HOTAIR have been shown in several studies to outperform conventional biomarkers such as neuron-specific enolase (NSE) and carcinoembryonic antigen (CEA) in terms of sensitivity and specificity in the diagnosis of NSCLC.

## 7.2 Classifications of non-coding RNAs

Techniques such as tilling arrays, cDNA libraries, and high-throughput sequencing technologies are used to find new ncRNAs. Finding new ncRNAs has been made much easier with the use of RNA sequencing methods, or RNA-seq. Conventional housekeeping non-coding RNAs include transfer RNA (tRNA), small nucleolar RNA (snoRNA), small-nuclear RNA (snRNA) and ribosomal RNA (rRNA). It takes both tRNAs and rRNAs to synthesize proteins. rRNAs make up the majority of the RNA part of ribosomes, whilst tRNAs transport the corresponding amino acid sequence to the codon to build the first peptide chain [9]. Spliceosomes, which catalyze the excision of introns for mRNA maturation, are primarily powered by snRNAs. Several kinds of RNA, such as rRNAs and snRNAs, undergo post-transcriptional alterations and maturation, which is facilitated by snoRNAs [10].

Short non-coding RNAs (sncRNAs), which have a length range of 20–30 nucleotides, include miRNAs, endogenous small interfering RNAs (endo-siRNAs), and PIWI-interacting RNAs (piRNAs). Through the formation of complexes with Argonaute family members, these sncRNAs engage in RNA interference (RNAi), a mechanism that selectively targets and mutes complementary mRNA transcripts. To be more specific, piRNAs associate with the PIWI clade of Aargonaute proteins to form regulatory complexes, whereas endo-siRNAs and miRNAs form RNA-induced silencing complexes (RISCs) with Argonaute proteins [11]. It has been established that miRNAs and siRNAs target distinct genes in various biological pathways, with functionally varying effects on cellular activity. piRNAs play highly specialized roles because they maintain genomic integrity to regulate germline growth and sustainability [12]. Long enhancer ncRNAs, transcribed ultra-conserved regions (T-UCRs), and long intergenic non-coding RNAs (lincRNAs) are examples of lncRNAs that are longer than 200 nucleotides. circRNAs, which are single-stranded closed chains with lengths ranging from 100 to 10 000 nucleotides, and pseudogenes derived from precoding transcripts, are two other ncRNAs that are frequently categorized as lncRNAs [13]. lncRNAs play a broader range of functions in the nucleus. They control the activity of the transcriptional machinery and chromatin assembly, respectively, to regulate gene expression at the transcriptional and epigenetic levels [14]. lncRNAs can regulate post-transcriptional mRNA processing inside the cytoplasm, post-translational protein modifications, and cell signaling pathways.

## 7.3 ncRNA biogenesis

Prior to being imported into the cytoplasm, RNA polymerase II transcribes miRNAs into primary miRNAs (pri-miRNAs), which are then cleaved into precursor miRNAs (pre-miRNAs) by the ribonuclease III enzyme Drosha, the double stranded RNA (dsRNA)-binding protein DGCR8, and the microprocessor complex (figure 7.1). Pre-miRNAs are converted into ds-miRNAs by cytoplasmic processing, and Argonaute proteins subsequently incorporate these ds-miRNAs into the RISC complex to repress or destroy mRNA [15].

Similar to transcripts that code for proteins, the nucleus is where lncRNAs are made. The transcription of lncRNAs, which undergo polyadenylation and capping at the post-transcriptional stage, is carried out by Poly II. RNase P cleavage, one of the RNA processing steps that some long primary transcripts go through to produce lncRNAs, creates a mature 3′ end for lncRNA stabilization [16]. Moreover, unique subnuclear structures referred to as 'paraspeckles' have been found during the biogenesis of several lncRNAs. During the synthesis of nuclear-enriched abundant transcript (NEAT), subnuclear structures called paraspeckles are produced. These structures may have an impact on the regulation of gene expression that is facilitated by lncRNAs, for example the nucleocytoplasmic transfer of mRNA [17].

The majority of circRNAs originate from genes that are known to code for proteins. When the pre-mRNA biogenesis slows down, these circRNAs reverse splice, connecting the 3′ and 5′ ends to become circular. Furthermore, research on the process of circularization was conducted, leading to the discovery of formation models such as 'intron-pair driven circularization' and 'lariat-driven circularization'. 'Lariat-driven circularization' generates an exon circle by forming a lariat structure that spans exons, skips exons, and deletes introns. Conversely, introns can be

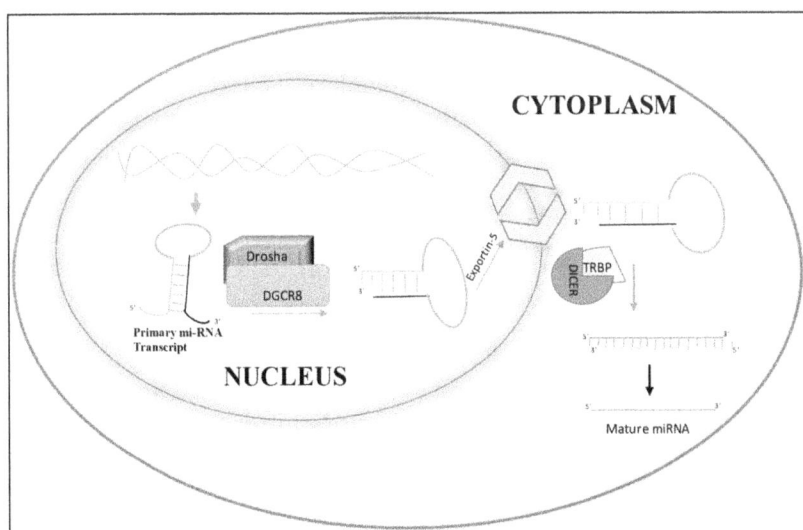

**Figure 7.1.** Biogenesis of miRNA.

removed to create exon–intron circRNA (EIciRNA) and exon circRNA (ecircRNA) by binding complimentary motifs to transcripts. Another work offered a fresh viewpoint on the procedure of circularity in circRNA biogenesis by describing the creation of circular intronic RNAs (ciRNAs) as a result of branching failure [18].

## 7.4 How ncRNAs enter the circulatory system and remain stable

An abundance of studies has demonstrated that circulating RNAs can be produced from sources other than blood cells [19]. A positive association was found by Turchinovich *et al* between increased levels of extracellular miRNA expression and accelerated cell death [20]. This might perhaps be attributed to a passive release pathway triggered by the apoptosis of cancer cells and necrosis. Apoptotic bodies have the ability to transfer ncRNAs into the bloodstream. One such ncRNA that is concentrated in apoptotic bodies is miR-126, which may be translocated when recipient cells absorb apoptotic particles. In addition to being crucial for cell-to-cell communication, EVs have the ability to package circRNAs, lncRNAs, and miRNAs.

An additional source of non-coding RNAs in circulation is RNA-binding proteins (RBPs). For example, high-density lipoprotein (HDL) was found to be associated with endogenous miRNA transit in plasma by Vickers *et al* [21]. Furthermore, Arroyo *et al* found that a population of circulating miRNA molecules has been detected in plasma carried by Argonaute 2 (Ago2) complexes, indicating that they may offer a reason for the long-term viability of plasma miRNAs [22].

According to studies, ncRNAs are comparatively stable in the bloodstream. It has been established that plasma contains RNase; nevertheless, endogenous miRNAs are stable in plasma whereas synthetic miRNAs break down quickly. Plasma GAS5 remained comparatively stable when it was repeatedly frozen, incubated at ambient temperature for 0 and 6 h, and then maintained at $-80$ °C [23]. The stability of plasma miRNA and lncRNA scans in extreme conditions may help preserve EV or other molecules such as RNA-protein complexes. circRNAs, which are RNA molecules with a distinct circular shape, have higher stability in the bloodstream and a half-life exceeding 48 h [24], making them promising candidates for use as biomarkers.

## 7.5 Non-coding RNA biomarkers as diagnosis tools for lung cancer

### 7.5.1 Micro RNAs

miRNAs, or single-stranded ncRNA fragments, have a length of about 20 ribonucleotides. Because miRNA is more resilient in biological fluids in comparison to free RNA molecules, it can be detected in both serum and plasma. miRNA generally controls post-transcriptional gene expression and is involved in the regulation of several biological processes, including cell division and apoptosis. Tumor suppressor genes and the oncogene are among the miRNA targets; dysregulation of miRNA can cause malignant cells to transform into a variety of tumor types.

Sozzi *et al* conducted a comprehensive retrospective investigation in this regard by utilizing a 24-miRNA classifier to analyse plasma samples from 939 volunteers from the Italian randomized MILD laparoscopic cholecystectomy diagnostic study (69 patients with LC and 870 normal individuals). The results demonstrated that the identified 24-miRNA classifier had a false-positive rate of 3.7% versus 19.4% with and without miRNA signature classifier (MSC) integration, and a greater sensitivity (87%) and similar specificity (81%) for LC identification when compared to LDCT alone (79% and 81%) [25].

An MSC was used to stratify patients into four distinct subgroups in a different prospective analysis carried out as part of the BIOMILD investigation: two MSC+ either with or without a positive CT scan and two MSC− alongside or without a positive CT scan [26]. The group with the lowest prevalence of LC was the one with a positive CT scan and no MSC. The shortest diagnosis intervals for both stage I and advanced cancer were also observed in this group, along with the lowest overall LC prevalence at four years and the lowest LC death rate at five years.

In a separate study, Shun *et al* employed a plasma signature panel consisting of three miRNAs (hsa-mir-486-5p, hsa-miRs-21, hsa-mir-210) on patients with benign pulmonary nodules (PNs), patients with malignant PNs, and healthy individuals. The testing cohort's area under the curve (AUC) for this method's identification of LC was 0.855. The panel of three miRNAs was then assessed in a separate cohort of 156 individuals with single PNs in order to provide further validation. The sensitivity and specificity of this miRNAs signature panel in differentiating benign from malignant solitary PNs were 76.32% and 85%, respectively [27].

Along with evaluating ten miRNAs that displayed differential expression in the sputum of lung cancer patients and healthy smokers, the same researcher combined two miRNAs (hsa-miR-210 and hsa-miR-31) to create a logistic regression model. The results of the study showed that, with an AUC of 0.83, LC patients could be identified from healthy smokers. Furthermore, an AUC of 0.95 was obtained when CT scans were combined with the two-miRNA combination. The specificity and sensitivity of the miRNA and CT scan combination were better than those of the CT scan alone, even though the AUC dropped to 0.79 in the additional validation group [27].

In a related study, Zheng *et al* used plasma samples to assess circulating small EV miRNAs in 208 individuals who had been diagnosed with PNs by CT. The characteristic panel of five miRNAs (hsa-mir-3168, hsa-miR-150-5p, let-7b-3p, miR-125b-5p, and hsa-miR-101-3p) is incorporated in the CirsEV-miR model. A testing cohort of 62 cases was used to validate the model after it had been tested on a small training sample of 47 patients. The AUC for detecting lung cancer was 0.920 and 0.760, respectively, according to the data. After that, the model's AUC was 0.781, and it was confirmed in 92 more patients who were not part of the trial [28].

In this instance, EVs and miRNAs were evaluated using next generation sequencing (NGS) analysis [29]. This group compared plasma from subjects with Lung-RADS4 PNs that were overdiagnosed or high-risk Lung-RADS2 screening controls to patients who's PNs were later confirmed to be LC. They discovered that the expression levels of microRNA hsa-miR-22-3p, let-7b-5p, and hsa-miR-184, suggesting that these genes could be utilized as biomarkers to distinguish individuals with cancer form high-risk controls. The combined integrated logistic regression analyses of the 3 EV miRNAs had a ROC AUC value of 92.4%, according to the results of this group investigation [30, 31].

In a study, Zaporozhchenko et al examined 179 miRNAs in plasma samples taken from either a cohort of healthy people who were cancer-free or from patients with hyper- or metaplastic endobronchitis (EB), a non-cancerous lung illness. The addition of samples from endobronchitis patients unexpectedly had no impact on the model's functioning, even though they found a 14-miRNA signature that set them apart from the LC group and controls [32]. Nadal et al evaluated blood samples from COPD patients using a similar methodology and discovered a 4-miRNA pattern for the detection of lung cancer. Furthermore, they separated the discovery set into two groups according to variations in metastasis-free survival (MFS) and overall survival (OS) [33].

As an alternative, Fehlmann et al conducted a large multicentered retrospective cohort analysis on 3046 samples of individuals with lung diseases, primarily COPD, and patients with LC (NSCLC and SCLC). Both in the testing set (accuracy of 92.5%, sensitivity of 96.4%, specificity of 88.6%) and the validation set (accuracy of 95.9%, sensitivity of 76.3%, specificity of 97.5%), a 14-miRNA signature derived from the training set was used to differentiate patients with lung cancer from patients with nontumor lung diseases [34]. In comparison to miR-944, which had an AUC of 0.982 for operable squamous cell carcinoma, miR-3662 had a greater diagnostic precision (0.926) for operable adenocarcinoma [35].

These single- or multi-biomarker-based methods produced comparable outcomes, but they are probably less trustworthy for clinical application in real-world settings due to the study's heterogeneity and lack of a validation cohort (table 7.1).

**Table 7.1.** miRNAs as diagnostic and prognostic biomarkers in NSCLC. (Adapted from Garbo et al 2023.)

| miRNA | AUC | Sample source |
|---|---|---|
| Two miRNAs (hsa-miR-31-5p, hsa-miR-210-3p) and three miRNAs (hsa-miR-486-5p, hsa-miR-21-5p, has-miR-210-3p) | 0.91 | Sputum and plasma |
| Two miRNAs (hsa-miR-21, -17) | Unknown | Serum |
| Four miRNAs (hsa-miR-450b-5p hsa-miR-106b-3p, hsa-miR-3615, hsa-miR-125a-5p) | 0.917 | Plasma |
| Two miRNAs (hsa-miR-944, -3662) | 0.881 | Plasma |
| Three miRNAs (hsa-miR-125a-5p, hsa-miR-25, miRNA-126) | 0.936 | Serum |
| Four miRNAs (miRNA-205-5p, -126-3p, -145, -210-3p) | 0.963 | Plasma |
| Five miRNAs (miRNA-223, miRNA-92, hsa-miR-140-5p, hsa-miR-331-3p, miRNA-374a) | 0.9865 | Serum |
| Six miRNAs (miRNA-26b, hsa-miR-190b, hsa-miR-17, miR-19a, miR-19b, miRNA-375) | 0.873 | Plasma |
| Two miRNAs (hsa-miR-942, -601) | 0.882 | Serum |

(*Continued*)

**Table 7.1.** (*Continued*)

| miRNA | AUC | Sample source |
|---|---|---|
| Three miRNAs (miRNA-205, hsa-miR-182, miR-200b) | 0.883 | Serum |
| Two miRNAs (miR-21, miRNA-141) | 0.804 | Serum |
| Four miRNAs (miRNA-301, hsa-miR-200b, miR-193b, hsa-miR-141) | 0.993 | Serum |
| Three miRNAs (hsa-miR-210, hsa-miR-21, hsa-miR-31) | 0.92 | Sputum |
| Two miRNAs (hsa-miR-1277-5p, hsa-miR-152-3p) | 0.791 | Plasma |
| Two miRNAs (miR-31, miRNA-210) | 0.83 | Sputum |
| Five miRNAs (miR-3168, let-7b-3p, miR-150-5p, miR-101-3p, miR-125b-5p) | 0.920 | Plasma |
| Three miRNAs (miRNA-486-5p, miRs-21, hsa-miR-210) | 0.855 | Plasma |
| Six miRNAs (hsa-miR-429, hsa-miR-205, miR-200b, miRNA-203, hsa-miR-125b, miRNA-34b) | 0.89 | Plasma |
| Three miRNAs (let-7b-5p, miR-22-3p, miR-184) | 0.924 | Plasma |
| Two microRNAs (miRNA-181a-5p, hsa-miR-1228-3p) | 0.711 | Serum |
| Six miRNAs (miR-409-3p, miRNA-584-5p, miRNA-19b-3p, miRNA-221-3p, miRNA-425-5p, miR-21-5p) | 0.84 | Serum |
| Seven miRNAs (hsa-miR-181-5p, hsa-mi-30a-3p, miRNA-30e-3p, hsa-miR-361-5p, hsa-miR-10b-5p, miRNA-15b-5p, miRNA-320b) | 0.899 | Plasma |
| Three miRNAs (miRNA-425-3p, miRNA-532, miR-628-3p) | 0.974 | Plasma |
| Four miRNAs (miRNA-448, miRNA-506, miRNA-4316, microRNA-4478) | 0.896 | Plasma |

### 7.5.2 Long non-coding RNAs

lncRNAs seem highly promising because they are frequently dysregulated in the pathophysiology of NSCLC and have been demonstrated to be stable in biofluids [36]. When Gupta *et al* examined lncRNAs from the sputum from individuals with LC and those without malignancy, they discovered that they could effectively identify between the two groups using a panel consisting of HOTAIR, SNHG1, and H19 (AUC 0.90) [37]. Using the second multi-lncRNA approach, Yuan *et al* gathered 528 plasma samples from patients with LC, other lung diseases, or healthy persons. The 4-lncRNA panel comprising TUG1, RMRP, MALAT1and NEAT1 was found to have a sufficient diagnostic value for NSCLC (AUC 0.85) with the cohort's continued development [38]. Li *et al* searched for lncRNAs in tumor-educated platelets (TEP) using a unique method. They discovered that an AUC of 0.895 [39] was obtained when lnc-ST8SIA4-12, linc-GTF2H2-1, and RP3-466P17.2 were combined. In a second study by Kamel *et al* the combination of SOX2-OT and GAS5 showed an AUC of 0.95 in differentiating patients with LC from normal controls [40]. Studies using single lncRNAs were carried out for several lncRNAs;

**Table 7.2.** lncRNAs as diagnostic and prognostic biomarkers in NSCLC.

| lncRNA | AUC | Sample source | Expression |
|---|---|---|---|
| AFAP1-AS1 | 0.759 | Serum | Up |
| SOX2-OT | 0.815 | Plasma exosome | Up |
| LINC00173 | 0.809 | Serum | Up |
| DLX6-AS1 | 0.806 | Serum, exosome | Up |
| XIST | 0.834 | Serum | Up |
| H19 | 0.73 | Plasma | Up |
| XLOC-009167 | 0.7398 | Whole blood | Up |
| ADAMTS9-AS2 | 0.957 | Plasma | Down |
| LINC00342 | 0.786 | Serum | Up |
| LINC00152 | 0.816 | Plasma | Up |
| RP11-438N5.3 | 0.814 | Plasma | Down |
| DLX6-AS1 | 0.806 | Serum, exosome | Up |
| SNHG15 | 0.856 | Serum exosome | Up |
| PCAT6 | 0.9213 | Plasma | Up |

the results showed inadequate performance, comparable to what has been seen with miRNAs thus far, which limited the possibility of any therapeutic application in a real-world scenario (table 7.2).

### 7.5.3 Circular-RNAs

Given that circRNAs are abnormally produced in early-stage lung adenocarcinoma (AC) and easily detectable in biofluids (plasma and saliva) and exosomes, they are a useful biomarker for lung cancer early detection [41]. Yang *et al* conducted a meta-analysis comparing the expression of circRNAs in tissue and plasma/serum samples. The findings showed that tissue had a greater level of diagnostic precision (AUC 0.85 versus 0.79), while another study suggests otherwise [42]. circRNAs (hsa_-circ_0001439, hsa_circ_0001492, hsa_circ_0000690, and hsa_circ_0001346) that were considerably more prevalent in the plasma exosomes of AC patients than in the controls who were in good health were confirmed by Falin *et al* in their validation of the collection [43].

Hang *et al* used qRT-PCR and RNA-seq methods to look into the expression of circRNAs linked to cancer. Their results showed that circFARSA was considerably more common in LC patients' plasma compared to controls, and it was more abundant in malignant tissues [44]. The other three circRNAs that have been investigated as potential biomarkers for LC early detection using liquid biopsy, CircFOXP1, Circ0023179, and Hsa_circ 0006423, showed good diagnostic accuracy [45] (table 7.3).

**Table 7.3.** circRNAs as diagnostic and prognostic biomarkers in NSCLC. (Adapted from Garbo *et al* 2023.)

| CircRNA | AUC | Expression | Sample source |
|---|---|---|---|
| circFOXP1 (circ-0008234) | 0.88 | Up | Serum |
| circ-0070354 | 0.660 | Up | Serum |
| circMAN1A2 | 0.645 | Up | Serum |
| circFARSA | 0.71 | Up | Plasma |
| circ-0013958 | 0.815 | Up | Plasma |
| circ-0048856 | 0.943 | Up | Serum exosome |
| circ-0000190 | 0.95 | Up | Plasma |
| circ-0086414 | 0.78 | Down | Plasma |
| circ-0005962 | 0.73 | Up | Plasma |
| circ-0056616 | NA | Up | Plasma exosome |

## 7.6 Additional non-coding RNAs and combinatorial approaches

Three studies assessing LC patients with controls looked at differences in small-nuclear RNAs. RNU2-1f was identified by Köhler *et al* from the serum of patients having LC, patients with chronic lung illness, and normal controls [46]. This result demonstrated that the LC group could be distinguished from other groups (AUC = 0.91). Additionally, in the study that followed, Mazières *et al* looked at the RNU2-1 and RNU2-2 isoforms and found the miR-U2-1 could distinguish between people who had COPD and people who had both COPD and LC (AUC 0.866) [47]. Using a tumor-platelet educated method, Dong *et al* discovered that early-stage LC patients have lower TEP U1, U2, and U5 levels than healthy participants [48].

Regarding piwiRNAs, a report by Li *et al* showing that serum exosome samples from AC patients had considerably higher levels of piR-hsa-5444 and piR-hsa-26925 than did healthy controls [49]. Peng *et al* created an miRNA and lncRNA MALAT1 panel that performed well in identifying NSCLC stages I, II, and III as well [50]. Dou *et al* examined a panel of seven small ncRNA pair ratios, which were capable to distinguish AC subjects from other lung conditions in high-risk controls [51].

## 7.7 RNA biomarker detection technologies

### 7.7.1 Amplification-based molecular-biology techniques

For the identification and study of ncRNA biomarkers, amplification-based nucleic acid discovery techniques including RNA-seq, microarrays, and RT-qPCR have been extensively employed. In most of these processes, the RNA template is reverse transcribed to complementary DNA (cDNA), using a reverse transcription (RT) enzyme. RT is a type of DNA polymerase that is dependent on RNA; it begins with mRNA and finishes with cDNA libraries. cDNA is then amplified once more using PCR or RNA-seq for detection purposes.

### 7.7.1.1 RT-qPCR

Since RT-qPCR has a relatively low starting RNA requirement, higher accuracy, and a large dynamic range, it is a sensitive and frequently used technique for RNA detection. Many RT-qPCR-based techniques for RNA analysis of expression have been developed over the past few years and are frequently employed in clinical investigations. One of the most used techniques for miRNA analysis, the TaqMan miRNA test, was created in 2005 by Chen *et al* using a special stem-loop reverse transcriptase; the five miRNAs that are present in mouse tissues overall were quantified using TaqMan PCR analysis after the cDNA conversion step. Since then, a variety of uses have been made of this technology to measure miRNAs. The capacity of this approach to distinguish between closely related miRNA sequences with just a single nucleotide variation is one of its outstanding features [52]. Mestdagh *et al* conducted a systematic comparison of the analytical powers of twelve widely available miRNA analysis platforms, including RT-qPCR, microarray, and RNA-seq [53]. The RT-qPCR technique provides the best sensitivity of all three approaches for miRNA analysis. RT-qPCR is limited in its ability to quantify RNAs in absolute terms, despite being sensitive and effective in determining the relative quantities of RNA compared to an internal standard. This method's preference for low-expression genes makes it unsuitable for high-throughput RNA screening, which is another possible issue. It is also critical to keep in mind that, although the RNA-seq and microarray methods are excellent for identifying and verifying novel RNA biomarkers, they are most effective when used to pre-identified and pre-validated RNA biomarkers.

### 7.7.1.2 Microarray-based methods

Microarray-based assays provide multiplexed analysis and may concurrently profile a large number of RNAs at a comparatively lower cost. A microarray typically consists of thousands of locations with numerous oligonucleotide probes on a platform; these probes hybridize with target RNAs to provide extensive expression profiling (figure 7.2). Numerous methods based on microarray technology have been created for RNA analysis throughout the genome.

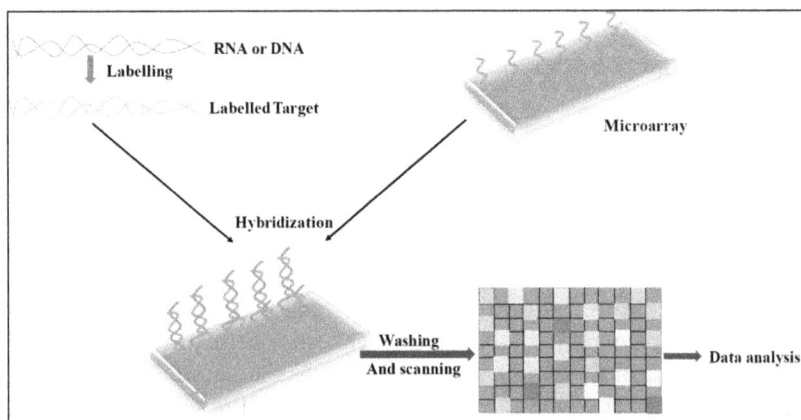

**Figure 7.2.** Schematic representation of a microarray.

A reverse format microarray known as an RNA expression microarray (REM) was created in 2004 by Rogler *et al* [54]. To create a cDNA library, whole RNAs were first reverse transcribed in REM. After that, Corning gamma amino propyl (GAP) slides were used as a dependable printing medium for these cDNAs. Using combined Cy3- and Cy5-labeled probes, a humidified hybridization chamber was built to allow concurrent hybridization of two genes. The potential of the REM to identify Igfbp-1, albumin, c-Myc, and Hnf-4expression in particular was investigated. Huang *et al* published the results of another microarray study to examine the function of miRNAs in resistance to gefitinib, an established EGFR inhibitor used to treat cancer [55]. They evaluated the miRNA activity of a gefitinib-resistant human cell line with that of the original, non-gefitinib-resistant cell line using commercialized Agilent miRNA-microarrays. The gefitinib-resistant cell line had changed miR-149-5p expression, according to the microarray profile. More research on biological activity and RT-qPCR confirmed the hypothesis that gefitinib resistance is influenced by overexpressed miR-149-5p. ZEB1-AS1 lncRNA differential expression in hepatocellular carcinomas (HCCs) was also discovered using the microarray technique, with ZEB1-AS1 lncRNA being mainly elevated in metastatic tumor tissues. Microarray profiling of lncRNAs in patients with colorectal cancer who had lymph node metastases was carried out by Rui *et al*. They found the dysregulation of 1133 lncRNA [56, 57]. In another microarray study, 2208 mRNAs and 3146 differentially expressed lncRNAs were discovered in sinonasal squamous cell carcinoma in comparison to non-cancerous tissues. Microarrays are a better option for discovery, according to these experiments [58, 59].

### 7.7.1.3 RNA-sequencing

One of the greatest substitutes for RT-qPCR and microarray technologies is massively parallel cDNA sequencing, or RNA-seq. It has garnered a lot of interest in both small- and large-scale studies of ncRNAs with improved sensitivity and specificity. In addition to having a somewhat broad spectrum of transcripts, it can detect non-coding RNA transcripts with single-nucleotide precision. However, in a sample with a highly distinct miRNA distribution pattern, the RNA-seq approach is not always able to accurately quantify circulating miRNAs [60, 61].

### 7.7.2 RNA detection by isothermal amplifications

When RNA sequences in living cells are being examined, RT-qPCR is not the best method since it uses repeated heating stages (also known as melting steps) to exponentially amplify up a small quantity of target RNA. There may be another option for RNA detection—isothermal nucleic acid amplification techniques. These techniques overcome the problems of heating by operating at biological temperatures. Many isothermal amplification-based RNA detection techniques have been successfully established in recent decades, such as reverse transcription loop-mediated amplification (LAMP), strand displacement amplification, RNA primed rolling circle amplification (RPRCA), and signal-mediated amplification of RNA technology. One target RNA sequence can often be amplified up to 108 times in an hour using RT-LAMP, a single-step isothermal amplification technique. It uses RT and DNA polymerase in conjunction with a set of specially designed primers, followed by a suitable readout method (such SYBR Green I stain visualization), and may be used to identify the amplified RNA products.

An RT-LAMP-based diagnosis was created by Katsuragi *et al* to detect metastases of lymph nodes in patients with stomach cancer. Employing this method, 92 lymph node tissues from nine stomach cancer patients had their RNA extracted, and then the mRNA for cytokeratin19 (CK19) was amplified isothermally. A nested RT-PCR test was used to demonstrate that fifteen of the ninety-two lymph node samples were positive for metastases. While RT-LAMP and RT-PCR have comparable sensitivity, RT-LAMP analysis is substantially quicker. In contrast to reverse transcriptase, the RPRCA method specifically uses primers made of RNA rather than DNA primers to detect small RNAs in a single tube [62]. In RPRCA, the target RNA usually hybridizes to the matching area on a circular DNA template, whereupon RNase H cleaves it at a temperature of 30 °C. After that, elongation (at 30 °C) is done, and amplification and detection techniques are used.

### 7.7.2.1 Loop-mediated isothermal amplification

High sensitivity DNA and RNA amplification may be achieved selectively using the isothermal process known as LAMP. Usually, four to six primers are used in this technique to hybridise to several target template sequences concurrently, resulting in concatemerization and exponential amplification. The process is started by the miRNA through auto-cycling displacement of strands of DNA synthesis and identifying specific primer binding sites in LAMP-based methods of miRNA identification. Many double stem-loop constructs with different stem lengths are produced at the end of this process, and they can start other LAMPs. Because each stem-loop product has several places where synthesis can begin, this process proceeds far more quickly than the product doubling observed in each PCR cycle. The same kinds of thermal cycling settings that are needed for PCR are not needed for this reaction as it can be finished at a single temperature. This could be utilized in forensics, with more portable and reasonably priced equipment, to offer precise identification of bodily fluids at a crime scene. The increased adaptability of LAMP detection techniques is partly attributed to their high amplicon yields. The identification of ten LAMP products by agarose gel electrophoresis, turbidity measurements, or real-time detection using intercalating or colorimetric dyes is made possible by massive volumes of DNA and amplification by-products. Gel electrophoresis is a widely used preliminary method to identify whether the test is operating as intended for the identification of LAMP products. LAMP end products are made up of stem-loop DNAs with inverted target repeats and a number of looping structures that resemble cauliflowers. When the products are recognized, they will arrange themselves in a ladder-like arrangement on a gel, symbolizing amplicons of various sizes. Magnesium pyrophosphate, a by-product of LAMP, accumulates and can be seen with the unaided eye or with a turbidimeter as a white precipitate. The visual approach of identifying LAMP products is specific to LAMP reaction chemistry, as PCR does not produce by-products of the same sort or size. Similarly, LAMP by-products can be identified using pH-indicating dyes such as phenol red or hydroxy-naphthol blue that change color as the quantity of available magnesium in the reaction decreases during the amplification process. To immediately identify products of double-stranded DNA, real-time PCR equipment is often used in conjunction with fluorescent intercalating dyes, such as SYBR Green [63].

### 7.7.3 RNA biosensors

New methods for biosensors have been developed as a result of nanotechnology's quick advances. A transducer, or signal-generating and amplifying element, which selectively detects the target analyte and transforms the bimolecular association into a detectable signal, and a receptor, or bimolecular recognition species, are usually the two primary parts of an effective biosensor. Nowadays, a number of innovative biosensors that employ optical, electrochemical, and nanopore readouts have recently been created in order to measure and assess ncRNA biomarkers.

#### 7.7.3.1 Optical sensors

Until now, the primary method used in optical biosensing approaches for miRNA, mRNA, and rRNA characterization and quantification has been surface plasmon resonance (SPR) and surface enhanced Raman spectroscopy (SERS) readouts. Target ncRNAs and specific bioreceptors have a surface-immobilized molecular interaction that results in the transducer's real-time determination of the refractive index in SPR. By examining binding kinetics, it can also provide an explanation for the molecular interaction of the ncRNA on the sensor. A portable, label-free SPR sensor was created by Sipova *et al* to identify has-miR-122 in mouse tissue from the liver. This method was relatively quick (35 min) and enhanced the assay's sensitivity by including an additional amplification stage when the miRNA was extracted and subsequently recognized by an antibody [58]. Huertas *et al* created a second SPR sensor to measure alternatively spliced variations of the Fas mRNA that are specific to cancer [64]. In terms of reproducibility and sensitivity, this method is identical to RT-qPCR. One reason for the approach's extraordinary specificity was the use of formamide that significantly decreased the possibility of cross-hybridization among Fas mRNA variants. It also featured a novel sample fragmentation procedure prior to the readout called RNA alkaline hydrolysis to minimize issues with long mRNA isoform accessibility. To evaluate the method's survivability even further, HeLa cancer cell lines were employed. In contrast, SERS-based techniques, which have been used to the investigation of numerous non-coding RNA biomarkers, including fusion mRNA, rely on measuring the level of surface plasmon excitation within the metallic nanostructures of SERS substrates. 'Molecular sentinel (iMS)' nanoprobes are used to identify multiplexed miRNAs. The 'OFF-to-ON' signal switch in this technique was caused by a change in conformation in stem-loop (hairpin) capturing probes after target attachment. The SERS probes used plasmonic-active nanostars as its sensing platform.

Combining the two differentially labeled nanoprobes enabled for the detection of microRNA-21 and microRNA-34a biomarkers, respectively, and assessed the assay's clinical usefulness in breast cancer cell lines.

### 7.7.3.2 Nanopore sensors

One of the most often used varieties of single molecule sensors is the nanopore sensing device. When a potential is maintained in the surroundings of a conducting fluid, charge transfer in the holes of nanopores frequently results in the production of electric current. The produced current depends critically on the pore's size and other physical properties. Thus, the target analyte (such as RNA) can be confined inside the pore after hybridization with a target-specific capture probe, enabling detectable current changes to be observed. The $\alpha$-hemolysin protein pore was utilized to construct a unique nanopore sensor; until now, nanopores have only been employed to explore miRNAs. The technique depended on single-stranded oligonucleotides translocating via a pore measuring 2 nm that was functionalized with a probe that could be programmed. After attaching a poly (dC)30 signal tag to both ends of the oligonucleotide probe, the target miRNA became highly specific to the probe, preventing cross-hybridization with nonspecific RNAs [65]. The existence of a particular miRNA determined the presence of a quantifiable signal. Additionally, the technique demonstrated a very precise limit for detection of $100 \times 10^{-15}$ M. Furthermore, the sensor's ability to distinguish between the relative amounts of miR-155 in healthy individuals and lung tumor patients was effectively verified.

### 7.7.3.3 Electrochemical biosensing of regulatory RNAs (non-coding RNAs)

DNA or ncRNA hybridization biosensors and miRNA electrochemical biosensing work on much the same principle. An instance of miRNA detection tactics is the examination of circulating miRNA bases by direct oxidation-based analysis [66]. In this method, hsa-miR-122 was hybridized to the inosine substitution capture probe using a carbon-based nanostructured electrode. In order to lower the electrical resistance and expand the electroactive surface, polymers with electroactive properties were also applied to the electrode. Then, during RNA hybridization, direct oxidation of guanine produced a detectable differential pulse voltametric (DPV) signal. This method significantly raised the detection limit of miRNAs that circulate in serum ($10 \times 10^{-15}$ m). By creating an ultrasensitive electrochemical approach based on DNA concatemers, the detection limit in patient serum was further enhanced to $100 \times 10^{-18}$ m [67]. This method involved the self-assembly of two auxiliary probes to create a one-dimensional DNA concatemer. An HP capture probe (sulfhydryl-hairpin probe) was immobilized over the surface of the gold electrodes printed on a screen. The HP probe maintained its loop shape when the target miR-21 was absent, preventing the DNA concatemers from adhering to it. Small electrochemical signals were generated by this. The HP capture probe's stem-loop structure, on the other hand, opened up in the presence of has-miR-21, enabling association with DNA concatemers. The electrochemical signal on the working electrode was then greatly magnified by the RuHex (ruthenium (III) hexamine) signal sensor binding to the negatively energized DNA concatemers, allowing for the detection. Sequence similarities exist between miRNAs and many phases of miRNA synthesis, including pre-miRNA, pri-miRNA, and other short ncRNAs such as rRNA. These nonspecific RNA molecules have the ability to cross-hybridize with the target miRNA during miRNA detection, causing a false-positive response. The sensor was modified to incorporate p19, a unique RNA-binding protein, in order to overcome this problem [68]. By functioning as a molecular calliper of short RNA with double strands (21–23 bp), the p19 protein often separates miRNAs based on size but not sequence. More specifically, p19 is unable to attach to dsDNA, single stranded ribonucleic acid (ssRNA), single stranded deoxyribonucleic acid (ssDNA), and mRNA; it can only bind to double-stranded miRNA. Therefore, adding p19 to the reaction mixture can drastically lower the possibility of nonspecific detection. Using this special property of the p19 protein, a three-mode electrochemical sensor has been created to detect circulating miRNAs. In the three-way analysis, one or more miRNAs are detected on screen-printed carbon electrodes enriched with gold nanoparticles using square wave voltammetry (SWV) in an incubation buffer made up of $[K_3(Fe(CN)_6]$ and $[Ru(NH_3)_6]Cl_3$. The target microRNA-21 hybridizes with its corresponding thiolated-immobilized probe to regulate the SWV signal in the first modality. It was found that there was a linear detection that ranged from $1 \times 10^{-15}$ m to $10 \times 10^{-12}$ m. In the second mode, the hybrid was exposed to the p19 protein dimer. The miR-21 can be detected ultrasensitively (i.e. having a linear range for detection of $10 \times 10^{-18}$ m to $10 \times 10^{-15}$ m) by connecting the bulky p19 protein dimer to the produced hybrid, therefore enhancing the SWV signal.

This enhances the SWV signal and permits an ultrasensitive identification of the miR-21 (i.e. linear detection range to $10 \times 10^{-18}$ m to $10 \times 10^{-15}$ m) by binding the bulky p19 protein and shielding the electrode surface. The final stage involves attaching the p19 to the resultant hybrid and using the self-assembled thiolated RNA probe connected to the concentration saturation from an miRNA as the basis for a universal displacement-based sensor. Next, a novel target microRNA (miR-200) and the corresponding nonthiolated-RNA probe are incubated with the p19-modified sensor. The p19 protein can be forced to separate from the immobilized hybrid on the electrode surface by a newly formed hybrid at a concentration that is relatively higher than the immobilized hybrids. This will cause the p19 protein to bind to the newly formed hybrid, reversing the SWV signal (i.e. the linear detection range to $100 \times 10^{-12}$ to $1 \times 10^{-6}$ m).

The reason for this is that the miR-200 sequence and the nonthiolated-RNA probe complement each other [69]. Therefore, any kind of miRNA may be detected using this displacement-based sensor without the requirement for a thiolated capture probe, and the p19-modified sensor is incubated with its corresponding nonthiolated-RNA probe. Additionally, the sensor can detect single base mismatches in miRNAs and discriminate between miRNAs with varying A/U and G/C contents. The increasing functional understanding of lncRNAs in gene regulation has led to an increase in investigations in the field of translational clinical research. Although lncRNAs have enormous therapeutic implications, little research has been done on their electrochemical detection. There have been very few papers of lncRNA electrochemical biosensing up to this point. The comparatively lengthy sequence and large molecular weight of lncRNA may help to explain this. Furthermore, because the RNA sugar contains an extra oxygen atom, lncRNAs prefer to form hydrogen bonds with the nucleic acid backbone, which can result in secondary or tertiary structures such as quadruplexes, hairpins, and triplexes. The most commonly employed RNA-hybridization-based electrochemical detectors are unable to recognize and effectively capture the necessary lncRNAs on the electrode surface when these issues are coupled. Liu *et al* detected nuclear paraspeckle assembly transcript 1 (NEAT1) lncRNA, which is allegedly overexpressed in HIV patients, by employing the catalyst-mediated amplifying abilities of carbon single-wall nanotubes covered via Au–Rh hollow nanospheres [70].

The advantages of gold's RNA-binding skills, single-wall carbon nanotubes' (SWCNTs) large edge-plane-to-basal-plane ratio, and Rh's superior catalytic qualities are all combined in the nanospheres. The gold (Au) electrode of this sensor was first altered using L-cysteine to produce a Au monolayer. Subsequently, a gold electrode containing L-cysteine was placed in a colloidal solution. The linked capture probe (an RNA fragment containing a (GGGG) nanomaterial (Au/Rh-HNP@SWCNT compound)) was then assigned to each potential AuNP binding site. In order to avoid nonspecific binding, hexanethiol was absorbed into the sensor. NEAT1 monitoring is made possible by soaking the sensor in hemin solution, which enables the quadruplex carrying target RNA to interact with hemin and provide a stronger (catalytic) redox output of hydrogen peroxide in the presence of HRP.

# References

[1] Liu C *et al* 2023 The effect of ambient PM2.5 exposure on survival of lung cancer patients after lobectomy *Environ. Health* **22** 23

[2] Herbst R and Morgensztern D 2018 The biology and management of non-small cell lung cancer *Nature* **553** 446–54

[3] Lo W C, Ho C C, Tseng E, Hwang J S, Chan C C and Lin H H 2022 Long-term exposure to ambient fine particulate matter (PM2.5) and associations with cardiopulmonary diseases and lung cancer in Taiwan: a nationwide longitudinal cohort study *Int. J. Epidemiol.* **51** 1230–42

[4] Schütte S, Dietrich D, Montet X and Flahault A 2018 Participation in lung cancer screening programs: Are there gender and social differences? A systematic review *Public Health Rev.* **39** 23

[5] Bowe B, Xie Y and Yan Y 2019 Burden of cause-specific mortality associated with PM2. 5 air pollution in the United States *JAMA Netw. Open* **2** e1915834

[6] Sang S, Chu C, Zhang T, Chen H and Yang X 2022 The global burden of disease attributable to ambient fine particulate matter in 204 countries and territories, 1990–2019: a systematic analysis of the Global Burden of Disease Study 2019 *Ecotoxicol. Environ. Saf.* **238** 113588

[7] Yang D, Liu Y, Bai C and Wang X 2020 Epidemiology of lung cancer and lung cancer screening programs in China and the United States *Cancer Lett.* **468** 82–7

[8] James S L *et al* 2018 Global, regional, and national incidence, prevalence, and years lived with disability for 354 Diseases and Injuries for 195 countries and territories, 1990–2017: a systematic analysis for the Global Burden of Disease Study 2017 *Lancet* **392** 1789–858

[9] Cech T R and Steitz J A 2014 The noncoding RNA revolution—trashing old rules to forge new ones *Cell* **157** 77–94

[10] Liang J, Wen J, Huang Z, Chen X P, Zhang B X and Chu L 2019 Small nucleolar RNAs: insight into their function in cancer *Front. Oncol.* **9** 587

[11] Carthew R W and Sontheimer E J 2009 Origins and mechanisms of miRNAs and siRNAs *Cell* **136** 642–55

[12] Moyano M and Stefani G 2015 PiRNA involvement in genome stability and human cancer *J. Hematol. Oncol.* **8** 38

[13] Kashi K, Henderson L, Bonetti A and Carninci P 2016 Discovery and functional analysis of lncRNAs: methodologies to investigate an uncharacterized transcriptome *Biochim. Biophys. Acta* **1859** 3–15

[14] Sabbih G, Kulabhusan P K, Singh R K, Jeevanandam J and Danquah M K 2021 Biocomposites for the fabrication of artificial organs *Green Biocomposites for Biomedical Engineering* (Cambridge: Woodhead) pp 301–28

[15] Pal S and Singh R K 2023 An overview of phytochemicals under clinical trials for various cancers *Phytochemicals as an Epigenetic Modifier in Cancer Prevention* (Bristol: IOP Publishing) pp 10-1

[16] Singh R K, Panigarhi B and Suryakant U 2023 Development of paper-based assay for detection of miRNA in various diseases *Paper-Based Diagnostic Devices for Infectious Diseases* (Bristol: IOP Publishing) p 8-1

[17] Naganuma T and Hirose T 2013 Paraspeckle formation during the biogenesis of long non-coding RNAs *RNA Biol.* **10** 456–61

[18] Zhang Y *et al* 2013 Circular intronic long noncoding RNAs *Mol. Cell.* **51** 792–806

[19] Sun Y, Zhang K, Fan G and Li J 2012 Identification of circulating microRNAs as biomarkers in cancers: what have we got? *ClinChem Lab. Med.* **50** 2121–6

[20] Turchinovich A, Weiz L, Langheinz A and Burwinkel B 2011 Characterization of extracellular circulating microRNA *Nucleic Acids Res.* **39** 7223–33

[21] Vickers K, Palmisano B, Shoucri B M, Shamburek R D and Remaley A T 2011 icroRNAs are transported in plasma and delivered to recipient cells by high-density lipoproteins *Nat. Cell Biol.* **13** 423–33

[22] Arroyo J D *et al* 2011 Argonaute2 complexes carry a population of circulating microRNAs independent of vesicles in human plasma *Proc. Natl Acad. Sci.* **108** 5003–8

[23] Liang W *et al* 2016 Circulating long noncoding RNA GAS5 is a novel biomarker for the diagnosis of nonsmall cell lung cancer *Medicine* **95** e4608

[24] Singh R K, Bhol P, Mandal D and Mohanty P S 2019 Stimuli-responsive photoluminescence soft hybrid microgel particles: synthesis and characterizations *J. Phys. Condens. Matter* **32** 044001

[25] Sozzi G *et al* 2014 Clinical utility of a plasma-based miRNA signature classifier within computed tomography lung cancer screening: a correlative MILD trial study *J. Clin. Oncol.* **32** 768–73

[26] Pastorino U *et al* 2022 Baseline computed tomography screening and blood microRNA predict lung cancer risk and define adequate intervals in the BioMILD trial *Ann. Oncol.* **33** 395–405

[27] Shen J *et al* 2011 Diagnosis of lung cancer in individuals with solitary pulmonary nodules by plasma microRNA biomarkers *BMC Cancer* **374** 11

[28] Zheng D *et al* 2022 Identification and evaluation of circulating small extracellular vesicle microRNAs as diagnostic biomarkers for patients with indeterminate pulmonary nodules *J. Nanobiotechnol.* **20** 172

[29] Vadla G P *et al* 2022 Combining plasma extracellular vesicle Let-7b-5p, miR-184 and circulating miR-22-3p levels for NSCLC diagnosis and drug resistance prediction *Sci. Rep.* **12** 6693

[30] Halvorsen A R *et al* 2016 A unique set of 6 circulating microRNAs for early detection of non-small cell lung cancer *Oncotarget* **7** 37250–9

[31] Panda S R, Singh R K, Priyadarshini B, Rath P P, Parhi P K, Sahoo T, Mandal D and Sahoo T R 2019 Nanoceria: a rare-earth nanoparticle as a promising anti-cancer therapeutic agent in colon cancer *Mater. Sci. Semicond. Process.* **104** 104669

[32] Zaporozhchenko I A *et al* 2018 Profiling of 179 miRNA expression in blood plasma of lung cancer patients and cancer-free individuals *Sci. Rep.* **8** 6348

[33] Nadal E *et al* 2015 A novel serum 4-microRNA signature for lung cancer detection *Sci. Rep.* **5** 12464

[34] Fehlmann T *et al* 2020 Evaluating the use of circulating microrna profiles for lung cancer detection in symptomatic patients *JAMA Oncol.* **6** 714–23

[35] Powrózek T, Krawczyk P, Kowalski D M, Winiarczyk K, Olszyna-Serementa M and Milanowski J 2015 Plasma circulating microRNA-944 and microRNA-3662 as potential histologic type-specific early lung cancer biomarkers *Transl. Res.* **166** 315–23

[36] Singh R K, Mishra S, Jena S, Panigrahi B, Das B, Jayabalan R, Parhi P K and Mandal D 2018 Rapid colorimetric sensing of gadolinium by EGCG-derived AgNPs: the development of a nanohybrid bioimaging probe *Chem. Commun.* **54** 3981–4

[37] Gupta C, Su J, Zhan M, Stass S A and Jiang F 2019 Sputum long non-coding RNA biomarkers for diagnosis of lung cancer *Cancer Biomarkers* **26** 219–27

[38] Yuan S *et al* 2020 Circulating long noncoding RNAs act as diagnostic biomarkers in non-small cell lung cancer *Front. Oncol.* **10** 537120

[39] Li X *et al* 2021 TEP linc-GTF2H2-1, RP3–466P17.2, and lnc-ST8SIA4–12 as novel biomarkers for lung cancer diagnosis and progression prediction *J. Cancer Res. Clin. Oncol.* **147** 1609–22

[40] Kamel L M, Atef D M, Mackawy A M H, Shalaby S M and Abdelraheim N 2019 Circulating long non-coding RNA GAS5 and SOX2OT as potential biomarkers for diagnosis and prognosis of non-small cell lung cancer *Biotechnol. Appl. Biochem.* **66** 634–42

[41] Zhao J, Li L, Wang Q, Han H, Zhan Q and Xu M 2018 CircRNA expression profile in early-stage lung adenocarcinoma patients *Cell. Physiol. Biochem.* **44** 2138–46

[42] Yang X, Tian W, Wang S, Ji X and Zhou B 2021 CircRNAs as promising biomarker in diagnostic and prognostic of lung cancer: an updated meta-analysis *Genomics* **113** 387–97

[43] Chen F, Huang C, Wu Q, Jiang L, Chen S and Chen L 2020 Circular RNAs expression profiles in plasma exosomes from early-stage lung adenocarcinoma and the potential biomarkers *J. Cell. Biochem.* **121** 2525–33

[44] Hang D *et al* 2018 A novel plasma circular RNA circFARSA is a potential biomarker for non-small cell lung cancer *Cancer Med.* **7** 2783–91

[45] Luo Y *et al* 2022 CircFOXP1: a novel serum diagnostic biomarker for non-small cell lung cancer *Int. J. Biol. Markers* **37** 58–65

[46] Köhler J *et al* 2016 Circulating U2 small nuclear RNA fragments as a diagnostic and prognostic biomarker in lung cancer patients *J. Cancer Res. Clin. Oncol.* **142** 795–805

[47] Mazières J *et al* 2013 Alternative processing of the U2 small nuclear RNA produces a 19–22nt fragment with relevance for the detection of non-small cell lung cancer in human serum *PLoS One* **8** e60134

[48] Dong X *et al* 2020 Small nuclear RNAs (U1, U2, U5) in tumor-educated platelets are downregulated and act as promising biomarkers in lung cancer *Front. Oncol.* **10** 1627

[49] Li J *et al* 2021 PIWI-interacting RNAs are aberrantly expressed and may serve as novel biomarkers for diagnosis of lung adenocarcinoma *Thorac. Cancer* **12** 2468–77

[50] Peng H *et al* 2016 A circulating non-coding RNA panel as an early detection predictor of non-small cell lung cancer *Life Sci.* **151** 235–42

[51] Dou Y *et al* 2018 Plasma small ncRNA pair panels as novel biomarkers for early-stage lung adenocarcinoma screening *BMC Genomics* **19** 545

[52] Chen C, Ridzon D, Broomer A, Zhou Z, Lee D H, Nguyen J T, Barbisin M and Xu N L 2005 Real-time quantification of microRNAs by stem–loop RT–PCR *Nucl. Acids Res.* **33** e179

[53] Mestdagh P, Hartmann N, Baeriswyl L, Andreasen D, Bernard N, Chen C and Cheo D 2014 Evaluation of quantitative miRNA expression platforms in the microRNA quality control (miRQC) study *Nat. Methods* **11** 809–15

[54] Rogler C E *et al* 2004 RNA expression microarrays (REMs), a high-throughput method to measure differences in gene expression in diverse biological samples *Nucleic Acids Res.* **32** e120

[55] Huang Y K and Yu J C 2015 Circulating microRNAs and long non-coding RNAs in gastric cancer diagnosis: an update and review *World J. Gastroenterol.* **21** 9863–86

[56] Rui Q, Xu Z, Yang P and He Z 2015 Long noncoding RNA expression patterns in lymph node metastasis in colorectal cancer by microarray *Biomed. Pharmacother.* **75** 12–8

[57] Gupta R *et al* 2022 Leveraging epigenetics to enhance the efficacy of cancer-testis antigen: a potential candidate for immunotherapy *Epigenomics* **14** 865–86

[58] Jit B P, Qazi S, Arya R, Srivastava A, Gupta N and Sharma A 2021 An immune epigenetic insight to COVID-19 infection *Epigenomics* **13** 465–80

[59] Jit B P, Bera R and Sharma A 2022 Mechanistic basis of regulation of host epigenetic landscape and its association with immune function: a COVID19 perspective *Epigenetics and Anticipation* (Cham: Springer International) pp 59–75

[60] Gupta R, Jit B P and Sharma A 2022 Epigenetic mediated regulation of cancer-testis/germline antigen and its implication in cancer immunotherapy: a treasure map for future anticipatory medicine *Epigenetics and Anticipation* (Cham: Springer International) pp 149–66

[61] Qazi S, Jit B P, Das A, Karthikeyan M, Saxena A, Ray M D and Sharma A 2022 BESFA: bioinformatics based evolutionary, structural and functional analysis of prostate, placenta, ovary, testis, and embryo (POTE) paralogs *Heliyon* **8** e10476

[62] Katsuragi K, Yashiro M, Sawada T, Osaka H, Ohira M and Hirakawa K 2007 Prognostic impact of PCR-based identification of isolated tumour cells in the peritoneal lavage fluid of gastric cancer patients who underwent a curative R0 resection *Br. J. Cancer* **97** 4

[63] Šípová H, Zhang S, Dudley A M, Galas D, Wang K and Homola J 2010 Surface plasmon resonance biosensor for rapid label-free detection of microribonucleic acid at subfemtomole level *Anal. Chem.* **82** 10110–5

[64] Huertas C S, Calvo-Lozano O, Mitchell A and Lechuga L M 2019 Advanced evanescent-wave optical biosensors for the detection of nucleic acids: an analytic perspective *Front. Chem.* **7** 724

[65] Henley R Y, Carson S and Wanunu M 2016 Studies of RNA sequence and structure using nanopores *Prog. Mol. Biol. Transl. Sci.* **139** 73–99

[66] Lusi E A, Passamano M, Guarascio P, Scarpa A and Schiavo L 2009 Innovative electrochemical approach for an early detection of microRNAs *Anal. Chem.* **81** 2819–22

[67] Hasan M R *et al* 2021 Recent development in electrochemical biosensors for cancer biomarkers detection *Biosens. Bioelectron.* X8 *100075*

[68] Wang M, Fu Z, Li B, Zhou Y, Yin H and Ai S 2014 One-step, ultrasensitive, and electrochemical assay of microRNAs based on t7 exonuclease assisted cyclic enzymatic amplification *Anal. Chem.* **86** 5606–10

[69] Topkaya S N, Ozkan-Ariksoysal D, Kosova B, Ozel R and Ozsoz M 2012 Electrochemical DNA biosensor for detecting cancer biomarker related to glutathione S-transferase P1 (GSTP1) hypermethylation in real samples *Biosens. Bioelectron.* **31** 516–22

[70] Liu F *et al* 2015 A novel label free long non-coding RNA electrochemical biosensor based on green L-cysteine electrodeposition and Au–Rh hollow nanospheres as tags *RSC Adv.* **5** 51990–9

[71] Garbo E, Del Rio B, Ferrari G, Cani M, Napoli V M, Bertaglia V and Passiglia F 2023 Exploring the potential of non-coding RNAs as liquid biopsy biomarkers for lung cancer screening: a literature review *Cancers* **15** 4774

# Chapter 8

## Emerging studies on the detection of cancer-associated exosomal bodies for the early diagnosis of cancer

**Pavitra Banan and Anushri Sharma**

Exosomes secreted by the process of endocytosis are linked with cancer and play a pivotal role in the tumor microenvironment. Their inherent capability to transport cargos of protein and nucleic acids, as well as serving various intercellular functions, makes them an important part of the cellular machinery. They can be exploited as an excellent diagnostic biomarker for early prognosis of different types of cancer due to their involvement in various pathways. Cancer-associated exosomal proteins play a significant role in cell proliferation, migration, differentiation, and immune responses, helping one to understand the tumor presence via a patient's serum. This review will deal with the past, present and future scope of research on exosomes associated with cancer, including their biological roles and detection techniques. Understanding their behavior and delving deep into these vesicles will pave the way for better diagnosis of cancers. The potential of exosomal proteins as cancer biomarkers is promising and this chapter will elucidate the available exosomal biomarkers for cancers. Improving patient outcomes is the prime directive in the fight to overcome cancer, and early diagnosis is the first step in the direction to achieve better results. Using exosomes as a diagnostic tool will be an important tool in the years to come.

## 8.1 Introduction

Worldwide death rates due to cancer are increasingly posing a severe hazard to humankind. Cancer cells proliferate and metastasize by interacting with the immune cells of the body. Extracellular vesicles form a major part of the environment that surrounds tumor cells, i.e. the tumor microenvironment (TME). Exosomes are one of the complex extracellular vesicles, containing RNAs, DNAs and lipid glycans and the TME can be altered either positively or negatively by these exosomes. The TME

doi:10.1088/978-0-7503-6234-4ch8
8-1

is made up of immune cells, stromal cells, and the extracellular matrix. The TME is essential to understanding tumor biology as it plays a part in tumor initiation, progression, and response to therapy. Exosomes are an essential component of the TME. They function as efficient messengers between cancerous cells and the surrounding TME cells [1], hence studying exosomes is important in order to fulfill unmet needs in the field of cancer biology.

Since exosomes contain various macromolecules in their lumen, an exosome derived from a tumor helps one understand the pathophysiological state of the parent tumor cells and hence the exosome serves as a cancer biomarker [2]. Exosomes are considered as attractive and sensitive diagnostic markers due to their presence in various biological fluids such as cerebrospinal fluid (CSF), blood, urine and *in vitro* in cell culture supernatants. Apart from serving as a diagnostic marker, exosomes also serve as therapeutic agents by playing a role in drug delivery systems because of their safety, low toxicity, low immunogenicity, ability to cross biological barriers, and targeted delivery [3].

Exosomes are also incredibly stable. Phosphorylation proteins can be isolated from exosomal samples that have been frozen for five years. Exosomal proteins are shielded from external proteases and other enzymes by the lipid bilayer [4]. Exosomes are therefore an ideal candidate for therapeutic applications [3]. When compared to proteins that can be found in the blood directly, exosomal proteins exhibit greater sensitivity. Nuclear transcription factors, X-box-binding protein 1 (NFX1), and cGMP-dependent protein kinase 1 (PKG1) exosomes are only found in plasma. Human blood contains about 109/ml exosomes, each of which exposes 10–100 surface antigens. However, certain proteins produced by cancer cells are diluted or mixed with other substances, such as protein-bound prostate specific antigen (PSA) in blood, which may alter the test findings. Furthermore, exosomal proteins are more selective than secretory proteins. Glypican-1 (GPC1), for example, has been shown to be selectively enriched on exosomes produced from cancer cells and exhibited superior specificity over serum-free GPC1 in differentiating between individuals without cancer and those with pancreatic cancer [4]. There is mounting evidence that exosomes produced from tumors are important players in cancer. The release and uptake of extracellular vesicles such as exosomes is an important way to mediate information exchange between tumor cells and their microenvironment. These exchanges and signal communication between the exosomes and the tumor cells are crucial in the maintenance of the dynamic balance of cancer stem cells. Exosomes have the capacity to regenerate stem cell phenotypes and then convert them to cancer stem cells by regulating the Hedgehog or Notch or Wnt pathway [5]. Since exosomes play a role in cross talk between cancer cells and cancer stem cells, exploring the contents of the exosomes becomes important. Exosomes and their contents could function as therapeutic targets, cancer prognostic indicators, or even anticancer drug carriers. Precise drug delivery to tumor cells is critically needed to increase the efficacy of cancer treatment. Exosomes are important molecular players in cancer biology that influence and modify the TME as well as its constituents, which include the tumor vasculature, the extracellular matrix, myofibroblasts, and a variety of immune cells. Specifically, tumor derived exosomes that are released from tumor cells are distinct in their origin and function based on the type of cancer. Exosomes appear to have two possible tumor-related functions, i.e. they can either promote or prevent tumor growth [6]. Clinically, one of the most promising methods to accomplish the latter is using drug delivery systems based on nanotechnology. Exosomes have been effectively employed as medication and functional RNA delivery vectors in the treatment of cancer due to their inherent delivery capabilities [1]. Researchers have projected that the exosome will not only prove to be a useful biomarker for early disease detection, but may also serve as a biomarker to predict a patient's reaction to medication. Thus, in other words, the detection of and response to a particular cancer in a patient can be successfully achieved with the help of exosomes [6].

This chapter aims to provide an overview of the bioactive exosomal research, with a particular focus on the process by which various exosomal bodies are involved in the early detection of cancer. It also explains the relationship between exosomes and the TME, explains how exosomes affect the epithelial–mesenchymal transition (EMT), and discusses potential exosome based approaches for future tumor suppression.

## 8.2 Formation, uptake, and secretion of exosomal bodies

Extracellular vesicles (EVs), released by different cells such as B-lymphocytes, cytotoxic cells, platelets, oligodendrocytes, dendritic cells, mast cells, adipocytes, neurons, glial cells, endothelial cells, epithelial cells, cancer cells and mesenchymal stem cells, help in cell–cell communication. They are broadly classified into three mainly classes, namely microvesicles (MVs) (100–1000 nm), exosomes (30–200 nm), and apoptotic bodies (>1000 nm) [7]. Microvesicles are larger sized heterogeneous classes of vesicles that bud directly from plasma membrane [8]. Exosomes make up a smaller sized homogeneous class of EVs [8]. Their clinical application as diagnostic and therapeutic markers, and their involvement in the regulation of the progression and metastasis in cancer make them an interesting subject of research [8, 9]. Further, understanding their biogenesis and uptake by cells is necessary in order to understand their overall theranostic mechanisms.

### 8.2.1 The formation of exosomes

Exosomes are formed as intraluminal vesicles (ILVs) by inward invagination of the limiting membrane of the late endosomes [1]. In this process, the early endosome, after its maturation into a late endosome, buds to form small vesicles known as ILVs that further generates multivesicular bodies (MVBs). During the formation of ILVs, cytoplasmic inclusions, and transmembrane and peripheral proteins are also integrated into them. The ILVs in MVBs have two different destinations: (i) either they fuse with the lysosomes causing the contents (bioactive factors, nucleic acid and proteins) of MVBs to degrade in order to down-regulate transmembrane receptors or (ii) they fuse with the plasma membrane, where ILVs are liberated into the extracellular space and are released as exosomes by the process of exocytosis [8]. The main proteins that help in the loading of cargoes into ILVS include Rab GTPase which controls the transport of endosomes, endosomal sorting complexes required for transport (ESCRT) that help in ILV formation, tetraspanins that help in curving of the membrane structure to enable the vesicle structures, and finally, the most important, lipid rafts inside endosomal membranes, in particular sphingolipids, that are converted to ceramide with the help of the enzyme sphingomyelinase to orchestrate the ESCRT-independent pathway and promote the formation of vesicles [8]. In addition to the loading of cargoes, proteins, Rab-GTPase and SNARE help in exosome secretion. Other proteins, Rab 11 and Rab 35, help in both the secretion and recycling pathways of exosomes [9]. In brief, coordinated efforts of several networks of proteins results in the formation and secretion of exosomes.

### 8.2.2 Uptake of exosomes

The uptake of exosomes, small extracellular vesicles engaged with cell-to-cell correspondence, is a complex process affected by a few variables. Studies have shown that the sort of cells included can affect the take-up of exosomes. Exosomes from different cell types can be taken up differently depending on the recipient cell type [10]. In addition, the assimilation of exosomes can vary depending on the physiological conditions of the microenvironment.

In addition, the mechanisms of exosome uptake are different. Although endocytosis is the main route of exosome internalization, studies have shown that other mechanisms such as phagocytosis may be involved in the cellular uptake of exosomes [11, 12]. In addition, the integrity of plasma membrane microdomains, especially cholesterol-rich lipid rafts, is associated with exosome uptake by target cells [13]. Certain molecules and proteins have been identified to facilitate the uptake of exosomes.

This assimilation of exosomes by recipient cells plays a crucial role in cell-to-cell communication, enabling the transfer of various bioactive substances. Taken together, exosome uptake is a dynamic process influenced by multiple factors, including the types of cells involved, the microenvironmental conditions and specific molecular interactions. Understanding the mechanisms and factors that regulate exosome uptake is crucial to clarify the role of exosomes in cell-to-cell communication and their potential applications in various physiological and pathological processes.

To summarize the exosome biogenesis and uptake pathway, figure 8.1 depicts the entire above process where the biosynthesis begins with cargo recruitment, membrane invagination of an MVB and formation of ILVs within the lumen of the MVB. Upon maturation of the ILVs, exosomes are discharged into the extracellular environment after the MVBs have merged with the plasma membrane [14].

Apart from proteins, exosomes also contain various RNAs such as microRNAs (miRNAs), messenger RNA (mRNA), ribosomal RNA (rRNA) and transfer RNA (tRNA). RNA that is predominantly transported by exosomes includes miRNAs and non-coding RNAs. The amount of RNA varies from one exosome to another, and this serves as a potential cancer biomarkers [8].

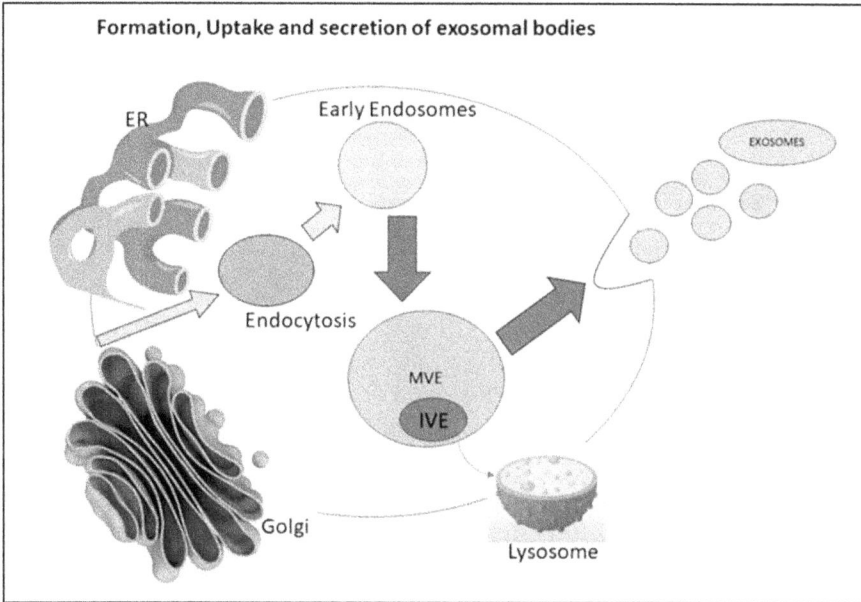

**Figure 8.1.** Formation, uptake, and secretion of exosomal bodies. (a) Formation of MVBs: plasma membrane invaginates to form an early endosome which further sprouts small vesicles forming MVBs. (b) The formation of exosomes: Internal vesicles in the MVEs lumen either fuse with lysosomes or fuse with the plasma membrane where ILVs are liberated into the extracellular space as exosomes.

### 8.2.3 Secretion of exosomes

The generation and secretion of exosomes is a multistep interlocking process that allows simultaneous control of multiple regulatory sites.

Three essential processes are involved in the secretion of MVBs outside the cell to produce exosomes: first MVBs are targeted for transport, they dock to the plasma membrane, and the MVB restriction membrane fuses with the plasma membrane. The MVB surface proteins are necessary for this mechanism to function properly. The receptor on the target membrane selectively recognizes and binds these proteins; the entire process works as a conveyor belt to move the MVB to the intended location. Numerous investigations have demonstrated the involvement of cytoskeletal proteins, tethering factors, the soluble N-ethylmaleimide-sensitive fusion attachment protein receptor (SNARE) protein family, and the RAB GTPase protein family in these regulatory processes. While SNARE proteins mediate the docking and fusing of MNBs with the plasma membrane, cytoskeletal proteins offer dynamic assistance during transport [15].

## 8.3 Exosome extraction

Exosomes are extracellular vesicles that originated from endocytic pathways. Exosomes are widely distributed in both sick and healthy species. It was established that exosomes were present in the urine, serum, plasma, lymph, and cerebrospinal

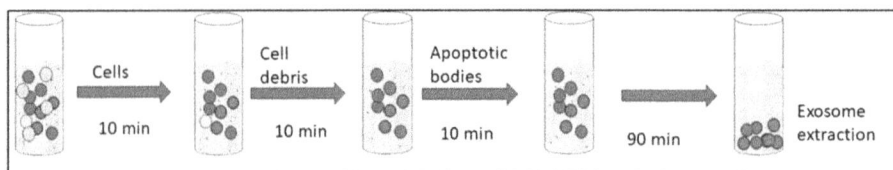

**Figure 8.2.** Schematic representation of the ultracentrifugation technique for exosome extraction.

fluid of both cancer patients and healthy individuals [4]. Several traditional methods, such as ultracentrifugation, ultrafiltration, and immunoaffinity capture based techniques have been reported for isolating exosomes from bodily fluids or cell culture supernatants. Of which the ultracentrifugation method, also known as the pelleting method, being both economical and taking less time, is the most commonly used technique. There are different types of ultracentrifugation techniques, i.e. differential and density gradient centrifugation (DGC), of which DGC is mostly commonly used for the extraction of exosomes [5]. Even though DGC takes 16 to 20 h, the exosome purity is higher [4]. DGC is considered the gold standard method for exosome isolation and plays a crucial role in exosome isolation. By rapid centrifugation with sequential centrifugation parameters, dead cells, cell debris, and apoptotic bodies are effectively removed (figure 8.2) and a variety of exosomes can be isolated based on their granulation characteristics.

## 8.4 Exosomes as therapeutic markers—the early detection of cancer

The most recent up-to-date listings on the exosome database show that exosomes are made up of a wide range of materials, including 1116 lipids, 3408 mRNAs, 2838 miRNAs, and 9769 proteins. Certain lipids, proteins, DNA, mRNAs, and non-coding RNAs are among its constituents and have the ability to function as autocrine and/or paracrine agents. These exosome contents may serve as graded indicators of cancer progression or as prognostic markers. In addition, they control angiogenesis, metastasis, tumor growth, and treatment resistance in tumor cells [1].

Numerous proteins, such as integrins, signaling molecules, and oncogenic proteins, are expressed by cancer exosomes. Exosomal protein packaging varies between cancer types and between malignancies with distinct potential for metastasis but comparable origins, according to the analysis of exosomes from cancer cells [8]. The exosomes detection method is represented in table 8.1.

### 8.4.1 Exosomes as breast cancer markers

Breast cancer is the most common cancer in women leading to mortality if not diagnosed in a timely fashion. Exosome biomarkers found by PCR, western blot, or flow cytometry can be utilized not only for diagnosis but also to predict a patient's prognosis if they have breast cancer. Higher levels of ubiquitin carboxyl terminal hydrolase-L1 (UCH-L1) and glutathione S-transferase P1 (GSTP1), for example, in exosomes are associated with a poorer partial or full remission ratio in

**Table 8.1.** Some of the examples of exosome biomarkers and their methods of detection.

| Exosome biomarker | Detection method |
| --- | --- |
| HER2 | Microfluidic chip/flow cytometry |
| CD47 | ELISA |
| CD44 | |
| CD49d | |
| CXCR4 | |
| | |
| miR-340-5p | qRT-PCR |
| miR-17-5p | |
| miR-130a-3p | |
| miR-93-5p | |
| GSTP1 | |
| | |
| TRPC5 | Flow cytometry/western blot |
| UCH-L1 | |

chemotherapy patients [16]. Exosomal proteins such as HER2, KDR, CD49d, CXCR4, and CD44 and miRNAs such as miR-340-5p, miR-17-5p, miR-130a-3p, and miR-93-5p are associated with tumor recurrence or distant organ metastasis. Another pair of proteins that control exosome synthesis in breast cancer cells are autophagy-related protein-5 (Atg5) and autophagy-related-16 like-1 (Atg16L1). The presence of T-SNARE, SNAP23, and syntaxin-4, which control exosome secretion, was demonstrated in HeLa cells. Additionally, tumors with distinct origins and metastatic tropisms exhibit differential and selective protein packing. The organs that internalize tumor exosomes are determined in part by the packaging of unique integrins in exosomes from various cancer types. The most prevalent integrins were a6b4 and a6b1 in breast cancer [9].

Figure 8.3 represents exosomal proteins that are mostly used for the diagnosis of different types of cancers. The expressions of exosome biomarkers in patients with breast cancer differ markedly from those in healthy donors or patients with benign breast tumors. One issue is that, when it comes to diagnostic tools, sensitivity and specificity are the two main criteria that need to be assessed, however, no study has shown what the sensitivity and specificity of an exosomal biomarker are. Therefore, more investigation is required to assess these two parameters [16].

### 8.4.2 Exosomes as lung cancer markers

Exosomes have also shown promise in lung cancer detection. Low-dose computed tomography (LDCT) is mostly used for lung cancer screening but repeated LDCT will, however, result in significant cumulative radiation exposure which could have various negative consequences. The gold standard for molecular detection and

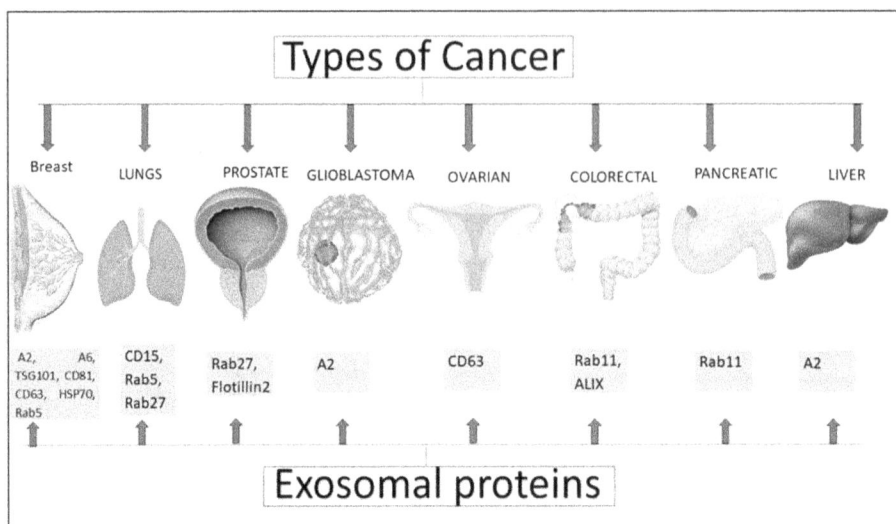

**Figure 8.3.** Exosomal proteins in different types of cancer (annexin proteins—A2, A6, A1, A2, A6; tetraspanin proteins—CD81, CD63, CD151; Rab GTPAse proteins—Rab5, Rab7, Rab11, Rab27; Flotillins—Flotillin2; programmed cell death 6-interacting protein—ALIX; tumor susceptibility protein—TSG101; heat shock protein—HSP70).

cancer diagnosis involves the identification of tumor tissue samples. However, there are quite a few drawbacks to this approach. For example, the quality and source of tissue samples might affect the accuracy of the results, and as tumors vary widely, even a good biopsy may only represent a small portion of them. Furthermore, the collection of tissues results in specific damage to patients, making it impossible to repeat the process. Due to these drawbacks, novel detection materials are desperately required for use in clinical settings. Individual chemicals released during the growth of cancer cells are known as tumor biomarkers, and they serve as indicators of the existence of tumors as well as a reflection of their unique biological features. Tumor marker detection is a highly desirable technology because it is easy to obtain, reproducible, and non-seminal when compared to tissue biopsy and LDCT. Prior to any clinical or radiological screening, the aforementioned indicators can identify cancer via hematological examination combined with a standard physical examination. Broad-spectrum tumor biomarkers, such as squamous cell carcinoma (SCC) antigen, carcinoembryonic antigen, carbohydrate antigen (CA125), etc, are currently the most common biomarkers used for lung cancer diagnosis. Exosomes have been linked to lung cancer progression in a growing number of studies, and they may have an impact on angiogenesis, metastasis, the EMT, and cell proliferation [17].

### 8.4.3 Exosomes as ovarian cancer markers

Exosomes are used as a prominent marker in multidrug resistant cancer where tumor cells post-chemotherapy release a lot of exosomes. These exosomes include the chemoresistance-related miRNAs and mRNAs of the cells, which change the susceptibility of the cells to chemotherapeutic medications such as cisplatin, trastuzumab, and doxorubicin [18]. The primary methods of diagnosing ovarian cancer include imaging and the biomarker CA125. However, blood CA125 levels are not always raised in the early stages of ovarian cancer. Confusion may also result from other conditions such endometriosis, pelvic inflammation, and breast cancer that have elevated CA125 levels. Finding novel biomarkers therefore becomes crucial and hence exosomes as biomarkers become of important prognostic value. For example, exosomes from ovarian cancer exhibit notably higher levels of TGF$\beta$1, melanoma-associated antigen (MAGE) 3 and MAGE6, in comparison to those from benign ovarian lesions. These findings could serve as possible biomarkers for differentiating between malignancy and benignity [19].

### 8.4.4 Exosomes as glioblastoma markers

As glioblastoma (GBM) is the most aggressive cancer, an effective treatment and a thorough molecular characterization of the tumor is necessary. Numerous compounds that have the potential to be important diagnostic and prognostic markers have been identified through research on exosomes from GBM patients. The IDH1 mutation is linked to the 'proneural' subtype of GBM, which is associated with better results, whereas EGFRvIII is associated with the 'classical' subtype of GBM, which tends to be extremely resistant to temozolomide. Moreover, researchers have identified syndecan-1 as an essential biomarker to distinguish between low- and high-grade gliomas. Additionally, the exosome number increases post radiotherapy, hence this rise in the level of exosome serves as a good diagnostic marker for the detection of GBM. It is also seen that exosomes released from irradiation cells upregulate pro-migratory molecular pathways, such as the focal adhesion kinase signaling pathway. Furthermore, a radiation-induced shift in GBM was seen towards the mesenchymal subtype, which is known for having a higher ability to invade through an EMT pathway [20].

Hence, exosomes are also of interest in the field of immunotherapy because of their previously noted impact on immune cells, which can strengthen the immune response to effectively combat cancer cells. However, further research is needed before scientists can make firm judgments about the clinical applicability of the above-mentioned hypothesis.

### 8.4.5 Exosomes as prostate cancer markers

Exosomes play a very significant role in prostate cancer, influencing various aspects of the disease. The analysis of urinary exosomes showed significant differences between metabolites in prostate cancer patients and healthy individuals, suggesting the potential of exosomal biomarkers for prostate cancer [21]. Research has also identified specific molecular components of exosomes that may act as prostate cancer biomarkers. For example, proteomic analysis of urinary exosomes identified differentially expressed proteins in prostate cancer patients, indicating their potential as diagnostic biomarkers [22]. In addition, exosomes have been implicated in promoting prostate cancer progression and treatment resistance. Exosomal miRNAs and lncRNAs have been found to play a crucial role in promoting castration resistance and metastasis in prostate cancer [23]. Exosomal proteins such as ITGA3 and integrin $\beta$4 have been associated with promoting cancer progression and taxane resistance in prostate cancer [24].

In general, prostate cancer exosomes act as carriers of various molecules that can influence tumor growth, metastasis, and response to therapy. Understanding the content and functions of exosomes in prostate cancer can provide valuable information about disease mechanisms and facilitate the development of new diagnostic and therapeutic strategies.

### 8.4.6 Exosomes as colorectal cancer markers

The role of exosomes in the treatment of colon cancer is rapidly evolving, and their potential as biomarkers and therapeutic targets is becoming increasingly clear. Exosome therapy holds great promise for improving the treatment of colon cancer.

Exosomes have become promising biomarkers and remedial focuses for colon and rectal disease because of their role in cell-to-cell communication and transport of tumor-derived particles. These extracellular vesicles, which have proteins, nucleic acids, and lipids, can be confined from biofluids and biopsied tissues, giving significant data to the diagnosis, prognosis, and therapy of colon malignant growth. Furthermore, studies have shown that exosome transport from colon disease cells can mirror the sub-atomic properties and hereditary changes of the tumor, making them a promising vehicle for customized medication and targeted treatments in the therapy of colon and rectal disease. Exosome-based treatments for malignant colorectal growths can possibly change the treatment of this disease. For example, exosomes can be designed to convey therapeutic atoms such as small interfering RNAs (siRNAs) that target explicit oncogenes or have tumor suppressing qualities. These exosome treatments enjoy the benefit of better reliability and targeted transport, reducing negative effects and improving therapeutic effectiveness [25].

Exosomes offer significant potential for the diagnosis, understanding, and treatment of colon disease. Utilizing their exceptional properties and transport, exosomes may alter the field of colon malignant growth research.

The role of the exosome in cancer can be well elucidated with the help of exosomal miRNAs. Exosomal miRNAs, for example, stimulate angiogenesis, fibroblast activation, migration, and osteoblast differentiation in prostate cancer (PrC), all of which supported the bone pre-metastatic niche (PMN). Tumor growth and metastasis are made possible by exosomal miR-1245 from colon cancer (CoC) cells, which reprogram macrophages to become tumor-associated macrophages (TAMs) with high transforming growth factor b (TGF-b) expression. Additionally, exosome miRNAs supported the metastatic niche. Exosomes from astrocytes carry miR-19a to breast cancer (BC) cells in the brain, which resulted in a decrease in *PTEN* expression. This, in turn, boosted proliferation, attracted myeloid cells, secreted CCL2, and ultimately accelerated brain metastasis. These investigations demonstrate the various functions of exosomal miRNAs in controlling the course of cancer [8].

### 8.4.7 Exosomes as pancreatic cancer markers

The cancerous disease known as pancreatic cancer (PC) still has a high death rate even with the advancements in imaging and therapeutic approaches. Treatment for pancreatic cancer with chemotherapy and surgery is no longer as successful due to chemotherapy resistance and tumor recurrence. The extracellular vesicles called exosomes allow close and distant cells to communicate intracellularly. The fact that early-stage PC illness is quiet is a major factor in the disease's dismal prognosis. Many cases of early PC are asymptomatic or manifest with widespread symptoms such as abdominal pain. Patients who receive therapy later than expected do not fully benefit from procedures such as surgery. Therefore, the development of non-invasive, sensitive, and specific biomarkers is essential to help with early PC diagnosis. Membrane-bound sacs containing molecules including RNA, proteins, and miRNA are known as EVs. Exosomes are a special kind of EV that transport molecular cargo from the cell of origin to specific locations inside the body. They range in size from 40 to 100 nm. Since exosomes originate from an endocytic origin, their vesicular contents are distinct to individual cells and may serve as an indicator of cellular pathology. Therefore, we suggest that exosomes found in from pancreatic juice could be used to identify a specific set of pathological indicators to help with PC diagnosis [26].

By connecting with the appropriate receptors on the cell membrane, exosomes released from PC cells and the related cells that surround them can communicate with one another. This results in tumor heterogeneity as well as alterations to the microenvironment and tumor-associated cells. As was previously noted, exosomes have a critical role in promoting carcinogenesis, proliferation, and metastasis as well as being engaged in a variety of pathogenic events and microenvironment modification. The focus of current clinical research has been on developing exosomes as markers for prognosis and early detection [27].

## 8.5 Effects of increased and decreased secretion of exosomes

Exosome secretion is enhanced when harmful or stimulating physiologically active chemicals are delivered to healthy cells. Exosomes with the same contents secreted more frequently can keep recipient cells overstimulated. For example, a high-fat diet may cause white adipose tissue to secrete more exosomes in order to improve liver tissue communication. These exosomes' increased CD36 enrichment promotes the liver's absorption of fat, which eventually results in fat deposits and the development of nonalcoholic fatty liver disease. Similar to this, papers have reported that the body of HIV positive patients experiences immunodeficiency due to stimulation from the HIV accessory protein negative factor (Nef), which travels on these exosomes and targets CD4 + T cells, inducing their death. Further, exosome secretion is also associated with neurodegenerative disorders such as Parkinsons, where it has been reported that alpha-synuclein-enriched MVBs in neuronal and glial cells cannot be broken down by the regular lysosomal pathway when lysosomal dysfunction takes place, leading to Parkinson's disease by secreting exosomes that go to neighboring neurons. Decreased secretion of exosomes may make it more difficult for beneficial, physiologically active compounds to reach healthy cells. Under physiological conditions, CD8þ T regulatory (Treg) cells actively carry out immunosuppressive actions [15].

### 8.5.1 Limitations of exosome secretion

While conventional exosome isolation techniques, such as ultra-centrifugation extraction and kit extraction, are widely used in scientific research, they do have some limitations, as shown in table 8.2, including low isolation yield, low purity, and time requirements.

### 8.5.2 Limitations of exosomes in cancer diagnosis and treatment

The development of novel, secure, and efficient drug carriers for cancer treatment has been in great demand. Recent research has demonstrated that exosomes can function as effective therapeutic carriers due to their low immunogenicity, high stability, innate and acquired targetability, and ability to stimulate immune responses against cancer [28]. The biggest concern while using exosomes as carriers in cancer treatment is that the amount of exosomes is low or insufficient for clinical application. There are some limitations such as unsatisfactory pharmacokinetic profile, involvement in tumor development and metastasis, and potential safety issues [29]. Malignant tumors continue to be difficult to treat, and more precise mechanisms of treatment resistance and immunosuppression need to be determined. Tumor spread is still unknown and in the early stages of research.

**Table 8.2.** The disadvantages of exosomal extraction methods.

| Sl. No. | Isolation method | Disadvantages |
|---|---|---|
| 1 | Ultracentrifugation | • Requires an ultracentrifuge machine<br>• Time consuming<br>• Low yield and requires a large sample volume |
| 2 | Density gradient centrifugation | • Low yield<br>• Exosome damage<br>• Complicated and time-consuming process |
| 3 | Size exclusion centrifugation | • Specialized instruments required<br>• High risk of contamination of small sized exosomes |
| 4 | Microfluidic isolation | A complex process which can lead to irreversible exosome damage |
| 5 | Immuno-isolation | • Expensive and low yield<br>• Gives high purity isolation but can also lead to contamination of exosomes |

Certain subpopulations of exosomes, each bearing a different cargo of biomolecules, can be released by different types of cancer cells [30]. Because of this variety, it is challenging to create standardized techniques for the detection and study of exosomes, which prevents them from being widely used as a diagnostic tool [31]. A second constraint is the low concentration of exosomes in physiological fluids. Accurately isolating and analysing exosomes is difficult due to their low concentration, particularly in early-stage cancer when circulating exosome levels may be significantly lower than in advanced stages [32].

One drawback of exosome detection is its lack of specificity. In a complicated biological sample, it might be challenging to discern between exosomes produced from cancer and those that are not. This is because exosomes can be released by both cancer cells and healthy cells. Moreover, dependable exosome detection and analysis are hampered by the absence of standard operating procedures for the separation and characterization of exosomes [33].

Exosomes have been proposed in numerous papers over the past few years as a viable drug delivery method for cancer treatment. Exosomes have several advantages over liposomes and nanoparticles, including good biocompatibility, minimal immunogenicity, facile permeability through biological barriers, and non-toxic accumulation. Consequently, creating a medication delivery system based on exosomes is extremely important from a scientific standpoint and may have future uses in therapeutic settings. Nonetheless, there are still certain difficulties in using exosomes as medication carriers in clinical applications [28].

## 8.6 Limitations of exosome extraction, secretion, and in cancer diagnosis and treatment

Exosome isolation has come to a consensus regarding the mechanisms underlying production, secretion, and uptake of exosomes. The subclass of small membrane extracellular vesicles known as exosomes holds great promise for both diagnosis and treatment; however, the implementation of exosomal technologies in clinical practice is hindered by the absence of standardized procedures for their effective isolation and analysis. Owing to their unique biological characteristics and complexity, the development of a straightforward, quick, and sensitive method for isolating exosomes remains the obstacle preventing their widespread use in medicine.

## 8.7 Conclusion

As important indicators for cancer screening in biological samples, exosomes have drawn a lot of attention. For tracking the advancement of cancer, exosome marker proteins such CD9, CD63, CD81, and TSG101 are essential. Information regarding the physiological and pathological states of cancer cells can be obtained from exosomes. Although there are numerous analytical methods, surface plasmon resonance (SPR), electrochemical, optical (fluorescent, colorimetric, etc), and electrochemiluminescence-based biosensors are most commonly employed.

Exosomes, which are naturally produced biological nanoparticles responsible for cell-to-cell communication, have shown potential as biomarkers for early cancer detection. Tumor microenvironment associated cells, cancer cells, and cancer stem cells all release exosomes linked to cancer. They are made up of several different types of material, including proteins, DNA, mRNA, miRNA, lncRNA, and circRNA. Since some of them function as biomarkers, we may use this to our advantage for early cancer diagnosis, prognosis, and the assessment of treatment efficacy. Some exosomes contribute to tumor growth, invasion, metastasis, and medication resistance by serving as mediators of signal transduction between cancer cells and other cancer cells or between cancer cells and cells associated with the tumor microenvironment. This allows us to create new tactics based on manufactured exosomes that contain targeted medications, nucleic acid compo-nents, or proteins that restrict tumor growth. These strategies are known as precision medicine.

Recent research has highlighted the involvement of exosomes in the processes by which brain tumors, in particular glioblastomas, grow, infiltrate surrounding tissue, develop resistance to therapy, and spread throughout the body. Furthermore, there has been a significant advancement in the use of exosomes as prognostic and diagnostic markers in brain tumors in recent years. They are currently being investigated as instruments to combat the aggressiveness of GBM through the creation of tailored medicines that precisely target the tumor because of their shape and ability to carry different chemicals. Notably, more investigation is needed before exosome subtyping and isolation can enable exosome based GBM diagnosis and therapy.

The research mentioned above serves as a foundation for the creation of therapeutic drugs and biomarkers based on exosomes. Exosomes are present in several body fluids, but they have a nanoscale volume, which makes it very difficult to separate them from bodily fluids in large quantities. Furthermore, the primary obstacle is in the lack of developed advanced instruments for the isolation of exosomes. Extensive research proving exosomes can be employed as a cancer diagnostic indication is lacking. Research and clinical trials are still needed before exosomes may be used to identify and cure cancer, however, the detection of cancer-associated exosomes in patient blood samples has shown promise for early cancer diagnosis and monitoring.

Even though a lot of research has been done to try and understand the molecular mechanisms underlying exosome production, endocytosis, and their biological roles in tumor progression, more work is still required to fully under-stand these issues in order to realize the therapeutic and diagnostic potential of exosomes. With continued research, we think we will soon be able to fully utilize exosomes' benefits as natural carriers while avoiding their drawbacks. By ana-lysing the molecular cargo carried by exosomes, it is possible to detect and monitor the molecular state of the tumor in real time. These advances in exosome analysis could revolutionize early cancer detection. For the benefit of countless cancer patients, significant advancements in exosome based cancer treatment approaches will be made.

# References

[1] Dai J, Su Y, Zhong S, Cong L, Liu B, Yang J, Tao Y, He Z, Chen C and Jiang Y 2020 Exosomes: key players in cancer and potential therapeutic strategy *Signal Transd. Targeted Ther.* **5** 145

[2] Shen M *et al* 2020 Progress in exosome associated tumor markers and their detection methods *Mol. Biomed.* **1** 1–25

[3] Sadeghi S, Tehrani F R, Tahmasebi S, Shafiee A and Hashemi S M 2023 Exosome engineering in cell therapy and drug delivery *Inflammopharmacology* **31** 145–69

[4] Li A, Zhang T, Zheng M, Liu Y and Chen Z 2017 Exosomal proteins as potential markers of tumor diagnosis *J. Hematol. Oncol.* **10** 1–9

[5] Budillon A, Curley S, Fusco R and Mancini R 2019 Identification and targeting of stem cell-activated pathways in cancer therapy *Stem Cells Int.* **2019** 8549020

[6] Bae S, Brumbaugh J and Bonavida B 2018 Exosomes derived from cancerous and non-cancerous cells regulate the anti-tumor response in the tumor microenvironment *Genes Cancer* **9** 87

[7] Xu R, Greening D W, Zhu H J, Takahashi N and Simpson R J 2016 Extracellular vesicle isolation and characterization: toward clinical application *J. Clin. Invest.* **126** 1152–62

[8] Wortzel I, Dror S, Kenific C M and Lyden D 2019 Exosome-mediated metastasis: communication from a distance *Dev. Cell* **49** 347–60

[9] Gurung S, Perocheau D, Touramanidou L and Baruteau J 2021 The exosome journey: from biogenesis to uptake and intracellular signalling *Cell Commun. Signal.* **19** 1–9

[10] Horibe S, Tanahashi T, Kawauchi S, Murakami Y and Rikitake Y 2018 Mechanism of recipient cell-dependent differences in exosome uptake *BMC Cancer* **18** 1–9

[11] Feng D, Zhao W L, Ye Y Y, Bai X C, Liu R Q, Chang L F, Zhou Q and Sui S F 2010 Cellular internalization of exosomes occurs through phagocytosis *Traffic* **11** 675–87

[12] Tian T, Wang Y, Wang H, Zhu Z and Xiao Z 2010 Visualizing of the cellular uptake and intracellular trafficking of exosomes by live-cell microscopy *J. Cell. Biochem.* **111** 488–96

[13] Plebanek M P, Mutharasan R K, Volpert O, Matov A, Gatlin J C and Thaxton C S 2015 Nanoparticle targeting and cholesterol flux through scavenger receptor type B-1 inhibits cellular exosome uptake *Sci. Rep.* **5** 15724

[14] Wang X, Tian L, Lu J and Ng I O 2022 Exosomes and cancer-diagnostic and prognostic biomarkers and therapeutic vehicle *Oncogenesis* **11** 54

[15] Xu M *et al* 2022 The biogenesis and secretion of exosomes and multivesicular bodies (MVBs): intercellular shuttles and implications in human diseases *Genes Dis* **10** 1894–907

[16] Wang M, Ji S, Shao G, Zhang J, Zhao K, Wang Z and Wu A 2018 Effect of exosome biomarkers for diagnosis and prognosis of breast cancer patients *Clin. Transl. Oncol.* **20** 906–11

[17] Xu K, Zhang C, Du T, Gabriel A N, Wang X, Li X, Sun L, Wang N, Jiang X and Zhang Y 2021 Progress of exosomes in the diagnosis and treatment of lung cancer *Biomed. Pharmacother.* **134** 111111

[18] Yousafzai N A, Wang H, Wang Z, Zhu Y, Zhu L, Jin H and Wang X 2018 Exosome mediated multidrug resistance in cancer *Am. J. Cancer Res.* **8** 2210

[19] Shen J, Zhu X, Fei J, Shi P, Yu S and Zhou J 2018 Advances of exosome in the development of ovarian cancer and its diagnostic and therapeutic prospect *OncoTargets Ther.* **2018** 2831–41

[20] Bălaşa A, Şerban G, Chinezu R, Hurghiş C, Tămaş F and Manu D 2020 The involvement of exosomes in glioblastoma development, diagnosis, prognosis, and treatment *Brain Sci.* **10** 553

[21] Fujita K and Nonomura N 2018 Urinary biomarkers of prostate cancer *Int. J. Urol.* **25** 770–9

[22] Valentino A, Reclusa P, Sirera R, Giallombardo M, Camps C, Pauwels P, Crispi S and Rolfo C 2017 Exosomal microRNAs in liquid biopsies: future biomarkers for prostate cancer *Clin. Transl. Oncol.* **19** 651–7

[23] Jiang Y, Zhao H, Chen Y, Li K, Li T and Chen J 2021 Exosomal long noncoding RNA HOXD-AS1 promotes prostate cancer metastasis via miR-361-5p/FOXM1 axis *Cell Death Dis.* **12** 1129

[24] Kawakami K, Fujita Y, Kato T, Mizutani K, Kameyama K, Tsumoto H, Miura Y, Deguchi T and Ito M 2015 Integrin $\beta$4 and vinculin contained in exosomes are potential markers for progression of prostate cancer associated with taxane-resistance *Int. J. Oncol.* **47** 384–90

[25] Zaborowski M P, Balaj L, Breakefield X O and Lai C P 2015 Extracellular vesicles: composition, biological relevance, and methods of study *Bioscience* **65** 783–97

[26] Zhang J, Li S, Li L, Li M, Guo C, Yao J and Mi S 2015 Exosome and exosomal microRNA: trafficking, sorting, and function *Genom. Proteom. Bioinform.* **13** 17–24

[27] Lan B, Zeng S, Grützmann R and Pilarsky C 2019 The role of exosomes in pancreatic cancer *Int. J. Mol. Sci.* **20** 4332

[28] Chen L, Wang L, Zhu L, Xu Z, Liu Y, Li Z, Zhou J and Luo F 2022 Exosomes as drug carriers in anti-cancer therapy *Front. Cell Dev. Biol.* **10** 728616

[29] Kim H, Jang H, Cho H, Choi J, Hwang K Y, Choi Y, Kim S H and Yang Y 2021 Recent advances in exosome-based drug delivery for cancer therapy *Cancers* **13** 4435

[30] Bastos N, Ruivo C F, da Silva S and Melo S A 2018 Exosomes in cancer: use them or target them? *Semin. Cell Develop. Biol.* **78** 13–21

[31] Ragusa M, Barbagallo C, Cirnigliaro M, Battaglia R, Brex D, Caponnetto A, Barbagallo D, Di Pietro C and Purrello M 2017 Asymmetric RNA distribution among cells and their secreted exosomes: biomedical meaning and considerations on diagnostic applications *Front. Mol. Biosci.* **4** 66

[32] Whiteside T L 2015 The potential of tumor-derived exosomes for noninvasive cancer monitoring *Expert Rev. Mol. Diagn.* **15** 1293–310

[33] Lane R E, Korbie D, Hill M M and Trau M 2018 Extracellular vesicles as circulating cancer biomarkers: opportunities and challenges *Clin. Transl. Med.* **7** 1

# Chapter 9

# Nanosensors: an overview of future utility in the biomedical domain

**Divya Bisht and Deena Prakash**

Nanotechnology has been utilized in several fields of medicine in different forms for its promising outcomes. Nanosensors are one such invention with great potential to revolutionize the biomedical domain due to their diverse applications in the diagnosis, monitoring, and management of various ailments in humans. This chapter focuses on the comprehensive use of nanosensors as a powerful tool to support medical science. The major highlights of this chapter include the fundamental workings of nanosensors and their various types and applications in the biomedical industry. Applications for nanosensors include target-specific drug delivery, disease detection and diagnosis, and monitoring of physiological parameters. Also, the challenges associated with the usage of nanosensors and their limitations are discussed. This chapter also elucidates the current advancements in the development and properties of nanosensors, mainly in the field of biomedicine. This chapter aims to illustrate the current and future prospects of nanosensors in healthcare management, better drug development, and precise delivery, with an overall improvement of medical sciences.

## 9.1 Introduction

The emergence of nanotechnology, with its development and advancement in various fields of science, has opened new avenues to explore with major achievements it the field of medicine. Nanotechnology has become an integral part of medicine and healthcare with its various tools and forms including nanosensors, nanoparticles, nanotubes/nanowires, nanocarriers, nanopores, nanorobots etc. Nanosensors are utilized in the biomedical, environmental, food safety, defense, industrial, electronic, structural, automotive, agriculture, energy, and space sectors for detecting and monitoring various substances and parameters (figure 9.1). In this chapter we are going to explore the diverse properties of nanosensors and their

doi:10.1088/978-0-7503-6234-4ch9

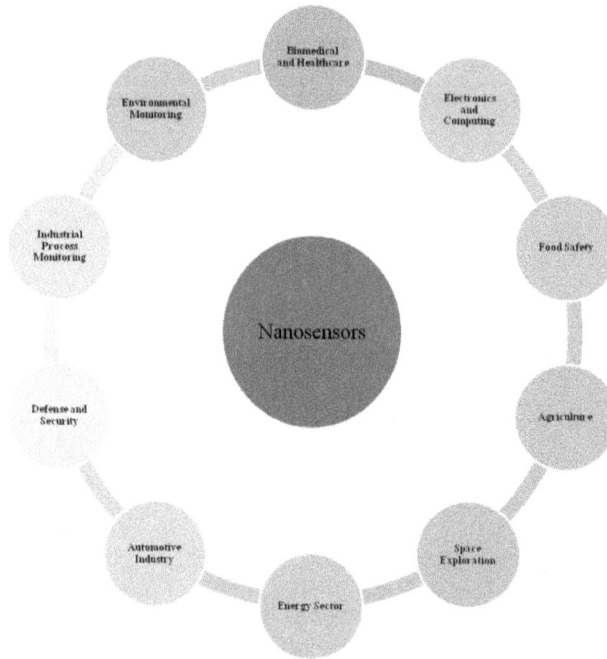

**Figure 9.1.** The diverse presence of nanosensors in multiple sectors.

multifaceted presence in biomedicine focusing on their remarkable precision and impact in disease diagnosis, monitoring and the progression of treatment regimes.

Nanotechnology explores and utilizes the physical, chemical and biological qualities of various materials at nanoscale ranging from 1 to 100 nm, thus tapping in to those properties of materials that are not fully expressed or utilized at the macroscopic level. Some of these properties that benefit nanotechnology are enhanced reactivity, increased strength and improved optical sensitivity. All these properties of nanosensors are greatly advantageous in the biomedical domain to evaluate various biological and chemical processes in the human body with an unprecedented level of sensitivity and specificity, making these nanosensors a reliable candidate for disease diagnosis and management (Nasrollahzadeh *et al* 2019).

Therefore the application of nanotechnology in medicine in the form of nanosensors is greatly encouraged worldwide. Nanosensors are very useful for the early detection and diagnosis of many deadly diseases. Their close interaction with biological systems at the molecular level helps in real-time physiological function monitoring, facilitating research into and analysis of various disease mechanisms and drug interaction pathways. Nanosensors work with high precision as excellent resources for point-of-care diagnostics and ongoing health monitoring due to their ability to produce precise and timely detectable signals in response to a variety of stimuli, including variations in pH, temperature, or the presence of particular biomolecules. This can expedite and personalize medical interventions and lower the need for invasive procedures (Debnath and Das 2020).

The remarkable characteristics of nanosensors are utilized in biomedicine in various ways. For example, the role of nanosensors in diagnostics is unique and significant in comparison to the currently available conventional methods due to the ability of nanosensors to detect various vital biomarkers at trace level concentrations that cannot be detected by current methods. This property works well for the early detection of diseases such as cancer, Alzheimers's, etc (Jeevanandam and Danquah 2020). Another popular application of nanosensors is in the treatment of diseases, due to their highly efficient and accurate drug-delivery systems. These systems are made to release drugs precisely in response to certain biological cues at predefined locations within the body. These delivery systems maximize therapeutic results by minimizing possible side effects and optimizing drug efficacy through the use of nanosensors (Gupta and Basu 2022).

Despite the wide range of beneficial applications of nanosensors in biomedicine there are various challenges that are important to be addressed while understanding nanosensors and their utility in medicine. Our biological system is diverse and dynamic in nature with an ever-changing acid–base balance, variation in pH, multiple interacting biomolecules, and many other conditions that significantly hamper the design and functionalization of nanosensors. Also quality assurance in terms of biocompatibility and the study of possible side effects is important before introducing nanosensors in a biological system to aid in diagnosis and treatment (Javaid *et al* 2021).

In addition to the challenges posed by complex biochemistry of biological system there are various technological and regulatory challenges in the path of development and integration of nanosensors in biomedicine. The concern of stability and reproducibility of particular nanosensors designed for specific purpose along with the challenges in large scale manufacturing of these nanosensors is a concern needs to be addressed. Following the development of these nanosensors for medical usage, appropriate screening, testing and validation is necessary to guarantee the safety and effectiveness of these tools in biomedicine before granting approval to be used clinically. Important steps in this direction include the creation of guidelines for clinical trials involving nanosensors and the development of standardized protocols for testing (Zielińska *et al* 2020).

The cost and capital associated with the research, development, clinical trials and manufacturing of these nanosensors is another obstacle to its widespread usage, in particular for less wealthy economies. Therefore it is important to create cost-effective nanosensors that are economical without compromising their quality and efficacy to deliver as tools in biomedicine. Furthermore, investment into nano-sensors can be encouraged using their potential to lower long-term healthcare costs through improved disease management and shorter hospital stays.

Despite all these challenges, nanosensors are worthy of attention due to their diverse properties and possibilities of application. Advanced innovations such as computational biology and new discoveries and developments in material science will aid the future of nanosensors, ensuring better outputs with high sensitivity, selectivity, and integration with other digital health technologies, making them unbeatable candidates in biomedicine (Kulkarni *et al* 2022).

In this chapter we will discuss various aspects of nanosensors in different sections addressing the role and future of nanosensors in medical technology. Even with their current contribution in facilitating early disease detection, enabling real-time monitoring, and supporting targeted therapy, nanosensors hold the potential to redefine the paradigms of healthcare. This chapter will illuminate their capabilities and challenges, and the future directions of this exciting field, underscoring their pivotal role in advancing medical science and improving patient outcomes.

## 9.2 The basic fundamentals of nanosensors

Nanosensors are pivotal tools in healthcare and use nanotechnology to detect and monitor crucial physical, chemical and biological changes happening in the human body at the nanoscale. To understand the wide presence and bright future of nanosensors in healthcare it is important to dive deeply into the fundamentals of these marvelous tools of nanotechnology. In this section we will learn about the basics of nanosensors, their working principles, their various types, and the technology involved.

### 9.2.1 The basics of nanosensors

Nanotechnology is the manipulation and development of various material on the nanoscale (1–100 nm), thus utilizing their properties at the molecular or atomic level in the creation of various devices and tools with novel functions. Nanosensors work on the same principle to sense and respond to various stimuli in a biological system when used in biomedicine. As the name suggests, a nanosensor contains a nanoscale sensor element and a transducer. The nanosensors interact with a physical or biological sample and the transducer converts this interaction into a measurable signal, sending it to the detector (figure 9.2). Because of their close interaction with biological systems and their nanoscale compatibility with a variety of biomolecules, nanosensors exhibit high sensitivity and precision (Javaid *et al* 2021).

### 9.2.2 Mechanisms and technologies involved in nanosensors

Nanosensors provide specific results because of the meticulously selected recognition element present in them, which is designed to detect specific chemicals, nucleotide sequences, proteins, and other biomarkers present in the human body and natural

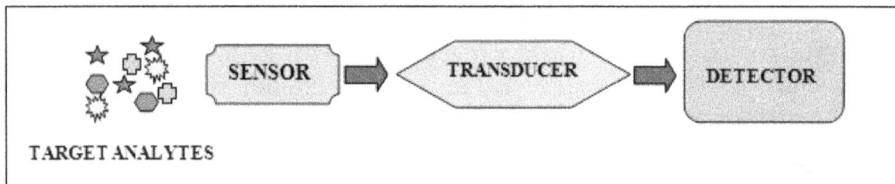

Figure 9.2. Basic components of nanosensors.

systems. This specificity is attained by adding particular chemical groups on the surface of a nanosensor, facilitating interaction with targeted analytes,and this process is known as surface functionalization. After recognizing and binding with the target, these nanosensors transform. This transformation is detected by the transducer and converted into electrical signals that are further amplified and processed into quantitative outputs of the intended analysis. This remarkable capability to analyse and record information from a nanoscale system is what makes these nanosensors great tools in medicine and healthcare (Agrawal and Prajapati 2012).

### 9.2.3 Types of nanosensors

There are several types of nanosensors classified on the basis of their detection mechanism (figure 9.3).

#### 9.2.3.1 Optical nanosensors
Optical nanosensors detect the variation in different properties of light in response to its interaction with the target analyte. Properties such as the intensity, wavelength, or polarization of light are monitored and recorded for analysis. Fluorescent dyes or quantum dots are used in optical nanosensors due to their property of emitting light of specific intensity on binding with specific molecules. In biomedicine, these nanosensors are popularly used in imaging and monitoring biochemical processes (Farmani *et al* 2020).

#### 9.2.3.2 Electrochemical nanosensors
As suggested by the name, these sensors detect changes in electrical properties including current, potential, or impedance in response to the chemical reaction that occurs at the surface of these nanosensors. Electrochemical nanosensors are mainly used for glucose monitoring in diabetes care (Barry and O'Riordan 2016).

#### 9.2.3.3 Mechanical nanosensors
These nanosensors are sensitive to changes in mechanical properties such as mass, viscosity, or force during their binding with target analytes. For example, the nanocantilever bends in response to molecular binding on its surface which is

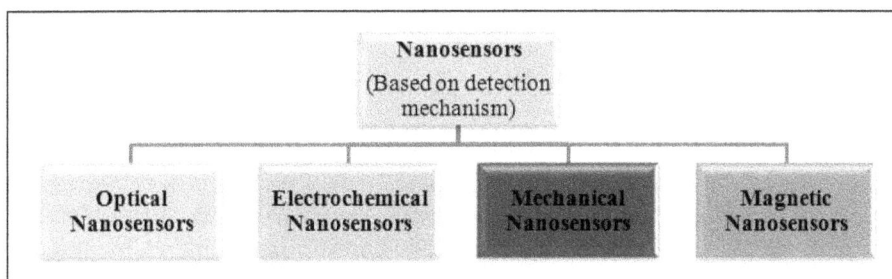

**Figure 9.3.** Different types of nanosensors based on the mechanism of detection.

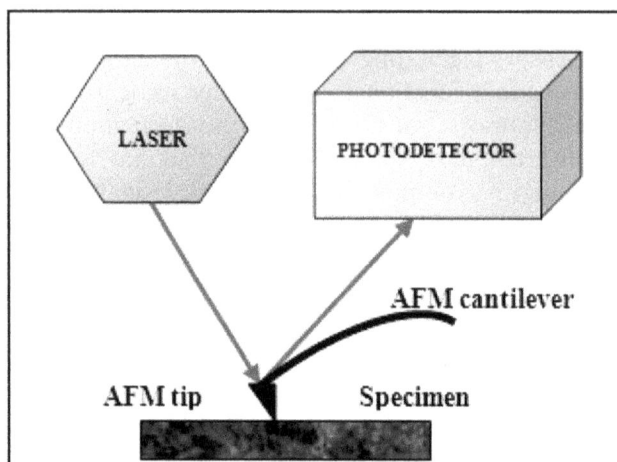

**Figure 9.4.** Mechanical nanosensors.

precisely measured to provide information about the molecular mass or mechanical properties of the target (Javaid *et al* 2021).

The atomic force microscope (AFM) is utilized for imaging surface structures at nanometer or even sub-nanometer scales and for measuring surface forces. Its functionality involves detecting the bending of a cantilever spring in response to applied forces on the surface (figure 9.4) (Ching and Lim 2014).

### 9.2.3.4 *Magnetic nanosensors*

These sensors are specifically used to identify any modifications in the magnetic fields that occur during molecular interactions. These magnetic nanoparticles have particular ligands on their surface that bind to target molecules and allow for magnetic field changes to be detected. Magnetic nanosensors can be used for diagnostic procedures where it is safe to apply external magnetic fields to the body, such as tracking cells *in vivo*. For example, magnetic nanosensors containing a chemotherapeutic agent were administered intravenously and guided by a magnet to the target tumor tissue, notably a liver tumor, enhancing drug concentration in the intended organ and potentially mitigating adverse effects by minimizing systemic drug dispersion (Doswald *et al* 2019).

There are various other types of nanosensors based on different parameters of functionality and composition. Some of these are mentioned briefly in tables 9.1 and 9.2.

### 9.2.4 Applications in the biomedical industry

Having covered the basics of nanosensors and their types along with the working principle of these nanoscale tools, it is time to learn about their role in the biomedical industry. Nanosensors are well known and utilized by scientists, researchers and healthcare professionals due to their diverse applications and close interaction with biological systems. Nanosensors are used in the medical field for a

**Table 9.1.** Types of nanobiosensors.

| Nanosensors | | |
|---|---|---|
| On the basis of reception molecules | On the basis of structure | On the basis of applications |
| • **Affinity-based nanosensors** Example: A versatile transduction platform employing impedimetric sensing without the need for labels, and integrating electrochemical affinity biosensors. <br> • **Catalytic-based sensors** Example: Glucose biosensors employ the enzyme glucose oxidase to catalyze the oxidation of glucose, producing hydrogen peroxide which can be detected electrochemically. | • **Optical nanosensors** Example: Plasmonic nanoparticles exploit the unique optical properties of metallic nanoparticles, such as gold or silver, to detect analytes with high sensitivity. <br> • **Electrochemical sensors** Example: Amperometry sensors measure the current generated from the electrochemical reaction between the target analyte and a sensing electrode. | • **Chemical sensors** Example: Gas sensors detect the presence of volatile organic compounds (VOCs) in the environment. <br> • **Deployable sensors** An example of deployable sensors includes those used in environmental monitoring systems. <br> • **Electrometers** Example: Field-effect transistor (FET) based sensor. <br> • **Biosensors** Example: Surface plasmon resonance biosensors utilize the interaction between light and a thin metal film, typically gold, to detect biomolecular interactions in real time. |

vast array of functions, ranging from drug discovery and development and the monitoring of vital parameters, to the diagnosis of diseases and tracking drug interaction in the human body (Agrawal and Prajapati 2012).

Understanding the variety of nanosensors in term of their composition and action confirms their vast range of applications depending on the specific requirements in different conditions based on the sensitivity, specificity, and operational environment. Nanosensors are selected for specific research or clinical needs depending on their feasibility in particular condition, expected sensitivity, response time, and interaction with other medical practices and modalities. These characteristics highlight the versatility of nanosensors and their immense potential to serve in the field of biomedicine (Mishra and Rajakumari 2019). In a further section we will discuss the detailed applications of nanosensors in healthcare with the associated challenges and future prospects these remarkable tools of nanotechnology in medicine.

## 9.3 Applications of nanosensors in biomedicine

Healthcare systems have improved tremendously in the past few decades owing to the advancements in various fields of science and technology. Nanotechnology has

**Table 9.2.** Summary of types of nano-biosensors (Cicek and Nadaroglu 2015).

| Nanobiosensors | Example | Advantages |
|---|---|---|
| Mechanical nanobiosensors | Nanocantilever; nanomechanical resonators | The smaller the size, the greater the sensitivity to changes in mass. |
| Optical nanobiosensors | Surface plasmon resonance | Exceptional sensitivity, noteworthy optical characteristics. |
| Nanowire biosensors | Boron-doped silicon nanowires (SiNWs) | Ultra-high sensitivity, providing real-time and quantitative measurements. |
| Electronic nanobiosensors | Carbon nanotube-based sensors; lab-on-a-chip | Each target DNA molecule from the same or different organisms can be selectively captured using independently addressed capture probes. |
| Viral nanobiosensors | Human immunodeficiency virus (HIV); herpes simplex virus (HSV) | Employed for the detection of clinically relevant viruses. |
| Probes encapsulated by biologically localized embedding (PEBBLE) nanobiosensors | Poly (decylmethacrylate)-based fluorescent PEBBLE | Effectively monitor real-time inter- and intra-cellular imaging of ions and molecules, exhibiting remarkable reversibility and stability against leaching. |
| Nanoshell biosensors | Gold-silica core–shell nanoparticles | Boost chemical sensing capability by up to 10 billion-fold. |
| Enzyme-based nanosensors | 4-hydroxyphenylpyruvate dioxygenase enzyme; glucose oxidase enzyme | Offers dependable, accurate, and cost-effective methods. |

contributed immensely in the transformation of the biomedical industry with nanosensors as a major tool offering significant aid, starting from precise early diagnosis to efficient treatment methods. In this section we will focus on the extensive presence of nanosensors in the medical industry reviewing in-depth studies of their various applications in healthcare for human welfare (figure 9.5).

### 9.3.1 Disease detection and diagnostics

Early diagnosis and detection of diseases is crucial for timely management of health conditions and nanosensors play a very important role in the field of medical diagnostics. In diseases such as cancer, where diagnosis in the initial stage of the disease can be life saving, with improved chances of proper treatment and

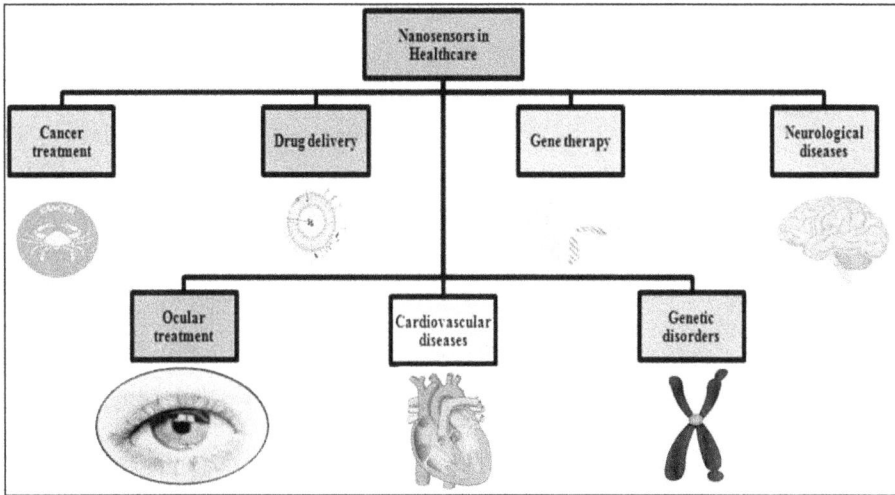

**Figure 9.5.** Various applications of nanosensors in biomedicine.

eradication of cancer in the patients, these miraculous nanotools can serve their purpose by detecting molecular level changes in the biochemical parameters much earlier than the appearance of physical symptoms. This allows for interventions that are much earlier and potentially more effective than traditional methods. Along with cancer diagnosis, nanosensors have the potential to transform the approach to a variety of other health conditions. By enabling precise and early diagnosis, nano-sensors facilitate better healthcare, improving patient outcomes. Additionally, the high sensitivity and specificity of these devices helps in designing more personalized treatment plans, catering to the unique biochemical composition of individual patients, and paving the way for advancements in personalized medicine (Anjum *et al* 2021). Some applications of nanosensors are as follows:

- *Cancer detection*: Even before clinical symptoms in patients, nanosensors are capable of detecting biomarkers associated with cancer at very early stages. Gold nanoparticle sensors are a popular example due to their application to identify specific proteins and microRNAs, which indicate the presence of cancer cells (Khazaei *et al* 2023).
- *Infectious diseases*: The precise and time-efficient detection of pathogens and their virulence factors with the use of nanosensors is vital for the management of serious infections and outbreaks. For example, genetic material from bacteria and viruses can be detected by electrochemical sensors without the use of sophisticated laboratory equipment (Deng *et al* 2020).
- *Genetic disorders*: Various critical genetic disorders can also be diagnosed by nanosensors as they identify particular genetic mutations in the DNA of humans. Using fluorescent labeling, optical nanosensors can detect DNA mutations linked to illnesses such as sickle cell anemia and cystic fibrosis (Falzarano *et al* 2018).

### 9.3.2 Monitoring physiological parameters

Real-time tracking of diverse physiological parameters is another vital application of nanosensors. This function is beneficial in various disease conditions and medical scenarios.

It is essential to monitored physiological parameters for the management of chronic diseases, the assessment of post-surgical recovery in patients, and overseeing the condition of patients in intensive care units. Nanosensors provide precise, up-to-date data helping healthcare professionals to make informed decisions choosing better treatment plans and interventions (Splinter 2018).

- *Diabetes management*: Continuous monitoring of blood glucose levels in diabetic patients is crucial and made possible by electrochemical glucose nanosensors incorporated into implants or wearable technology. This real-time feedback and alert system helps in the management of diabetes more effectively (Pathak *et al* 2023).
- *Cardiovascular health*: Cardiovascular diseases are serious health concerns and nanosensors contribute as efficient tracking and monitoring tools for crucial parameters associated with the cardiovascular system. Magnetic nanosensors monitor blood flow and signs of arterial plaques, whereas mechanical nanosensors track blood pressure and heart rate in patients, assessing the risk of atherosclerosis and heart attacks (Tang *et al* 2022).
- *Neurological monitoring*: Nanosensors serve as safeguards against various neurological disorders by measuring brain activity and neurotransmitter levels. For example, optical nanosensors can provide vital information for the treatment of neurological disorders such as epilepsy and Parkinson's disease (Liu *et al* 2020).

### 9.3.3 Target-specific drug delivery

Drug delivery is a crucial factor deciding the efficacy and success of any particular treatment plan. Target-specific drug delivery enhances the therapeutic effects of drugs many-fold, eliminating any side-effects or contraindications of that drug in human body. Nanosensors also play a pivotal role in enhancing the efficiency of drugs by aiding target specific delivery within the body in response to specific physiological conditions. Some examples of nanosensors in target-specific drug delivery are as follows:

- *Chemotherapy*: Target-specific drug delivery is crucial in cancer treatment where preserving the non-cancer tissues is as important as the eradication of the tumor. Nanosensors enhance the targeting of chemotherapeutic agents, ensuring that medications are activated only upon reaching a tumor site, thus minimizing the side effects. pH-sensitive nanoparticles release the anti-cancer drug only after identifying the acidic environment of tumor tissues (Salvati *et al* 2015).
- *Immunotherapy*: Nanosensors improve the outcomes of treatment against autoimmune diseases and allergies by ensuring precise delivery of

immunomodulatory agents. This reduces the risk of adverse effects of these treatments in healthy regions of the body (Nguyen-Le *et al* 2022).

- *Smart pills*: 'Smart pills' are innovative nanosensors that are ingested by patients. They track gut health and release medication at the best sites of the gastrointestinal system. This is especially helpful for conditions such as ulcerative colitis and Crohn's disease that need specialized care (Senturk *et al* 2022).

All these applications of nanosensors in biomedical systems have revolutionized the healthcare system and mitigated the challenges of various deadly diseases by improving the accuracy and efficiency of medical treatments, along with minimally-invasive to non-invasive diagnostics and customized therapy regimens specific to the needs of individual patients. Nanosensors are paving the way for a new era of advanced, patient-centric healthcare, reducing the social and economical burden of various diseases.

## 9.4 Challenges and limitations

There are various challenges in the path of nanosensor based medical systems, with several limitations that are required to be addressed in order to achieve the maximum potential of this remarkable tool of nanotechnology. These obstacles range from technical and material complexities to ethical and regulatory concerns in terms of the manufacturing and usage of various nanosensors (Kulkarni *et al* 2022). This section delves into major challenges associated with nanosensors, providing information of these hurdles that are required to be overcome.

### 9.4.1 Biocompatibility and toxicity

Biocompatibility is the ability of a material to interact with a specific host, providing an appropriate biological response and not causing any adverse reactions when introduced into the body. It is one of the most important prerequisites when developing any nanosensors for biomedical usage. Nanosensors that aim to serve in healthcare are essentially required to be safe, non-toxic, and non-carcinogenic with no adverse effect on the immune system. Nanosensors must not release any harmful by-products during their interaction or degradation in the body (Perdomo *et al* 2021). The following factors are important to create biocompatible and non-toxic nanosensors:

- *Material safety*: The choice of material to create nanosensors plays crucial role in maintaining the non-toxic nature of these devices as nanosensors made of heavy metals such as cadmium, zinc, etc, can cause toxicity with prolonged exposure or high concentrations in the body.
- *Immunogenicity*: The human body detects foreign material, thus triggering an immune response, which can cause inflammation and other harmful reactions hampering the medicinal benefits of these nanosensors. Therefore it is important to design nanosensors that cannot be recognized by the immune system as a threat to avoid by adverse immunoreactions.

- *Degradation products*: Anything that enters human body is metabolized and bioassimilated, leading to complete breakdown before excretion from the body. Nanosensors are to be designed while considering that the by-products of the breakdown process must not be toxic. All the components of nano-sensors should be biocompatible throughout their lifecycle.

### 9.4.2 Manufacturing challenges

Once the biocompatibility and non-toxicity of the nanosensors is established, keeping all the important factors in consideration, the next challenge is the large scale production of these nanosensors. Their manufacture involves various complex fabrication techniques and is required to be handled carefully for the production of identical nanosensors in terms of composition and functionality. The production methods should also be cost-effective and scalable to compete well with the alternatives available in the biomedical industry (Kulkarni *et al* 2022, Singh *et al* 2022). The following points need to be focused on during the mass production of nanosensors:

- *Scalability*: The techniques used to develop the initial prototype of nano-sensors in research using a large laboratory set-up with various resources are generally expensive with a small output. The same methods cannot be considered for the large scale production of nanosensors.
- *Quality control*: Uniformity of production and high quality standards are essential during the manufacturing of nanosensors. Any malfunctioning or defect in these sensors can cause significant discrepancies in sensor perform-ance, thus impacting its medical benefits.
- *Integration and packaging*: After successful production of premium nano-sensors, the next crucial step is their compact biocompatible packaging that can shield the delicate components of nanosensors from the complex and dynamic environment of the body without interfering in their interaction with the target analytes.

### 9.4.3 Accuracy and reliability

It is important to ensure the accuracy and reliability of nanosensors due to their vital role in medical decision-making. The sensors must have consistency in their outputs with uniform precision throughout the biological system (Javaid *et al* 2021). The following factors are to be kept in consideration to ensure the accuracy and reliability of nanosensors:

- *Signal interference*: The biological fluids in the human body are composed of a complex mixture of substances that can interfere with the accuracy of nanosensors in terms of pH or other biomarkers.
- *Calibration*: Nanosensors require regular recalibration to maintain the uni-formity and precision of outputs. It is difficult to recalibrate them once they are inside the body of a patient.

- *Drift*: The accuracy and output response can change over time due to changes in the material of the nanosensors or variations in the biological system, leading to the inefficient functioning of these sensors.

### 9.4.4 Regulatory and ethical issues

Ethical and regulatory issues arise simultaneously with the emergence of any new medical technology or treatment option to ensure the quality, safety, privacy, equity and societal impact of these innovations. Nanosensors, as novel tools in the biomedical industry, undergo such scrutiny to fulfill all the following factors before introducing them to the public (Maria *et al* 2019):

- *Regulatory approval*: To gain approval from esteemed regulatory bodies such as Food and Drug Administration (FDA) is essential. It is a laborious and time-consuming process that requires documentation substantiating the safety and efficacy of nanosensors along with lengthy clinical trials.
- *Privacy concerns*: Nanosensors are designed to continuously monitor and collect data from patients. It is important to handle the personal information of patients with confidentiality and to follow data protection laws to avoid the potential misuse of collected data.
- *Informed consent*: Ethical considerations mandate that patients should be completely aware of both the advantages and disadvantages along with potential risks associated with the use of nanosensors.

### 9.4.5 Market and economic factors

The development and dispersal of nanosensors for public usage in healthcare is also crucially dependent on the economy as well as market dynamics. The following factors can both support or hinder the promotion of nanosensors in the biomedical industry (Perdomo *et al* 2021):

- *Cost*: The difference in the economy of various regions can hinder the production and utilization of these nanosensors limiting their medical benefits. Therefore it is important to make them cost-effective and accessible to the mass population.
- *Reimbursement*: Due to the novel nature of nanosensors in the field of medicine they do not fit in the classical definition and policies of healthcare reimbursement systems. Such policies must evolve to cover innovative technologies to provide benefits to the patients.
- *Market acceptance*: For nanosensors to be successfully introduced and employed into healthcare plans, they must be accepted by medical practitioners along with the regulatory bodies and patients.

To summarize, there are various challenges to overcome before global acceptance and implementation of nanosensors, with their numerous applications for developing medical research and enhancing patient care with further advancements in biomedicine. The following sections will dive into the recent developments and potential paths for the field, emphasizing the continuous efforts to attain their full potential in healthcare.

## 9.5 Current advancements and future prospects

Nanosensors are evolving continuously with better approaches toward medical problems with collective development in the field of nanotechnology, material science as well as digital technology. These changes help in enhancement of all the existing features of nanosensors with the addition of new innovations improving treatment methods and healthcare as a whole. In this section the aim is to explore current developments in the field of nanosensor technology, some recent break-throughs and advancements, and potential future developments that can overcome all the limitations with enhanced performance of these sensors.

### 9.5.1 Recent technological advancements

In the past few years nanosensor technology has seen some remarkable innovations with enhanced features and functionalities improving and expanding the application of these tools in the biomedical industry. These advancements include improved sensitivity and specificity, and faster and better output with the incorporation of better materials, technology and overall features. All these changes in nanosensors improved the diagnosis, monitoring and treatment sector in medicine (Perdomo *et al* 2021). The following are the important factors adding to the major advancements in nanosensors technology:

- *Material innovations*: As the materials of nanosensors play a crucial role in its performance and durability, various new nanomaterials have been developed in the past few years, including graphene, carbon nanotubes, and quantum dots. These new materials have considerably overcome the limitations associated with the functioning of nanosensors with major enhancement in their electrical, optical, and mechanical properties. One such recent advance-ment is graphene-based sensors with exceptional sensitivity to the target analyte and high stability in biological systems that allows the detection of biomarkers in trace amounts at the early disease stages, helping patients and saving lives.
- *Integration with digital technology*: Over the years, digital technology has become an integral part of human life. Researchers have combined this digital advancement with nanosensors by connecting these sensors with smartphones and the Internet of Things (IoT). This integration has revolutionized the monitoring aspect of nanosensors with real-time data collection and analysis. This has helped tremendously in the timely management of diseases with proper treatment execution.
- *Multiplexing capability*: There have been several improvements in the specificity and action of nanosensors through advancements in multiplexing capabilities to identify and act on multiple target analytes at once, thus improving the functioning of these sensors, particularly benefiting the monitoring, detection and treatment of complex diseases such as cancer,

where multiple biomarkers need to be evaluated to understand the disease progression and response to treatment.

### 9.5.2 Enhancements in manufacturing and scalability

Considerable progress has been made in addressing the problem of scaling up the production of nanosensors while maintaining their functionality and consistency. Technological advancements in manufacturing are propelling this field's affordability and accessibility. The use of 3D printing, which makes precise and adaptable sensor designs suited to particular biomedical applications possible, is one noteworthy strategy. Furthermore, the fabrication of flexible, wearable nanosensors is becoming more efficient thanks to the adoption of roll-to-roll production, which was adopted from the electronics sector. This is resulting in lower costs and higher production rates. Furthermore, by enabling the automatic assembly of molecular components into functional structures, self-assembly techniques are streamlining the production of nanosensors. These developments highlight the ways in which nanosensors have become more widely available and reasonably priced, which has led to their increasing use in biomedicine (Yang and Duncan 2021).

### 9.5.3 Challenges in clinical integration

Even with these significant advancements, there are still a number of issues that need to be resolved before nanosensors can be safely and effectively used in clinical settings. The most important of these challenges is the need to deal with safety and biocompatibility concerns. In order to ensure acceptance in medical applications, it is imperative that the potential long-term effects of nanomaterials within the body be thoroughly studied in order to reduce any potential risks of toxicity or adverse immune reactions. Moreover, because the technologies involved are complex and innovative, overcoming regulatory barriers is a difficult challenge. Facilitating the market entry of these innovative solutions and expediting the approval process require clear and streamlined regulatory pathways. Furthermore, the protection of data security and privacy becomes imperative, especially in light of the widespread acquisition of private medical data by nanosensors. Ensuring the confidentiality and integrity of sensitive medical information is crucial for fostering trust between patients and healthcare providers. This can be achieved by implementing strict protocols and strong encryption techniques. Realizing the full potential of nanosensors to improve healthcare delivery while maintaining safety and privacy standards requires tackling these issues in their entirety (Javaid *et al* 2021).

### 9.5.4 Future prospects and emerging trends

Given the number of new developments that are anticipated to spur additional innovation and market expansion, the future of nanosensors in biomedicine appears bright. The idea of personalized medicine is at the forefront, and nanosensors are essential to adjusting medical care to each patient's unique genetic profile and set of medical conditions. Future research will concentrate on developing sensors that can adjust to the specific requirements of each patient, allowing for more personalized treatment plans. The fusion of artificial intelligence (AI) and nanosensors is another noteworthy development, enhancing data analysis capacities for improved predictive analytics and diagnostics. By using AI algorithms to decipher complex data streams from nanosensors, medical practitioners can more precisely anticipate the course of diseases and tailor their treatments accordingly. Furthermore, as sustainability becomes more popular, research efforts are being directed towards creating environmentally friendly nanosensors. In line with international sustainability goals, the objective is to develop biodegradable sensor materials that lessen their negative effects on the environment without sacrificing functionality. Theranostics, an emerging field that combines diagnostic and therapeutic functions into a single platform, is also gaining momentum. Because they can simultaneously diagnose diseases and deliver precise therapies at the molecular level, nanosensors are well suited for theranostic applications. All things considered, these new developments highlight how much more can be done with nanosensors to improve healthcare and open the door to future treatments that are more effective, efficient, and long-lasting (Gupta and Basu 2022).

### 9.5.5 Vision for the future

Nanosensors have promising features to completely transform healthcare systems at the molecular level in the field of biomedicine. These sensors provide a vision of early disease detection and diagnosis using nanoscale biomarker changes, crucially in conditions such as cancer, diabetes, and neurodegenerative disorders, which is difficult with current medical technology. Real-time monitoring and output of data through these sensors by integration of wearable nanosensors with digital technology could provide 24-7 observation of patients to provide proactive treatment in a customized manner. Therefore successful advancements in the field of nanosensor technology with more integrated, efficient, and patient-friendly healthcare solutions can be predicted in the near future. The convergence of nanotechnology with biotechnology, information technology, and cognitive sciences holds the potential to change the treatment system with enhanced disease management. Continued research and collaboration across disciplines are vital to overcome existing challenges and to fully harness the potential of nanosensors in enhancing health outcomes. The next decade could see nanosensors becoming ubiquitous in clinical practices and everyday health management (Kaushik *et al* 2022).

## 9.6 Conclusion

Scientific fields, including biomedicine in particular, have been revolutionized by the advancements in nanotechnology and development of nanosensors. These powerful and versatile nanotools have sparked a new era of medical science with improved diagnosis and treatment systems benefitting mankind against a large number of deadly diseases. This chapter explored nanosensors in detail, starting from the fundamental structure and working principle, variants of nanosensors, and their diverse uses in biomedicine, emphasizing on their critical functions in healthcare of providing remarkable detection tools to monitor the vital physiological parameters and biomarkers present in the human body. There are several types of nanosensors, such as mechanical, optical, and electrochemical sensors, each designed to serve a particular medical application with utmost accuracy and precision.

Among the major applications of nanosensors in the biomedical industry, the primary uses are in the fields of disease detection and diagnosis, where nanosensors have demonstrated exceptional efficacy in the early detection of diseases, thereby improving treatment strategies and outcomes. Moreover, nanosensors provide real-time data acquisition in the monitoring of physiological indicators, such as glucose levels in diabetes or neurotransmitter fluctuations in neurological conditions, helping in the management of chronic diseases. Nanosensors have also made a significant contribution in drug delivery systems, allowing and improving the target therapies that improve treatment efficacy while reducing side effects. All these applications of nanosensors highlight the versatility and adaptability of these nanotools to cater to various clinical needs, suggesting a future of biomedicine with nanosensors in all fields of healthcare.

The introduction of nanosensors into medical systems has progressed the treatment approach toward preventive, precise, and personalized care. Additionally, the integration of nanosensors promises lower healthcare costs and affordable treatment options by reducing overly extensive interventions and optimizing resource allocation with the early detection of diseases and customized treatment plans as per the patient's needs.

However, there is huge scope of improvement and advancement in nanosensor technology. For the seamless integration of nanosensors in routine medical practice, careful consideration of challenges such as biocompatibility, data privacy, and ethical considerations are required, although the enormous possibilities in biomedicine with these nanosensors outweigh the associated hurdles and limitations.

Therefore nanosensors should be credited with a revolution in healthcare with their unparalleled sensitivity, specificity, and adaptability. These sensors have the potential to completely transform the medical field further and make healthcare affordable and effective. Nanosensors will obviously continue to play a significant role in influencing the direction of biomedicine, improving patient care, and improving health outcomes all around the world as research advances and new innovations arise.

## References

Agrawal S and Prajapati R 2012 Nanosensors and their pharmaceutical applications: a review *Int. J. Pharm. Sci. Technol.* **4** 1528–35

Anjum S, Ishaque S, Fatima H, Farooq W, Hano C, Abbasi B H and Anjum I 2021 Emerging applications of nanotechnology in healthcare systems: grand challenges and perspectives *Pharmaceuticals* **14** 707

Barry S and O'Riordan A 2016 Electrochemical nanosensors: advances and applications *Rep. Electrochem.* **2016** 1–14

Ching R C M and Lim T C 2014 Mechanical nanosensors ed D Li *Encyclopedia of Microfluidics and Nanofluidics* (Boston, MA: Springer)

Cicek S and Nadaroglu H 2015 The use of nanotechnology in the agriculture *Adv. Nano Res.* **3** 207

Debnath N and Das S 2020 Nanobiosensor: current trends and applications *Nanobiomedicine* ed S Saxena and S Khurana (Springer: Singapore) pp 389–409

Deng J, Zhao S, Liu Y, Liu C and Sun J 2020 Nanosensors for diagnosis of infectious diseases *ACS Appl. Bio Mater.* **4** 3863–79

Doswald S, Stark W J and Beck-Schimmer B 2019 Biochemical functionality of magnetic particles as nanosensors: how far away are we to implement them into clinical practice? *J. Nanobiotechnol.* **17** 73

Falzarano M S, Flesia C, Cavalli R, Guiot C and Ferlini A 2018 Nanodiagnostics and nanodelivery applications in genetic alterations *Curr. Pharm. Design* **24** 1717–26

Farmani A, Soroosh M, Mozaffari M H and Daghooghi T 2020 Optical nanosensors for cancer and virus detections *Nanosensors for Smart Cities* (Amsterdam: Elsevier) pp 419–32

Gupta S L and Basu S 2022 Smart nanosensors in healthcare recent developments and applications *Nanosensors for Futuristic Smart and Intelligent Healthcare Systems* (Boca Raton, FL: CRC Press) pp 3–18

Javaid M, Haleem A, Singh R P, Rab S and Suman R 2021 Exploring the potential of nanosensors: a brief overview *Sens. Int.* **2** 100130

Jeevanandam J and Danquah M K 2020 Nanosensors for better diagnosis of health *Nanofabrication for Smart Nanosensor Applications* (Amsterdam: Elsevier) pp 187–228

Kaushik S, Soni V and Skotti E (ed) 2022 *Nanosensors for Futuristic Smart and Intelligent Healthcare Systems* (Boca Raton, FL: CRC Press)

Khazaei M, Hosseini M S, Haghighi A M and Misaghi M 2023 Nanosensors and their applications in early diagnosis of cancer *Sens. Bio-Sens. Res.* **41** 100569

Kulkarni M B, Ayachit N H and Aminabhavi T M 2022 Recent advancements in nanobiosensors: current trends, challenges, applications, and future scope *Biosensors* **12** 892

Liu J *et al* 2020 A sensitive and specific nanosensor for monitoring extracellular potassium levels in the brain *Nat. Nanotechnol.* **15** 321–30

Maria L, Moses J A and Anandharamakrishnan C 2019 Ethical and regulatory issues in applications of nanotechnology in food *Food Nanotechnology* (Boca Raton, FL: CRC Press) pp 67–92

Mishra R K and Rajakumari R 2019 Nanobiosensors for biomedical application: present and future prospects *Characterization and Biology of Nanomaterials for Drug Delivery* (Amsterdam: Elsevier) pp 1–23

Nasrollahzadeh M, Sajadi S M, Sajjadi M and Issaabadi Z 2019 An introduction to nanotechnology *Interface Science and Technology* **vol 28** (Amsterdam: Elsevier) pp 1–27

Nguyen-Le T A *et al* 2022 Nanosensors in clinical development of CAR-T cell immunotherapy *Biosens. Bioelectron.* **206** 114124

Pathak K, Saikia R, Sarma H, Pathak M P, Das R J, Gogoi U, Ahmad M Z, Das A and Wahab B A A 2023 Nanotheranostics: application of nanosensors in diabetes management *J. Diabetes Metab. Disorders* **22** 119–33

Perdomo S A, Marmolejo-Tejada J M and Jaramillo-Botero A 2021 Bio-nanosensors: fundamentals and recent applications *J. Electrochem. Soc.* **168** 107506

Salvati E, Stellacci F and Krol S 2015 Nanosensors for early cancer detection and for therapeutic drug monitoring *Nanomedicine* **10** 3495–512

Senturk S, Kok I and Senturk F 2022 Internet of nano, bio-nano, biodegradable and ingestible things: a survey arXiv: 2202.12409

Singh S, Kumar A, Behura S K and Verma K 2022 Challenges and opportunities in nano-manufacturing *Nanomanufacturing and Nanomaterials Design* (Boca Raton, FL: CRC Press) pp 17–30

Splinter R 2018 The physics of nanosensor systems in medicine and the development of physiological monitoring equipment *Computational Approaches in Biomedical Nano-Engineering* (Hoboken, NJ: Wiley) pp 89–111

Tang X, Zhu Y, Guan W, Zhou W and Wei P 2022 Advances in nanosensors for cardiovascular disease detection *Life Sci.* **305** 120733

Yang T and Duncan T V 2021 Challenges and potential solutions for nanosensors intended for use with foods *Nat. Nanotechnol.* **16** 251–65

Zielińska A *et al* 2020 Nanotoxicology and nanosafety: safety-by-design and testing at a glance *Int. J. Environ. Res. Public Health* **17** 4657

# Chapter 10

## Paper-based point of care diagnostic systems for cancer

**Neha Sharma, Khushboo Joshi, Raghvendra Kumar Mishra, Sharmistha Banerjee and Shuchi Kaushik**

Cancer is one of the leading causes of death worldwide because of the fast proliferation of cancer cells and lack of timely detection systems. There is thus a requirement for early and easy detection of cancer progression at an initial stage. Early and minimal invasive detection can not only reduce cancer mortality rates but also helps in reducing healthcare costs and improving the patient's condition. A paper-based point-of-care (PoC) system is a portable device used for the analysis and detection of disease outside a traditional laboratory and can provide early and rapid diagnosis of patients. Paper-based PoC devices are a new approach and necessity for the detection of biomarkers and infectious agents. Numerous remarkable characteristics of paper, such as cost-effectiveness, easy availability, simplicity, ease of use, portability, disposability, ecofriendliness and easy storage, make it a strong candidate for PoC devices. Paper-based analytical devices have been used widely in various fields such as biomedicine (e.g. cancer diagnosis, pregnancy test kits, urine analysis), environmental remediation, and food quality testing. The use of a paper-based device does not require expensive instruments, special procedures, or trained medical staff. This chapter will focus on different PoC paper-based diagnostic systems that are used for the detection of cancer biomarkers (such as proteins, nucleic acids, exosomes, and secondary metabolites). These may reduce the current challenges in the diagnosis of different cancers and give future prospects for the safe and easy detection of multiple cancers or enhance the sensitivity of specific cancer detection. The associated advantages and challenges are summarized.

## 10.1 Introduction

Unhealthy lifestyles and the changing environment because of industrialization and urbanization pose a significant global public health challenge in which cancer is second most common cause of death globally (Siegel *et al* 2019, Alba *et al* 2020). Cancer arises from a combination of mutations and environmental factors leading to uncontrolled cell growth and the formation of abnormal masses known as tumors. These tumors can grow further by creating new blood vessels and can metastasize, spreading to other parts of the body. The primary global challenge lies in early detection and effective treatment. Various imaging techniques such as mammography, magnetic resonance imaging (MRI), computed tomography (CT) scans, x-rays, ultrasound, and mass spectroscopy, along with biomarker detection, are used for cancer diagnosis (Shankaran *et al* 2018). Biomarkers are molecules that are expressed in normal as well as diseased cells, and encompass a wide range of substances, including genes, DNA, RNA, microRNA (miRNA), proteins, enzymes, lipids, exosomes, and secondary metabolites. These molecules serve various roles in the body, such as storage of genetic information, biological activity regulation, and substance transportation, and can be found in normal and tumor tissues, and bodily fluids such as blood, urine, and oral fluid (Tothill *et al* 2015, Mahmoudi *et al* 2020).

Biosensors are specialized devices comprising two essential components: a recognition element or bioreceptor, such as enzymes or antibodies, which identifies a specific target, and a transducer, such as optical or electrochemical components, which converts this identification into a measurable signal (Tothill *et al* 2015). These biosensors possess the capability to detect and identify individual biomarkers or groups of biomarkers accurately, even in minute quantities. Consequently, researchers are focusing on developing biosensor techniques for various applications, particularly in cancer detection, with an emphasis on their potential deployment in point of care (PoC) settings outside traditional laboratory environments.

Figure 10.1 shows the different types of samples and biomarkers, the types of papers used in PoC testing, the binding or recognition elements, the different types of nanoparticles (NPs), and the detectors used for signal detection.

Different types of materials are absorbed by paper to make it a portable paper-based device. When samples such as blood or urine are allowed to interact with recognition elements, signals are generated which in turn are detected by various detectors. Paper, being a versatile material (Ratajczak *et al* 2020, Suntornsuk *et al* 2020), serves as the foundation for devices such as flow assays and microfluidic paper-based analytical devices (µPADs), facilitating the movement of samples through various channels on the paper. Materials such as filter paper, nitrocellulose (NC), or other porous substances with suitable properties are utilized in constructing these devices. Capillary action propels fluid through the porous paper, orchestrating all the processes on the device, thereby enabling individuals to obtain test results without requiring advanced skills or additional equipment (Mahmoudi *et al* 2020, Chauhan *et al* 2023). Paper serves as an excellent platform for both chemical and biological analysis. The pores of cellulose paper facilitate the immobilization of reagents and subsequent drying, making it suitable for the development of various devices. The hydrophilic nature of paper, combined with the capillary pressure induced by liquids within cellulose fibers, avoids the need for pumps to transport fluids. As a result, paper-based analytical devices (PADs) function effectively in the form of lateral flow assays (LFAs) and spot tests without requiring external power

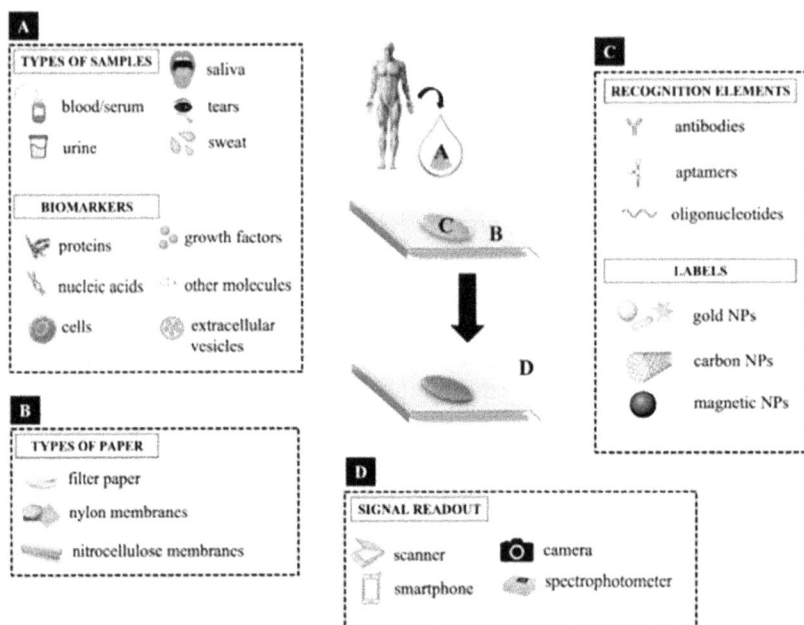

**Figure 10.1.** (A) Types of samples and biomarkers, (B) types of paper, (C) recognition elements and labels, and (D) signal readouts used in paper-based sensors (Reproduced from Carneiro *et al* (2022). CC BY 4.0.).

sources (Carrell *et al* 2019, Kasetsirikul *et al* 2020). Optical and electrochemical methods are commonly employed in tandem with PADs to detect various substances (Liu *et al* 2019). Furthermore, the integration of smartphones, operating systems, and wireless connectivity enables real-time analysis (Aydindogan *et al* 2020).

Consequently, incorporating nanoparticles made from diverse materials into PADs enhances sensitivity, and these particles can be easily tailored with biorecognition elements to ensure specificity. PADs are user-friendly as they require minimal invasive samples and provide easily interpretable results, eliminating the need for specialized personnel or sophisticated equipment. The swift response of PADs is facilitated by cellulose properties such as porosity and capillary forces, expediting the assay process. Additionally, the components of PADs contribute to their resilience. Lastly, the deliverability of these devices enables patients to conduct self-testing at home, eliminating the need for hospital visits (Kasetsirikul *et al* 2020, Mahmoudi *et al* 2020, Suntornsuk *et al* 2020).

## 10.2 Types of paper-based analytical devices

Various types of paper are utilized in the fabrication of PADs depending on the sensor's construction and its intended application. The most commonly used paper is Whatman® paper and NC paper because of their pore size and effective retention capabilities. NC membranes, which feature a smooth surface and a pore size of 0.45 $\mu$M, find widespread use in LFAs. Their versatility allows for modification with biomolecules and efficient substance retention. Additionally, bioactive paper, modified with biomolecules, nylon membranes, and common papers such as printing paper and paper towels, serves as a viable options for PAD fabrication (Singh *et al* 2018).

In certain scenarios, bacterial cellulose based nanopaper is employed due to its flexibility and remarkable optical transparency (Ratajczak *et al* 2020). Various types of PADs have been developed for clinical diagnosis and monitoring purposes, including spot tests, LFAs, μPADs, and dipsticks. The details of these assays are discussed in the following sections.

### 10.2.1 Spot tests

Spot tests are based on chemical reactions that result in the production of any distinctive generally colored product, either in the form of a spot on white paper, or in a droplet on a spot plate. (Spinola *et al* 1995). The most quick and affordable devices are spot tests and were used initially around 1940s for detecting the presence of metal ions through colorimetric ligands (West *et al* 1945). This has laid the foundation for the creation of other on-site analysis devices.

Spot tests are often used in many areas such as quality control, in food and pharmaceutical analysis, environmental and water analysis, metal and mineral analysis, conservation and restoration of cultural heritage, forensic sciences, and screening tests in clinical analysis (Jungreis 1996).

### 10.2.2 Flow assays

Flow assays have gained significant importance in the detection of various analytes in complex samples within a short period. They have been categorized into two main types, i.e. LFAs and vertical flow assays (VFAs) depending on the directionality of the flow of the sample due to the capillary mode of action

#### 10.2.2.1 Lateral flow assays

A typical LFA designed to detect a single biomarker consists of four primary components: a sample pad, conjugate pad, reaction membrane, and adsorbent pad, as outlined by Kasetsirikul *et al* (2020). Positioned sequentially with some overlap, these pads facilitate the flow of the liquid sample through the device. The sample pad receives the liquid sample, pre-loaded with necessary compounds, while the conjugate pad contains capture-ligand-conjugated nanoparticles that bind to the analyte as the sample progresses. The reaction membrane features two parallel lines: a test line with biomarker-specific detection ligands and a control line capturing nanoparticles. The adsorbent pad collects liquid, aiding in sample flow through the device. Encased within a cassette, these components enable ease of use (Koczula *et al* 2016, Liu *et al* 2019) (figure 10.2).

There are two primary formats of LFAs: sandwich LFAs (sLFAs) and competitive LFAs (cLFAs). The sLFA is effective for detecting high-weight molecular compounds and involves two distinct recognition steps to enhance specificity and sensitivity. Initially, the analyte is captured by a primary antibody on the conjugate pad, forming a complex that is subsequently captured by a transducer, often a

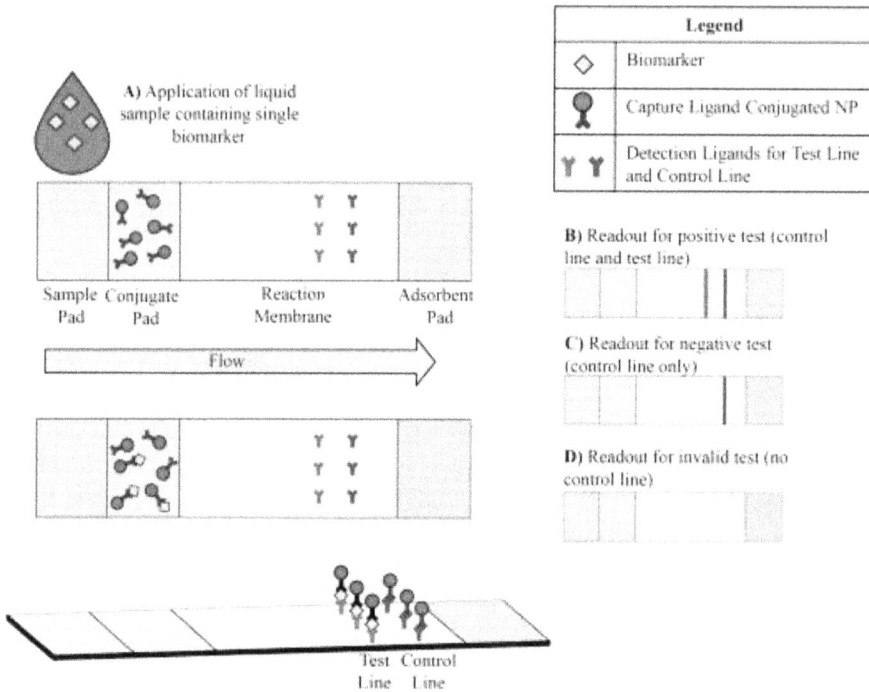

**Figure 10.2.** A diagram illustrating a prevalent sandwich format LFA set-up and its utilization for the detection of a single biomarker (Yonet *et al* 2021. John Wiley & Sons. © 2021 Wiley-VCH GmbH.).

colorimetric probe, immobilized with a secondary antibody at the test line. Higher concentrations of the target result in a more intense positive signal at the test line. On the other hand, cLFA is preferred for detecting small molecules with single antigenic determinants. In this set-up, the analyte competes with and obstructs test line binding sites, leading to a decrease in signal intensity with higher target concentrations (Hu *et al* 2014, Shankaran *et al* 2018).

Regarding biorecognition elements, LFAs are classified into lateral flow immunoassays (LFIA), which commonly utilize labeled antibodies coupled with colorimetric or fluorescent readouts, and aptamer-based LFAs that employ aptamers for target recognition. Colloidal gold nanoparticles (AuNPs) are frequently employed as colorimetric probes in LFAs due to their unique optical properties and ease of functionalization for target recognition (Kasetsirikul *et al* 2020, Ratajczak *et al* 2020). Multiplex LFAs which utilize a multi-test line format have been explored for detecting biomarkers associated with various cancer types. Li and colleagues introduced a multiplex LFA using fluorescent latex beads to detect two gastric cancer biomarkers, pepsinogen I (PG I) and pepsinogen II (PG II). Two test lines, one for each biomarker, were printed on the reaction membrane, enabling simultaneous detection.

LFAs are NC strips assembled in a plastic (e.g. polyvinyl chloride) carrier card, which contain different parts such as the sample pad, conjugate pad, flowing membrane or test pad, and adsorbent pad (Lim *et al* 2017, Liu *et al* 2019, Mahmoudi *et al* 2020, Kasetsirikul *et al* 2020, Yu *et al* 2020). The sample and adsorbent pads are generally made of cellulose paper or glass fibers, while the flowing membrane is usually an NC membrane and the conjugate pad is commonly made of glass fibers (Mahmoudi *et al* 2020). The pads are placed adjacently in order to provide a continuous lateral flow of the solutions once they are added to the sample pad (Yu *et al* 2020).

The sample pad facilitates proper interaction of an analyte of interest with the molecules present on the conjugate pad and the NC membrane. The conjugate pad contains immobilized analyte-specific antibodies bound to colored or fluorescent particles and subsequently allows the release of conjugated molecules toward the test pad. The test line depicts the interaction through color change, which can be correlated to the concentration of the target analytes whereas the control line depicts the positive capillary flow of the sample. The absorbent pad helps in maintaining the rate of capillary action and prevents sample backflow (Bhardwaj *et al* 2024).

### *10.2.2.2 Vertical flow assay*

The VFA follows the same principle as the LFA but differs in the direction of the flow of the sample, which is applied vertically in the presence of an external force (Jiang *et al* 2019). Unlike LFAs, VFAs can minimize concentration associated agglutination (Hooke's effect) of the analytes, e.g. antibodies and cross-reactivity issues associated with multiplexed detection of analytes (Jiang *et al* 2019, Jiao *et al* 2020).

### 10.2.3 Microfluidic paper-based analytical devices

The concept of $\mu$PADs originated in 2007, emerging from Whiteside's lab, for colorimetric glucose detection in urine using photolithography (Martinez *et al* 2007). $\mu$PADs have found applications across various fields, including medical diagnostics, environmental monitoring, food safety, and forensic analysis. Unlike LFAs and spot tests, $\mu$PADs allow sample flow through hydrophilic channels, enabling multiplex detection (Lim *et al* 2017). Two-dimensional (2D) $\mu$PADs create channels via hydrophobic barriers using techniques such as photolithography, wax printing, screen-printing, inkjet printing, and plasma oxidation. In contrast, three-dimensional (3D) $\mu$PADs involve layering patterned paper (Liu *et al* 2019). Whatman® filter paper No.1 is commonly selected for its consistent thickness and wicking properties. Requiring minimal fluid (5–10 $\mu$l), $\mu$PADs provide rapid responses compared to laboratory techniques, offering advantages such as miniaturization, disposability, multiplex analysis, and on-site capability, particularly beneficial for resource-limited regions (Ozer *et al* 2020, Alahmad *et al* 2021) (figure 10.3).

### 10.2.4 Dipsticks

A dipstick, a simplified version of a PAD, involves a paper strip infused with reagents that undergo color changes when exposed to the analyte, yielding a qualitative response (Hu *et al* 2014). The initial dipstick, developed in 1956, aimed

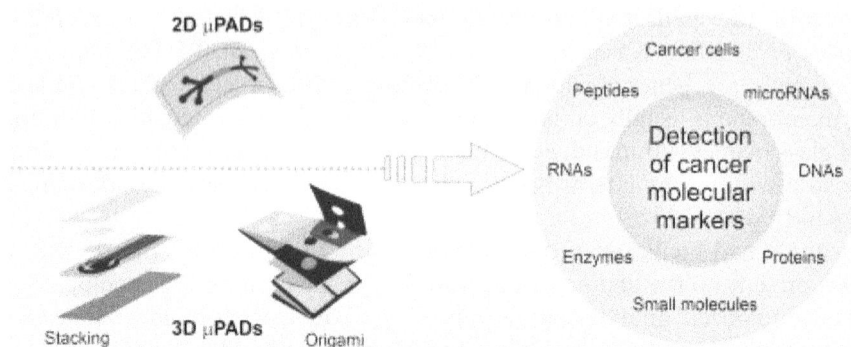

**Figure 10.3.** A diagram illustrating PADs used for quantitative sensing of oncomarkers as 2D and 3D devices (Reprinted from Ebrahimi *et al* (2023), Copyright (2023), with permission from Elsevier.).

to quantify glucose in urine. Dipsticks are easy to manufacture, providing results easily interpreted by the naked eye. However, they exhibit drawbacks such as low accuracy, extended analysis time, and offering only a qualitative response (Singh *et al* 2018). Common examples include pH strips or urine test strips, simultaneously screening for various conditions such as diabetes and kidney disease. This approach can potentially be used in cancer detection with the help of biorecognition elements (Kuswandi *et al* 2019).

## 10.3 Detection mechanisms of cancer biomarkers

Analysing molecular biomarkers using biosensor platforms provides early diagnosis and monitoring of pathological conditions, especially cancer disease, and may significantly improve prognosis and survival rates, thereby reducing the disease burden and helping social development and expanding access to healthcare for people all over the world. Possible disease biomarkers include a wide range of DNA and biomolecules that can be detected by a variety of biosensor detection techniques (Meyer *et al* 2007, Gopinath *et al* 2015, Murillo *et al* 2019, Zhang *et al* 2019).

Recognition elements such as antibodies (Abs), aptamers, or specific ligands are affixed to the surface of the paper. These elements exhibit high affinity and selectivity for the targeted cancer biomarkers. The sample containing the suspected cancer biomarkers is administered onto the PAD. The sample engages with the immobilized recognition elements through interactions such as antigen–antibody or ligand–receptor interactions. The interaction between the recognition elements and the target biomarkers induces a discernible color change. This transformation can arise from enzymatic reactions, alterations in pH, or other chemical processes that generate visible chromogenic reactions. Visual assessment involves comparing the PAD's appearance before and after the reaction to observe the color change. Alternatively, quantification of color intensity or hue can be accomplished using a straightforward handheld device or smartphone app for more objective measurements (Wei *et al* 2022).

The selection of recognition elements depends on the target to be detected. Abs and aptamers are the most common receptors used in the development of PADs for cancer biomarker detection. The immobilization of the receptors should take place on the paper surface either by physical or chemical methods. For immobilization of receptors as Abs on tags, adsorption techniques or covalent binding are usually employed.

### 10.3.1 Colorimetric detection

Paper-based colorimetric biosensors use paper as a substrate, and are ideal for field use because they are easy to use and require a minimal amount of sample (Cheng *et al* 2019).

Colorimetric assays detect the absence or presence and respective concentration of the analyte of interest through the evaluation of color production or color change. This production or change of color could be induced by dyes, enzymes or NPs such as AuNPs (Singh *et al* 2018). Colorimetric assays evaluate the absorbance or reflectance intensity changes due to chemical or biochemical reactions between the target and chromogenic substances used as probes. Absorbed or reflected light intensity generally results from optical property changes due to SPR or structural shifts (Aydindogan *et al* 2020, Suntornsuk *et al* 2020). This is one of the most common detection techniques used in PADs as it enables a simple, cost-effective, real-time, and on-site detection of several molecules (Shende *et al* 2019). In addition, paper provides a bright background with high contrast over color development (Agarwal *et al* 2019). Additionally, the samples to be analysed using colorimetric PADs can be obtained by invasive collection, such as blood, serum, or synovial fluid, or by the minimally invasive or non-invasive methods, such as tears, saliva, urine, or sweat (Shende *et al* 2019).

Colorimetric detection in PADs for cancer diagnosis relies on color alterations that occur upon specific interactions between the target cancer biomarkers and immobilized recognition elements. This method is particularly advantageous for PoC applications due to its simplicity, cost-effectiveness, and straightforward interpretation. The foundational principle of colorimetric detection centers on the alteration of color, readily visible to the naked eye, as a consequence of the binding interaction between the target cancer biomarkers and the recognition elements immobilized on the paper (Singh *et al* 2018). This binding event initiates a distinct reaction that leads to a color shift, facilitating qualitative or semi-quantitative analysis (Suntornsuk *et al* 2020).

### 10.3.2 Fluorescent detection

Fluorescent detection in PADs for cancer diagnosis involves employing fluorescent dyes or quantum dots. Immobilized recognition elements on the paper interact with cancer biomarkers, triggering a fluorescent signal. This emitted light, upon excitation, is then quantified using a fluorescence reader. This technique offers sensitivity and specificity, enabling rapid and precise cancer detection at the PoC, enhancing its utility for resource-limited settings (Liang *et al* 2017).

### 10.3.3 Chemiluminescent detection

Chemiluminescent detection in PADs for cancer detection utilizes chemical reactions to produce light signals indicative of specific biomarkers (Guo *et al* 2019). Recognition elements, immobilized on the paper, interact with cancer biomarkers, initiating enzymatic or chemical reactions that generate luminescence. The emitted light is then quantified using a luminometer. Despite its potential, ongoing research aims to address challenges such as stability issues and enhance the performance of chemiluminescent PADs for robust and reliable cancer diagnostics in diverse healthcare settings.

### 10.3.4 Electrochemical detection

Electrochemical detection in PADs for cancer diagnosis involves immobilizing recognition elements on paper electrodes. When cancer biomarkers interact with these elements, they induce changes in electrical properties, such as current or voltage. These changes are measured using electrodes, providing a quantitative signal. This technique offers advantages such as sensitivity and specificity, making it suitable for PoC cancer detection but it includes the need for stable electrode modifications and to address few other challenges associated with this technique (Wang *et al* 2019).

### 10.3.5 Surface-enhanced Raman scattering

Surface-enhanced Raman scattering (SERS) in PADs for cancer detection is an advanced technique leveraging the unique spectral characteristics of Raman scattering, enhanced by nanostructured surfaces (Raman *et al* 1928).

Nanostructured surfaces, often composed of silver or gold NPs, are immobilized on the paper. These surfaces possess unique optical properties that enhance the Raman scattering signal. Recognition elements, such as antibodies or aptamers specific to cancer biomarkers, are functionalized onto the nanoparticles. This allows for selective binding with the target molecules. The patient's sample, containing the cancer biomarkers, is applied to the PAD. The interaction between the target molecules and the functionalized nanoparticles enhances the Raman signal. The enhanced Raman signal is then analysed using Raman spectroscopy. This allows for the identification and quantification of the cancer biomarkers based on their unique spectral fingerprints. It has high sensitivity and specificity but requires stability of the nanostructured surfaces and specialized instrumentation (Han *et al* 2021).

### 10.3.6 Surface plasmon resonance

Surface plasmon resonance (SPR) in PADs for cancer detection exploits the phenomenon of SPR to monitor changes in refractive index, providing label-free and real-time detection. SPR occurs when polarized light interacts with a thin metal film, causing a resonance condition that is sensitive to changes in the surrounding refractive index. Recognition elements, such as antibodies or aptamers specific to cancer biomarkers, are immobilized on the paper. The sample containing cancer biomarkers is applied to the PAD. Binding events cause changes in refractive index on the metal surface. The SPR signal proportional to biomarker concentration is monitored in real-time and quantified. This signal transduction technique allows label-free detection and continuous real-time monitoring (Nguyen *et al* 2015, Das *et al* 2023).

## 10.4 Application of paper-based devices in detecting cancer biomarkers

Certain proteins such as carcinoembryonic antigen (CEA) and cancer antigen 125 (CA-125) are recognized biomarkers for cancers such as breast, liver, gastric, and ovarian cancer. Alpha-fetoprotein (AFP) serves as a marker for conditions and cancers, particularly liver cancer. Prostate-specific antigens (PSAs) play a crucial role in prostate cancer diagnosis, screening, and monitoring. Additionally, sarcosine, an amino acid, holds promise as a non-invasive indicator for prostate cancer, detectable in urine samples.

The exploration of circulating tumor cells (CTCs) has been undertaken in the realm of cancer detection. CTCs, rare cellular entities shed into circulation by primary tumors, have the potential to infiltrate the bloodstream and initiate new tumor growth elsewhere in the body. Detecting and quantifying CTCs in the bloodstream holds significant promise as a biomarker for cancer diagnosis, treatment management, and patient monitoring.

Tumor-derived exosomes carry tumor antigens and immunosuppressive proteins such as FasL, TRAIL, and TGF-$\beta$, playing crucial roles in tumor development, metabolism, and migration. For example, exosomes released from breast cancer cells that overexpress CXCR4 contain notable stemness-related markers and metastasis-related messenger ribonucleic acids (mRNAs), influencing cancer cell invasiveness and metastatic potential (Huang *et al* 2019). Additionally, exosomes from cells overexpressing CD184 contribute to enhanced stemness markers, increased invasiveness, and heightened metastatic potential. Similarly, exosomes from adipose-derived mesenchymal stem cells promote cancer migration and proliferation through the Wnt/$\beta$-catenin signaling pathway (Lin *et al* 2013). In colorectal cancer, exosomes from cancer-associated fibroblasts activate cancer stem cells, fostering resistance to radiotherapy and chemotherapy via the Wnt signaling pathway.

### 10.4.1 Carcinoembryonic antigen

CEA, a cell surface glycoprotein, is widely recognized as a biomarker for various cancers, including breast, liver, gastric, and colorectal cancers (Suntornsuk *et al* 2020). Wang *et al* developed a colorimetric CEA detection method for diagnosing gastric cancer using a sandwich immunoassay on a multilayer $\mu$PAD fabricated via wax printing (Wang *et al* 2020).

### 10.4.2 Cancer antigen 125

A colorimetric paper-based immunosensor targeting CA-125, a mucin-like glyco-protein crucial for monitoring epithelial ovarian cancer was developed by Hosu *et al* (2017). Their approach involved a sandwich strategy where a primary antibody was immobilized on an NC membrane, gold nanoparticles were labeled with a secondary antibody, and silver enhancement solution was utilized.

### 10.4.3 Alpha-fetoprotein

Aydindogan and his coworkers developed an immunosensor for AFP, a well-known marker for liver cancer (Aydindogan *et al* 2020). The sensor utilized cysteamine-conjugated AuNPs on an NC membrane along with cross-linked antibodies specific to AFP. Visual colorimetric changes were captured using a smartphone and analysed with ImageJ software.

In another targeted experiment focusing on liver cancer diagnosis, researchers created an electrochemical PAD for detecting AFP, a prominent biomarker associated with liver cancer. The methodology involved using graphene-modified electrodes to immobilize antibodies specific to AFP. The binding of AFP to the immobilized antibodies induced noticeable changes in the electrochemical signal, forming the basis for detection. The results demonstrated the electrochemical PAD's effectiveness in detecting AFP in serum samples. This innovative approach offers a sensitive and selective method for liver cancer diagnosis, presenting a potential PoC solution (Kim *et al* 2018, Liu *et al* 2022).

### 10.4.4 Prostate-specific antigens

PSAs play a crucial role in diagnosing, screening, and monitoring prostate cancer (Nie *et al* 2012). Fu and colleagues introduced a photothermally responsive poly (methyl methacrylate) (PMMA)/paper hybrid disk (PT-disk) for PSA detection on a paper substrate. The method involves a sandwich immunoreaction on aldehyde-modified cellulose paper, where anti-PSA antibodies recognize PSA. $Fe_3O_4$ nano-particles labeled with anti-PSA are introduced to form an immunocomplex. The innovative aspect lies in the colorimetric detection, where the conversion of iron oxide to Prussian blue nanoparticles (PBNPs) induces a visible color change from brown to blue. This change serves as an indicator of PSA presence, offering a simple and effective means for detection. Fu's work demonstrates the potential of this paper-based system for sensitive and specific PSA detection, providing a promising tool for prostate cancer diagnosis and monitoring (Fu *et al* 2020).

### 10.4.5 HER2

HER2 is a biomarker for various cancers including breast and lung cancer and is detected using a colorimetric LFIA. An aptamer attached to AuNPs prevents their aggregation, resulting in a red solution. In the presence of HER2, AuNPs are released (figure 10.4).

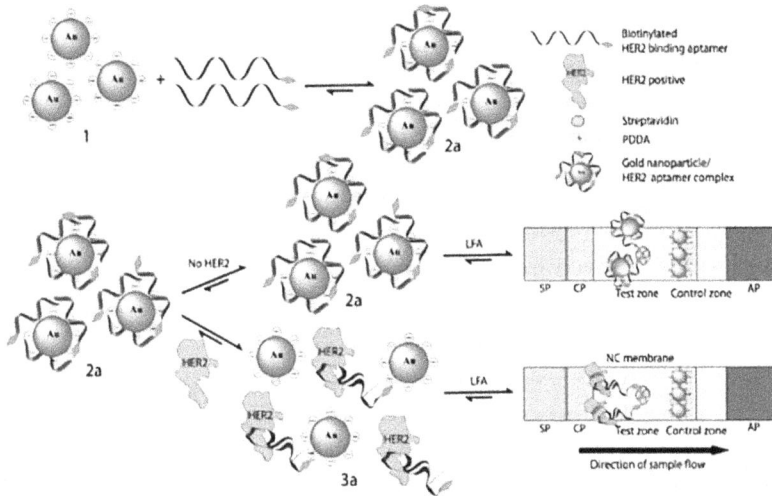

**Figure 10.4.** A diagram illustrating HER2 detection by an adsorption–desorption colorimetric LFA (Reprinted from Ranganathan *et al* (2020), Copyright (2020), with permission from Elsevier.).

A novel experiment aimed at detecting breast cancer markers, specifically HER2, involved the development of a PAD utilizing chemiluminescence. The method entailed immobilizing enzyme-functionalized AuNPs onto a paper substrate. Detection relied on the interaction between these functionalized nanoparticles and the target biomarkers, triggering a chemiluminescent reaction. The successful outcome demonstrated the PAD's effectiveness in detecting HER2 within serum samples. This chemiluminescent detection method shows promise for breast cancer diagnosis due to its sensitivity and specificity in identifying these biomarkers. By using gold nanoparticles as the detection platform and incorporating the chemiluminescent reaction, the sensitivity of the PAD is enhanced, offering potential for early and accurate breast cancer detection. This development represents a significant advancement in PoC diagnostics, providing a rapid and cost-effective means to assess breast cancer markers (Ranganathan *et al* 2020).

### 10.4.6 Alkaline phosphatase

Alkaline phosphatase (ALP) is an enzyme crucial for hydrolyzing phosphoric acid esters and serves as a biomarker in diagnosing various illnesses, including breast and prostate cancers (Resmi *et al* 2018). A colorimetric PoC paper-based device for ALP detection was produced. Employing a commercial wax printer the paper was patterned and para-nitrophenyl phosphate (PNPP) was immobilized as a colorimetric probe in the reagent zone. Upon the addition of ALP inducing a dephosphorylation reaction, the reagent zone transformed to a yellow color. The color intensity, indicative of the ALP concentration, was captured using a digital camera, and MATLAB software was employed for Red, Green, Blue (RGB) and Hue, Saturation, Brightness (HSB) calculations, enabling the extrapolation of target concentrations (Ma *et al* 2024).

### 10.4.7 NSCLC-derived exosome

Yu and colleagues devised an LFIA using a competitive strategy to detect exosomes derived from non-small cell lung cancer (NSCLC) (Yu *et al* 2020). They opted for an aptamer targeting CD63 protein on exosome membranes as the biorecognition element due to its high affinity and stability. Streptavidin-biotin-CD63 aptamer was immobilized on the NC membrane, competing with AuNPs functionalized with CD63 aptamer as colorimetric probes. This LFIA offers a promising approach for detecting exosomes derived from NSCLC.

## 10.5 Conclusion and future perspectives

Early detection, diagnosis, and monitoring of cancer are crucial for reducing mortality rates and healthcare costs. Paper-based analytical devices have emerged as cost-effective platforms for rapid and sensitive detection of multiple cancer biomarkers in body fluids. Novel LFAs and $\mu$PADs offer easy-to-use, sensitive diagnostic tools with semi-quantitative and quantitative capabilities. PADs are an alternative for cancer biomarker detection compared to complex laboratory methods making them user-friendly and they also do not require specialized training. PDAs provide rapid results, contributing to timely diagnosis and facilitating prompt initiation of cancer treatment; moreover the compact and lightweight nature of PADs enhances their portability and allow for on-site testing (Koczula *et al* 2016). Despite having numerous advantages, there are some challenges in using PADs such as high limits of detection and limited specificity. PADs may face stability issues, affecting their shelf life and reliability, especially in diverse environmental conditions (Carrell *et al* 2019, Kasetsirikul *et al* 2020, Murray *et al* 2020).

To make these paper-based point of care diagnostic systems for cancer more user-friendly and compact, research is focussing on making 'all-in-one' paper-based devices. This focuses on capturing and amplifying a target analyte present in different samples directly on paper, enabling interaction with specific biomarkers for detection. In the future, the incorporation of nanomaterials in PADs will gain significance as nanoparticles enhance the performance of biosensors by increasing specificity of interaction.

## References

Agarwal C and Csóka L 2019 Recent advances in paper-based analytical devices: a pivotal step forward in building next-generation sensor technology *Sustainable Polymer Composites and Nanocomposites* (Cham: Springer) pp 479–517

Alahmad W, Sahragard A and Varanusupakul P 2021 Online and offline preconcentration techniques on paper-based analytical devices for ultrasensitive chemical and biochemical analysis: a review *Biosens. Bioelectron.* **194** 113574

Alba-Bernal A, Lavado-Valenzuela R, Domínguez-Recio M E, Jiménez-Rodriguez B, Queipo-Ortuño M I, Alba E and Comino-Méndez I 2020 Challenges and achievements of liquid biopsy technologies employed in early breast cancer *EBioMedicine* **62** 103100

Aydindogan E, Ceylan A E and Timur S 2020 Paper-based colorimetric spot test utilizing smartphone sensing for detection of biomarkers *Talanta* **208** 120446

Bhardwaj P, Arora B, Saxena S, Singh S, Palkar P, Goda J S and Banerjee R 2024 Based point of care diagnostics for cancer biomarkers *Sens. Diagn.* **3** 504–35

Carneiro M C, Rodrigues L R, Moreira F T and Sales M G F 2022 Colorimetric paper-based sensors against cancer biomarkers *Sensors* **22** 3221

Carrell C, Kava A, Nguyen M, Menger R, Munshi Z, Call Z and Henry C 2019 Beyond the lateral flow assay: a review of paper-based microfluidics *Microelectron. Eng.* **206** 45–54

Chauhan P S, Sharma N and Tomar R S 2023 Sensing technologies used in microfluidic paper-based analytical devices (μPADs) *Paper-Based Diagnostic Devices for Infectious Diseases* (Bristol: IOP Publishing) p 12-1

Cheng N, Du D, Wang X, Liu D, Xu W, Luo Y and Lin Y 2019 Recent advances in biosensors for detecting cancer-derived exosomes *Trends Biotechnol.* **37** 1236–54

Das S, Devireddy R and Gartia M R 2023 Surface plasmon resonance (SPR) sensor for cancer biomarker detection *Biosensors* **13** 396

Ebrahimi G, Pakchin P S, Mota A, Omidian H and Omidi Y 2023 Electrochemical microfluidic paper-based analytical devices for cancer biomarker detection: from 2D to 3D sensing systems *Talanta* **257** 124370

Fu G, Li X, Wang W and Hou R 2020 Multiplexed tri-mode visual outputs of immunoassay signals on a clip-magazine-assembled photothermal biosensing disk *Biosens. Bioelectron.* **170** 112646

Gopinath P, Anitha V and Mastani S A 2015 Microcantilever based biosensor for disease detection applications *J. Med. Bioeng.* **4** 34

Guo X, Guo Y, Liu W, Chen Y and Chu W 2019 Fabrication of paper-based microfluidic device by recycling foamed plastic and the application for multiplexed measurement of biomarkers *Spectrochim. Acta* A **223** 117341

Han X X *et al* 2021 Surface-enhanced Raman spectroscopy *Nat. Rev. Methods Primers* **1** 87

Hosu O, Ravalli A, Piccolo G M L, Cristea C, Sandulescu R and Marrazza G 2017 Smartphone-based immunosensor for CA125 detection *Talanta* **166** 234–40

Hu J, Wang S, Wang L, Li F, Pingguan-Murphy B, Lu T J and Xu F 2014 Advances in paper-based point-of-care diagnostics *Biosens. Bioelectron.* **54** 585–97

Huang T and Deng C X 2019 Current progresses of exosomes as cancer diagnostic and prognostic biomarkers *Int. J. Biol. Sci.* **15** 1

Jiang R, Ahmed, Damayantharan M, Una H and Yetisen K 2019 Lateral and vertical flow assays for point-of-care diagnostics *Adv. Healthcare Mater.* **8** e1900244

Jiao Y, Du C, Zong L, Guo X, Han Y, Zhang X and Huang W 2020 3D vertical-flow paper-based device for simultaneous detection of multiple cancer biomarkers by fluorescent immunoassay *Sens. Actuators* B **306** 127239

Jungreis E 1996 *Spot Test Analysis: Clinical, Environmental, Forensic, and Geochemical Applications* **vol 2** (New York: Wiley)

Kasetsirikul S, Shiddiky M J and Nguyen N T 2020 Challenges and perspectives in the development of paper-based lateral flow assays *Microfluid. Nanofluid.* **24** 1–18

Kim D H, Oh H G, Park W H, Jeon D C, Lim K M, Kim H J and Song K S 2018 Detection of alpha-fetoprotein in hepatocellular carcinoma patient plasma with graphene field-effect transistor *Sensors* **18** 4032

Koczula K M and Gallotta A 2016 Lateral flow assays *Essays Biochem.* **60** 111–20

Kuswandi B and Ensafi A A 2019 Perspective—Paper-Based Biosensors: Trending Topic in Clinical Diagnostics Developments and Commercialization *J. Electrochem. Soc.* **167** 037509

Liang L, Lan F, Yin X, Ge S, Yu J and Yan M 2017 Metal-enhanced fluorescence/visual bimodal platform for multiplexed ultrasensitive detection of microRNA with reusable paper analytical devices *Biosens. Bioelectron.* **95** 181–8

Lim W Y, Goh B T and Khor S M 2017 Microfluidic paper-based analytical devices for potential use in quantitative and direct detection of disease biomarkers in clinical analysis *J. Chromatogr.* B **1060** 424–42

Lin R, Wang S and Zhao R C 2013 Exosomes from human adipose-derived mesenchymal stem cells promote migration through WNT signaling pathway in a breast cancer cell model *Mol. Cell. Biochem.* **383** 13–20

Liu L, Wang H, Xie B, Zhang B, Lin Y and Gao L 2022 Detection of alpha-fetoprotein using aptamer-based sensors *Biosensors* **12** 780

Liu L, Yang D and Liu G 2019 Signal amplification strategies for paper-based analytical devices *Biosens. Bioelectron.* **136** 60–75

Ma B L and Zhang Z L 2024 A point-of-care solid-phase colorimetric sensor based on the enzyme-induced metallization for ALP detection *Talanta* **268** 125365

Mahmoudi T, de la Guardia M and Baradaran B 2020 Lateral flow assays towards point-of-care cancer detection: a review of current progress and future trends *TrAC, Trends Anal. Chem.* **125** 115842

Martinez A W, Phillips S T, Butte M J and Whitesides G M 2007 Patterned paper as a platform for inexpensive, low-volume, portable bioassays. *Angew. Chem.* **119** 1340–2

Meyer M H, Stehr M, Bhuju S, Krause H J, Hartmann M, Miethe P and Keusgen M 2007 Magnetic biosensor for the detection of *Yersinia pestis J. Microbiol. Methods* **68** 218–24

Murillo A E, Melo-Maximo L, Garcia-Farrera B, Martínez O S, Melo-Máximo D V, Oliva-Ramirez J and Oseguera J 2019 Development of AlN thin films for breast cancer acoustic biosensors *J. Mater. Res. Technol.* **8** 350–8

Murray L P and Mace C R 2020 Usability as a guiding principle for the design of paper-based, point-of-care devices—a review *Anal. Chim. Acta* **1140** 236–49

Nguyen H H, Park J, Kang S and Kim M 2015 Surface plasmon resonance: a versatile technique for biosensor applications *Sensors* **15** 10481–510

Nie J, Zhang Y, Lin L, Zhou C, Li S, Zhang L and Li J 2012 Low-cost fabrication of paper-based microfluidic devices by one-step plotting *Anal. Chem.* **84** 6331–5

Ozer T, McMahon C and Henry C S 2020 Advances in paper-based analytical devices *Annu. Rev. Anal. Chem.* **13** 85–109

Raman C V and Krishnan K S 1928 A new type of secondary radiation *Nature* **121** 501–2

Ranganathan V, Srinivasan S, Singh A and DeRosa M C 2020 An aptamer-based colorimetric lateral flow assay for the detection of human epidermal growth factor receptor 2 (HER2) *Anal. Biochem.* **588** 113471

Ratajczak K and Stobiecka M 2020 High-performance modified cellulose paper-based biosensors for medical diagnostics and early cancer screening: a concise review *Carbohydr. Polym.* **229** 115463

Resmi P E, Stanley J, Kumar S, Soman K P, Ramachandran T and TG S B 2018 Fabrication of paper microfluidics POCT device for the colorimetric assay of alkaline phosphatase *2018 15th IEEE India Council Int. Conf. (INDICON)* (Piscataway, NJ: IEEE) pp 1–4

Shankaran D R 2018 Nano-enabled immunosensors for point-of-care cancer diagnosis *Applications of Nanomaterials* (Cambridge: Woodhead) pp 205–50

Shende P, Prabhakar B and Patil A 2019 Color changing sensors: a multimodal system for integrated screening *Trends Anal. Chem.* **121** 115687

Siegel R L, Miller K D and Jemal A 2019 Cancer statistics, 2019 *CA: A Cancer J. Clin.* **69** 7–34

Singh A T, Lantigua D, Meka A, Taing S, Pandher M and Camci-Unal G 2018 based sensors: emerging themes and applications *Sensors* **18** 2838

Spinola A, Pinto M S and Neto C C 1995 Fritz Feigl (1891–1971): The centennial of a researcher *Bull. Hist. Chem.* **17** 31–9

Suntornsuk W and Suntornsuk L 2020 Recent applications of paper-based point-of-care devices for biomarker detection *Electrophoresis* **41** 287–305

Tothill I and Altintas Z 2015 Molecular biosensors: promising new tools for early detection of cancer *Nanobiosen. Dis. Diagn.* **4** 1–10

Wang Y, Luo J P, Liu J T, Sun S, Xiong Y, Ma Y Y, Yan S, Yang Y, HB Y and Cai X X 2019 Label-free microfluidic paper-based electrochemical aptasensor for ultrasensitive and simultaneous multiplexed detection of cancer biomarkers *Biosens. Bioelectron.* **136** 84–90

Wang K, Yang J, Xu H, Cao B, Qin Q, Liao X and Cui D 2020 Smartphone-imaged multilayered paper-based analytical device for colorimetric analysis of carcinoembryonic antigen *Anal. Bioanal. Chem.* **412** 2517–28

Wei Z, Zhou Y, Wang R, Wang J and Chen Z 2022 Aptamers as smart ligands for targeted drug delivery in cancer therapy *Pharmaceutics* **14** 2561

West P W 1945 Selective spot test for copper *Ind. Eng. Chem. Anal. Ed.* **17** 740–1

Yonet-Tanyeri N, Ahlmark B Z and Little S R 2021 Advances in multiplexed paper-based analytical devices for cancer diagnosis: a review of technological developments. *Adv. Mater. Technol.* **6** 2001138

Yu Q, Zhao Q, Wang S, Zhao S, Zhang S, Yin Y and Dong Y 2020 Development of a lateral flow aptamer assay strip for facile identification of the ranostic exosomes isolated from human lung carcinoma cells *Anal. Biochem.* **594** 113591

Zhang Z, Zhou J and Du X 2019 Electrochemical biosensors for detection of foodborne pathogens *Micromachines* **10** 222

IOP Publishing

Nano Biosensors for Non-Invasive Diagnosis of Cancer

Nidhi Puranik and Shiv Kumar Yadav

# Chapter 11

## Utility of various types of nanoparticles as potential materials for biosensors

Arun Sharma, Surabhi Singh, Nidhi Puranik, Kavita Shukla and Bharti Sahu

Point-of-care biosensor devices have a lot of capacity to expand owing to recent developments in nanomaterials and nanostructured materials, which might completely change how personalized healthcare is diagnosed and treated in the future. The usage of nanoparticle (NP)-based biosensors is the main topic of this chapter. It examines a variety of NPs, describing how they are synthesized and emphasizing how crucial they are to building highly effective biosensing systems. The chapter also explores several transducer elements and explains how they work in biosensors, including electrochemical, optical, piezoelectric, thermal, and surface plasmon resonance. To fabricate biosensors, the critical step of immobilizing bioreceptors on NPs is addressed. This provides a methodical illustration and clarifies the conjugation of nanomaterials with biomaterials. NPs may immobilize a greater number of bioreceptor units at lower volumes and even function as transduction elements themselves. Moreover, nanomaterials present exciting opportunities for higher sensitivities and lower detection limits in early diagnosis. Gold NPs (AuNPs), silver NPs (AgNPs), bimetallic (Cu–Au)/(Pd–Au)/(Ag–Pt)/(Au–Pt) NPs, polymer NPs, semiconductor quantum dots (QDs), multiwalled carbon nanotubes (MWCNTs), nanodiamonds (NDs), and graphene are among the nanomaterials that have been the subject of substantial research. The chapter also examines the broad range of uses for biosensors, including clinical diagnostics, healthcare, microbiology, environmental monitoring, industrial process control, and military.

## 11.1 Introduction

The detection of pathogens/viruses/toxins is essential in diagnosing the cause of a disease. Various methods are used, such as radioimmunoassays, ELISA, fluorescence, chemiluminescence and biosensors (Sharma *et al* 2020). The advantage of biosensor technology is that it can enhance the sensitivity and limit of detection for

doi:10.1088/978-0-7503-6234-4ch11          11-1

pathogens/viruses/toxins. According to the International Union of Pure and Applied Chemistry (IUPAC) recommendations, a biosensor is a self-contained integrated receptor–transducer device, which is capable of providing selective quantitative or semi-quantitative analytical information using a biological recognition element (Harold 1996). Nanomaterials have the potential for improving sensitivities and achieving lower thresholds for detection because they enable the immobilization of a larger number of bioreceptor units in smaller quantities. They can also serve as transduction components.

In various technological domains, nanomaterials such as semiconductor QDs, AuNPs, carbon nanotubes (CNTs), polymer NPs, bimetallic NPs, NDs, and graphene have proven to be suitable for biosensing applications. A key challenge in biosensor development is the immobilization strategy used to formulate these transducing elements to conjugate intimately with the bio-specific entity (Holzinger *et al* 2014). Biomolecules are attached to the nanomaterials using coupling, covalent conjugation, and non-covalent conjugation to prepare 'bio-nanoconjugates'. These bio-nanoconjugates comprise the properties of both the biomolecule and nano-material. Uncontrolled anchoring may affect the recognition event and alter the reversibility and reproducibility, which can cause severe deviation in the results. In the practical application of a developed biosensor, it is essential to regenerate the transducer element as needed.

Based on their chemical composition, nearly all nanomaterials can acquire suitable functions through direct functionalization, sometimes even during synthesis, or by applying coatings of functional polymers without altering their inherent properties. This type of functionalization not only facilitates the consistent immobi-lization of bioreceptor units but also has the potential to enhance the biocompat-ibility of these materials (Biju 2014). In this chapter all variety of available biosensors based on different transducing techniques, e.g. electrochemical, piezo-electric, optical, and liquid crystal based biosensors (figure 11.1), as well as those that depend on different bioreceptor units, e.g. enzymes, DNA, antibodies, etc, are discussed in detail (Sharma *et al* 2016a, Asal *et al* 2018). At the same time, a diverse range of NPs, including inorganic, organic, polymeric, magnetic, nanocomposite, and carbon nanotubes, is showcased in the development of various biosensor types (Eissa *et al* 2018).

These biosensors are mostly used in the environmental, biomedical, defense, and pharmacy fields because of their many advantages, including compatibility with miniature and portable technologies, heightened sensitivity, cost-effectiveness, and rapid response capabilities. Biosensors have many benefits but their design has several drawbacks. The high cost of biomolecules, their sensitivity to environmental factors including pH, temperature, devitalizers, and air pollutants, their reduced long-term stability, difficult immobilization techniques, and instability toward certain compounds are a few of these. Electrochemical biosensors, which use non-biological recognition components such transition metal oxides (MXenes), have been developed to circumvent these limitations. MXenes have become more well-known recently because of their remarkable stability, and excellent selectivity and

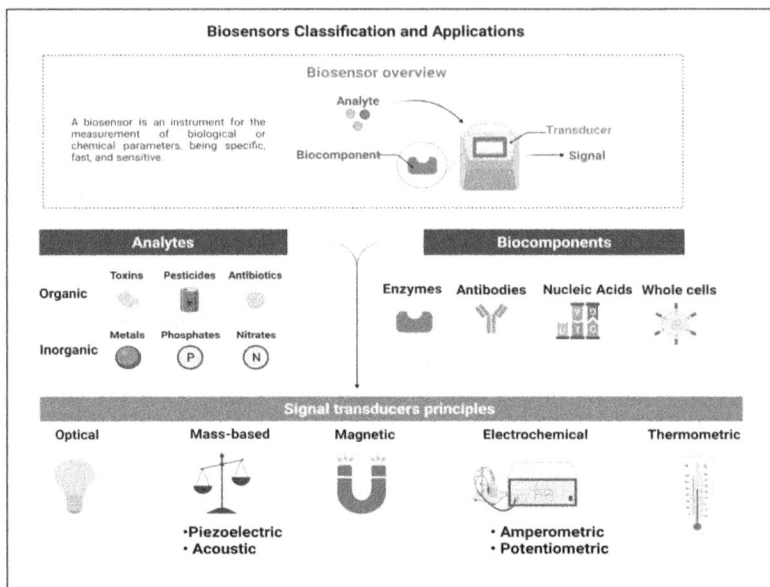

**Figure 11.1.** Biosensor classification and applications based on various analytes, biocomponents, and transducing platforms. (Created using Biorender.com.)

sensitivity, which help them overcome the drawbacks of conventional biosensors (Liu *et al* 2022).

In this chapter the utility of various nanostructured materials, such as zero-dimensional (0D), one-dimensional (1D), two-dimensional (2D), and three-dimensional (3D) NPs, and their role in the development of potential biosensors is mainly discussed (Mekuye and Abera 2023). The utilization of nanomaterials can enhance the efficiency of biosensors, particularly in achieving a low detection limit and heightened sensitivity. Their widespread application in biosensing is attributed to their elevated surface-to-volume ratio, chemical reactivity, mechanical robustness, electrocatalytic characteristics, improved diffusivity, and fluorescence properties. In biosensors, nanomaterials play a crucial role by bridging the space between the transducer and the bioreceptor (Malhotra and Ali 2018). The recent progress in nanomaterials and nanostructured materials has opened up the possibility of significant advancements in point-of-care biosensor devices, with the potential to transform the landscape of personalized healthcare diagnostics and therapeutic approaches in the future.

## 11.2 Synthesis of nanoparticles

Nanomaterials in a variety of forms, such as colloidal forms of NPs, QDs, nanoclusters, nanotubes, nanocubes, NDs, nanorods, nanowires, nanopowders, thin films, and more, may be produced using a variety of techniques. Nanomaterials may be made using conventional methods with the right adjustments.

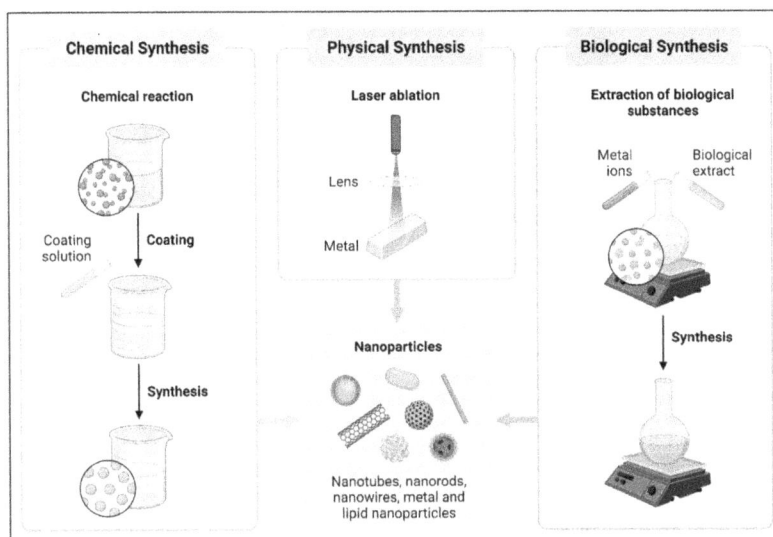

**Figure 11.2.** Schematic representation of different techniques that can be used for the synthesis of NPs, including chemical, physical, and biological methods. (Created with Biorender.com.)

A flowchart of several synthesis methods suitable for NPs is shown in figure 11.2. Technological developments in the physical, chemical, biological, and hybrid fields have improved the formulation of nanomaterials. There are different methods of NP synthesis. Two main approaches are used: (i) top-down approaches and (ii) bottom-up approaches.

These methods are compared in figure 11.3.

In a typical top-down approach, a large-scale object is gradually reduced until its size or dimensions comes to the nanometer regime. These methods are generally called physical methods. Simply put, in the top-down method, bulk material is first ground mechanically, and nanosized particles are obtained. These particles are stabilized by the addition of protecting agents. Photolithography, high-energy ball milling, melt mixing, physical vapor deposition, laser ablation, laser pyrolysis, sputtering, ion beam techniques, and electron beam lithography are the commonly used top-down techniques for the synthesis of nanomaterials (table 11.1). In the bottom-up approach, the atoms that are produced by the reduction of their ions are assembled in controlled conditions to produce nanostructured materials (Cao 2004). The bottom-up method includes collecting, consolidating, and arranging individual atoms and molecules into different structures, which can be carried out by a sequence of chemical reactions with or without catalysts. There are various bottom-up techniques such as chemical bath synthesis, electrochemical deposition, the sonochemical approach, the hydrothermal method, and the photochemical reduction method (table 11.1). Bottom-up techniques are usually followed by the addition of capping agents during the growth of nanomaterials to prevent aggregation and precipitation of the NPs out of the solution. A capping agent may be a unifunctional, bifunctional ligand, polymer, or surfactant that is used to stabilize the

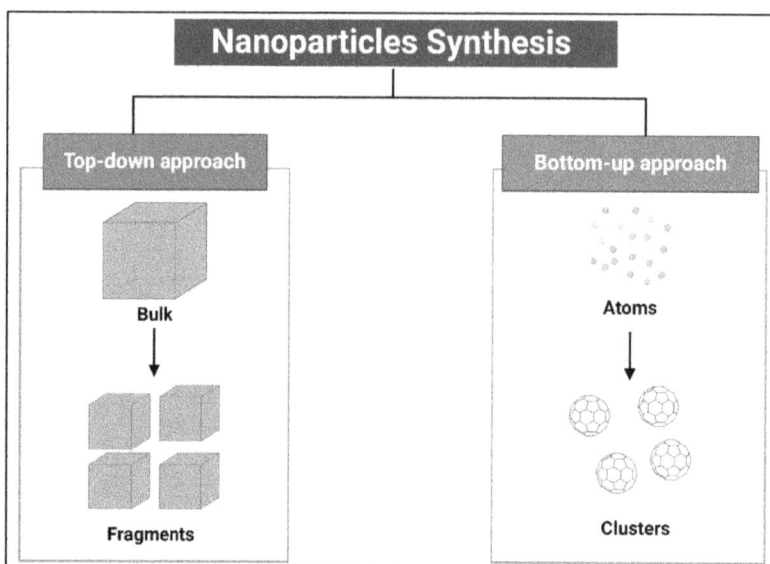

**Figure 11.3.** The top-down approach versus the bottom-up approach. (Created with Biorender.com.)

**Table 11.1.** Comparison of top-down and bottom-up processes.

|  | Top-down processes | Bottom-up processes |
|---|---|---|
| **Principles** | Bulk material is ground mechanically and quantum dots are obtained. | Atoms are produced by the reduction of their ions and assembled in controlled conditions to produce NPs. |
| **Methods** | Physical methods: energy ball milling, melt mixing, physical vapor deposition, laser ablation, laser pyrolysis, sputtering, ion beam techniques and lithography, etc. | Chemical methods: chemical bath synthesis, electrochemical deposition, the sonochemical approach, the hydrothermal method, and the photochemical reduction method, etc. |
| **Advantages** | Produces very fine particles at a large scale in a short time. | A simple way to produce homogeneous nanomaterials with fewer defects and contamination, a more economical process. |
| **Disadvantages** | Imperfections of the surface structure, crystallographic damage, broad size distribution, varied particle shape, difficulty to design and control process, very expensive, impurities and defects on the nanomaterial surface. | Controlled conditions are needed during the synthesis procedure such as temperature, duration, pH of the medium, concentration of precursors, etc. Requires well-trained personnel. |

nanomaterials (Sharma *et al* 2016a). The size and shape of the NPs can be controlled and depend on the technique which is used for the synthesis, the reaction temperature, and the choice of capping material (Sharma *et al* 2016b). Nanomaterials can be synthesized of various shapes, i.e. spheres, rods, cubes, disks, wires, tubes, triangular prisms, flowers, stars, and tetrahedral NPs (Shevchenko *et al* 2003). The size and shape of NPs are tunable by altering the duration, temperature, and ligand molecules (Andrea and Horst 2002). The choice of synthesis method is contingent upon the specific material of interest, the type of nanomaterial (0D, 1D, 2D, 3D), their respective sizes, and the desired quantity (Malhotra and Ali 2018).

## 11.2.1 Classification of nanomaterials based on their dimensions

Nanomaterials can be categorized based on their dimensions and size. Nanomaterials come in four different varieties: 0D, 1D, 2D, and 3D structures.

### 11.2.1.1 Zero-dimensional nanomaterials

All three material dimensions are within the nanoscale range in 0D nanomaterials, such as gold, palladium, platinum, silver, or quantum dots, which are examples of NPs (Sharma *et al* 2014b). These NPs can have a diameter of 1–50 nm and a spherical form. Interestingly, 0D nanomaterials also include certain cube and polygonal forms (figure 11.4). Examples of 0D carbon nanomaterials are CDs and fullerenes. There are more active edge sites per unit mass due to the intrinsic structural properties of 0D, which are defined by ultra-small diameters and high surface-to-volume ratios. These nanomaterials have unique or improved features such as increased chemiluminescence (CL) and photoluminescence (PL) quantum efficiency due to their edge and quantum confinement effects (Chen *et al* 2019).

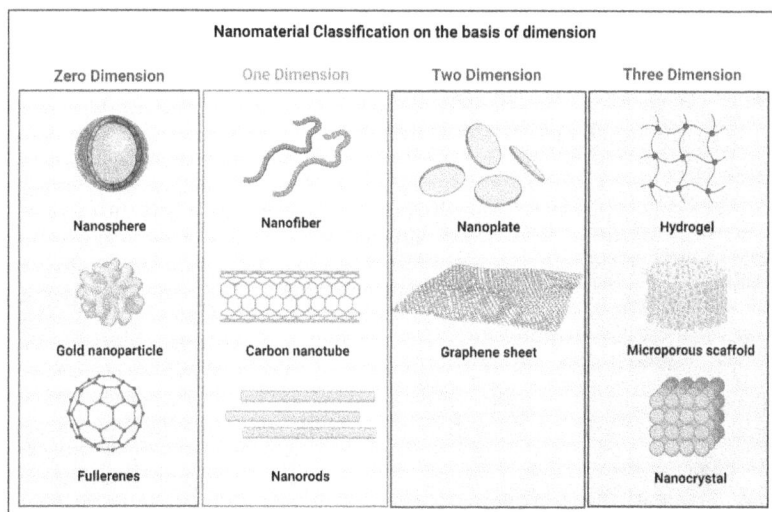

**Figure 11.4.** Classification of nanomaterials based on their dimensions. (Created with Biorender.com.)

A structure created by reshaping NPs into 0D structures can have special characteristics that set it apart from materials with greater dimensions (Liang *et al* 2014). Zero-dimensional nanomaterials are mostly spherical or quasi-spherical NPs having a diameter of less than 100 nm, in contrast to bulk high-dimensional nanomaterials. Zero-dimensional nanomaterials exhibit remarkable versatility for biomedical applications, such as nanomedicine, cosmetics, bioelectronics, biosensors, and biochips. These applications are made possible by their unique attributes, which include optical stability, wavelength-dependent photoluminescence, chemical inertness, cellular permeability, and biocompatibility (Yao *et al* 2018). The main focus of this chapter is on the use and potential applications of 0D NPs in biosensors.

### 11.2.1.2 One-dimensional nanomaterials
Nanomaterials with a single dimension falling within the 1–100 nm range, while the remaining two dimensions can extend into the macroscale, are classified as 1D nanomaterials. One-dimensional nanomaterials may exist either in a chemically pure form or as impure entities, as seen in doped semiconductors (Bashir and Liu 2015). These materials can manifest independently or be incorporated within another medium. In the context of 1D materials, their length surpasses their width. Examples of such 1D nanomaterials include nanofilaments, nanowires, nanofibers, nanorods, and nanotubes (figure 11.4). Certain metals (such as Au, Ag, Si), carbon nanotubes, and metal oxides (such as ZnO, $TiO_2$, $CeO_2$) are capable of forming these one-dimensional nanostructures. Their widespread development and utilization across various fields stem from their distinctive linear morphology, offering a substantial specific surface area, efficient separation of electron–hole pairs, robust light absorption capacity, abundant exposed active sites, and other noteworthy characteristics (Linares *et al* 2014). In this chapter, the potential application of 1D nanomaterial is emphasized in the field of biosensing.

### 11.2.1.3 Two-dimensional nanomaterials
In this class of nanomaterials, two dimensions are in the nanoscale and one dimension is in the macroscale. Nano thin films, thin-film multilayers, nanosheets, or nanowalls are 2D nanomaterials (figure 11.4). The area of 2D nanomaterials can be several square micrometers, keeping the thickness always in the nanoscale range. Two-dimensional nanomaterials have garnered a lot of attention lately because of their unique properties and their applications in a variety of fields. In contrast to traditional bulk materials, which have three dimensions, two-dimensional nanomaterials have one or two nanometer-sized dimensions and are characterized by an incredibly thin, sheet-like structure. Their exceptional mechanical, electrical, and optical properties stem from their unusual structure, which makes them extremely promising for a wide range of applications, including electronics, energy storage, medicinal devices, and environmental cleanup.

Graphene is one of the most well-known and researched 2D nanomaterials. It is a single sheet of carbon atoms arranged hexagonally. Its mechanical strength is remarkable, and it has excellent thermal and electrical conductivity as well as extraordinary optical clarity. These characteristics have made it a mainstay in a wide range of applications, including flexible electronics, sensors, and transparent conductive films. Transition metal dichalcogenides (TMDs), which are composed of two layers of chalcogen atoms (such as tellurium, selenium, or sulfur) and transition metal atoms, are another interesting type of two-dimensional nano-material. TMDs have a bandgap, which makes them suited for optoelectronic uses including solar cells, light-emitting diodes (LEDs), and photodetectors, in contrast to graphene. Other two-dimensional nanomaterials are insulators such as boron nitride (BN), which is perfect for protective coatings and high-temperature applications due to its remarkable chemical inertness and thermal stability. A layered substance with a tunable bandgap, black phosphorus (BP) has shown promise as in energy storage devices, photodetectors, transistors, and biosensors.

### 11.2.1.4 Three-dimensional nanomaterials

In 3D nanomaterials, there are no dimensions on the nanoscale, and all dimensions are on the macroscale (figure 11.4). A family of materials known as 3D nano-materials has at least one dimension in the nanometer scale, which usually ranges from 1 to 100 nm. These materials' small size, high surface area-to-volume ratio, and quantum effects all contribute to their distinctive characteristics. They have drawn a lot of interest from a variety of industries, such as electronics, energy storage, and biological applications.

3D nanomaterials can completely change how electronic devices are designed and manufactured. For example, high-performance transistors, sensors, and memory devices with enhanced functionality and lower power consumption can be made using 3D nanostructures. Furthermore, 3D nanomaterials can be incorporated into stretchy and flexible circuits, opening up new possibilities for wearable and implantable medical devices. 3D nanomaterials have great potential for tissue engineering, medication delivery, and diagnostic imaging in the biomedical industry. For instance, 3D nanostructured scaffolds can encourage tissue regeneration and cell proliferation by imitating the extracellular matrix of tissues. Furthermore, targeting ligands and imaging agents can be functionalized into 3D nanomaterials to facilitate targeted drug delivery and non-invasive tissue imaging.

## 11.3 Utility and applications of zero-dimensional nanoparticles in biosensors

Zero-dimensional nanomaterials are powerful sensing agents that play a key role as probes to increase biosensor sensitivity and enhance analytical performance. Their unique optical features and conductive qualities are responsible for this improvement (Sondhi *et al* 2020). Various 0D nanomaterials, including carbon QDs (CQDs), graphene QDs (GQDs), inorganic QDs, polymer dots (Pdots), fullerenes, magnetic NPs (MNPs), upconversion NPs (UCNPs) and noble metal NPs have garnered a great deal of attention in biosensing research in recent years.

Owing to their exceptional physical and chemical characteristics, ultra-small size, quantum confinement effect, and strong biocompatibility, 0D nanomaterials show great promise in fields such as pathogen detection, ion detection, biomolecular recognition, and disease diagnosis. Zero-dimensional nanomaterials exhibit an increased photoluminescence quantum yield attributed to the quantum confinement effect, making them pivotal in various fluorescence sensing systems. This section delves into the biosensing applications of 0D nanomaterials, specifically in detecting diverse biomarkers and ions. The realm of biosensing is experiencing a rapid expansion of 0D nanomaterial applications, and this section highlights recent advancements in their composition, properties, and biosensing applications (Byakodi *et al* 2022) (table 11.2).

Notably, the major focus of biosensing research continues to be on carbon-based nanomaterials (such as CQDs, GQDs, and fullerenes), MNPs, inorganic QDs, and noble metal NPs (such as AgNPs and AuNPs). Furthermore, novel nanomaterials with interesting uses include Pdots, silicon quantum dots (SiQDs) and UCNPs. To sum up, 0D nanomaterials have a remarkable affinity for biomolecules, which makes it easier to immobilize proteins, enzymes, antibodies, nucleic acids, and other compounds that are important to clinical practice. Their different physical and chemical qualities, such as high surface-to-volume ratios, adjustable optical characteristics, and outstanding binding capabilities with biomolecules, are conferred by their unique 0D architectures. The widespread use of 0D nanomaterials highlights their potential to improve the sensitivity and adaptability of biomolecular detection techniques, as covered in this chapter. Without question, 0D nanomaterials are set to make significant strides in biosensing and may soon find their way into clinical research and real-world applications.

## 11.4 Utility and applications of one-dimensional nanoparticles in biosensors

One-dimensional NPs such as nanowires, nanotubes, and nanorods, have unique properties that make them suitable for biosensor applications. These characteristics include their large surface area, high aspect ratio, and flexible mechanical, optical, and electrical characteristics. Because of these characteristics, 1D NPs may interact with biological molecules, such as proteins and DNA, with remarkable sensitivity and specificity, making them ideal for use in biosensor applications (table 11.3).

Moreover, 1D NPs can bind to poisons and contaminants in the environment with remarkable sensitivity and specificity. Their mechanical, optical, and electrical characteristics can also be adjusted, which makes it easier to create biosensors with great selectivity and sensitivity. In general, 1D NPs can be used in biosensors for a variety of tasks, such as the identification of poisons, environmental contaminants, and biomolecules. They are perfect candidates for use in biosensors because of their special qualities, which include their high aspect ratio, huge surface area, and tunable electrical, optical, and mechanical capabilities.

**Table 11.2.** The role of 0D nanomaterials in biosensing applications.

| Sl. No. | Chemical formulation of 0D nanomaterials | Size in nanometers (nm) | Outstanding features | Targeted antigen/foreign species with limit of detection (LOD) | References |
|---|---|---|---|---|---|
| 1 | Graphene quantum dots (GQDs) | <10 nm | Tunable photoluminescence (PL), functionalization, biocompatibility and conductivity | Metal ions | Chung et al (2021) |
| 2 | Au@SCX8-rGO-TB | <500 nm | Electrochemical properties | SARS-CoV-2 (LOD 200 RNA copies/ml) | Zhao et al (2021) |
| 3 | Magnetic graphene oxide quantum dots (Fe-GOQDs) | <10 nm | Fluorescence | Arsenic ions (LOD 5.1 ppb) | Pathan et al (2019) |
| 4 | Aptamer probe and GOQDs | <10 nm | Excellent biocompatibility, optical properties and high quantum yield | Lead ions (LOD 0.6 nm) | Qian et al (2015) |
| 5 | GQDs | 7.06 nm | Fluorescence | Ascorbic acid (LOD 0.32 $\mu$M) | Liu et al (2017) |
| 6 | Carbon quantum dots (CQDs) | <10 nm | Highly photoluminescence (PL), chemiluminescence (CL) and electrochemiluminescence (ECL) | Selenol | Wang et al (2017) |
| 7 | Nitrogen-doped CQDs (N-CQDs) | <10 nm | Fluorescence | $\beta$-glucuronidase (GLU) (LOD 0.3 U L$^{-1}$) | Lu et al (2016) |
| 8 | Co$_3$O$_4$-fullerene | <10 nm | Photoelectrochemical (PEC) properties | DNA p53 gene (LOD 20 aM) | |
| 9 | 4-MPBA@n-C$_{60}$-PdPt | <100 nm | High rate of electron transferability and sensitivity | α2,3-sialylated glycans (LOD 3 fg ml$^{-1}$) | Yuan et al (2018) |
| 10 | Lead sulfide quantum dots (PbSQDs) | 15–30 nm | Excellent fluorescence and electrochemical properties | Staphylococcal enterotoxin B (LOD 0.01 ng ml$^{-1}$ by QD-ELISA and 0.03 ng ml$^{-1}$ by QD-FLISA) | Sharma et al (2014b) |
| 11 | Gold nanoparticles (AuNPs) | <100 nm | Good biocompatibility and unique photoelectric properties | Aflatoxin B1 (carcinogen) (LOD 33 fg ml$^{-1}$) | Li et al (2021) |

| # | Nanomaterial | Size | Properties | Target (LOD) | Reference |
|---|---|---|---|---|---|
| 12 | Zinc sulfide quantum dots (ZnSQDs) | ~5–10 nm | Excellent fluorescence and electrochemical properties | *Staphylococcal enterotoxin* B (LOD 0.02 ng ml$^{-1}$ by fluorescence assay and 1.0 ng ml$^{-1}$ by electrochemical assay) | Sharma *et al* (2015) |
| 13 | High-luminance quantum dots (QDs) and magnetic nanoparticles (MNPs) | <100 nm | High magnetic susceptibility and high PL quantum yields | H1N1 (LOD 0.21 nM), H3N2 (LOD 0.16 nM) and H9N2 (LOD 0.12 nM) | Zhang *et al* (2018) |
| 14 | AuNPs | <100 nm | Optical properties | Aflatoxin B1 (carcinogen) (LOD 10 nM) | Kasoju *et al* (2020b) |
| 15 | Water-dispersible Ag$_2$S QDs with AuNPs | <100 nm | PEC properties | Living cells (LOD 100 cells/ml) | Li *et al* (2018b) |
| 16 | AuNPs | <25 nm | Catalytic and optical properties | Aflatoxin M1(carcinogen) (LOD 3 pM) | Kasoju *et al* (2020a) |
| 17 | CdSe@ZnSQDs | <100 nm | ECL properties | miRNA-141 in cancer cells (LOD 33 aM) | Li *et al* (2017b) |
| 18 | V&A@Ag$_2$S QDs | <10 nm | Fluorescence | Prodromal biomarker of traumatic brain injury | Li *et al* (2020) |
| 19 | SiQDs | <50 nm | High quantum yield and strong resistance to photobleaching | Zn$^{2+}$ ions (LOD 0.17 $\mu$M) | Li *et al* (2018c) |
| 20 | 0D MNPs | <50 nm | High saturation magnetization and superparamagnetism | Prostate-specific antigen (LOD 0.8 fM) | Chuah *et al* (2019) |
| 21 | Gold-coated MNPs | <100 nm | Supersensitivity | miRNA (LOD 10 aM) | Tavallaie *et al* (2018) |
| 22 | MNP–antibody conjugates (MNPs-ABS) | <100 nm | Fluorescence | Ovarian cancer biomarkers, CA-125, β-2 M and ApoA1 (LOD 0.26 U ml$^{-1}$, 0.55 ng ml$^{-1}$ and 7.7 ng ml$^{-1}$) | Pal *et al* (2015) |
| 23 | MNPs | <50 nm | Magnetic properties | *Pseudomonas aeruginosa* (LOD 10$^2$ cfu ml$^{-1}$) | Alhogail *et al* (2019) |
| 24 | Au@Fe$_3$O$_4$ core–shell MNPs | <50 nm | Magnetic properties | Asthma biomarker eosinophil cationic protein (LOD 0.3 nM) | Lee *et al* (2018) |
| 25 | AuNP/MNP hybrid nanocomposite with CdSeS QDs | <50 nm | Fluorescence and magnetic properties | Norovirus (NoV) (LOD 0.48 pg ml$^{-1}$) | Takemura *et al* (2019) |
| 26 | Au–Cu bimetallic nanocrystals | 2–3 $\mu$m | High surface area and excellent electrochemical sensitivity | Carcinoembryonic antigen CEA (LOD 0.5 pg ml$^{-1}$) | Tran *et al* (2018) |

(Continued)

**Table 11.2.** (*Continued*)

| Sl. No. | Chemical formulation of 0D nanomaterials | Size in nanometers (nm) | Outstanding features | Targeted antigen/foreign species with limit of detection (LOD) | References |
|---|---|---|---|---|---|
| 27 | AuNPs | <100 nm | Excellent electrical conductivity, high sensitivity and electrocatalytic performance | Levodopa (LOD 0.5 $\mu$M) | Ji et al (2019) |
| 28 | AuNPs | <100 nm | CL | Hepatitis B surface antigen (LOD 14 pg ml$^{-1}$) | Sabouri et al (2014) |
| 29 | AuNPs | 6.1–11.0 nm | High surface area and high conductivity | Zika virus (ZIKV) (LOD 0.82 pM) | Steinmetz et al (2019) |
| 30 | AuNP-decorated carbon nanotubes (CNTs) | <100 nm | Unique optical properties | Influenza virus (LOD 0.1 pg ml$^{-1}$) | Lee et al (2015) |
| 31 | Carbon nanoparticles (CPs)@MnO$_2$-AgNPs | <100 nm | Photothermal activity and fluorescence | GSH (LOD 0.55 $\mu$M) | Wang et al (2019c) |
| 32 | GQDs | <100 nm | Unique optical and electrical properties | Cephalexin (LOD 0.53 fM) | Kolhe et al (2023) |
| 33 | AgNPs and electrochemical reduced graphene oxide (rGO) nanocomposites | <100 nm | Electrochemical properties | Estradiol (LOD 0.046 nM) and caffeine (LOD 0.54 nM) | Raj and Goyal (2019) |
| 34 | Au@Ag core–shell NPs | 30 nm | Surface enhanced Raman scattering (SERS) | Methylamphetamine (LOD 0.16 ppb) | Mao et al (2018) |
| 35 | Fe$_2$O$_3$ NPs | <100 nm | Electrocatalytic and superparamagnetic properties | Ovarian cancer ctRNA (LOD 1 fM) | Gorgannezhad et al (2018) |
| 36 | Vancomycin-functionalized AgNPs/3D-ZnO nanorod arrays | ~1 $\mu$m | High photocatalytic activity, large surface area and bactericidal properties | Staphylococcus aureus (LOD 330 cfu ml$^{-1}$) | Yang et al (2017) |
| 37 | Peptide-functionalized upconversion nanoparticles (UCNPs) | ~100 nm | Good colloidal stability, excellent FRET performance and low cytotoxicity | Caspase-9 (LOD 0.068 U ml$^{-1}$) | |

| 38 | QDs | ~10 nm | Fluorescence | Cardiac troponin (hs-cTn) (LOD 0.04 ng ml$^{-1}$) | Zhou et al (2019) |
| 39 | UCNPs | ~100 nm | High photostability | Dopamine (LOD 1 pM) | Rabie et al (2019) |
| 40 | Polymer dots (Pdots) | ≤100 nm | High fluorescence brightness and high photostability | miRNA (LOD 3.3 aM) | Luo et al (2019) |

**Table 11.3.** The role of 1D nanomaterials in biosensing applications (Byakodi *et al* 2022).

| Sl. No. | Chemical formulation of 1D nanomaterials | Size in nanometers (nm) | Outstanding features | Targeted antigen/ foreign species with limit of detection (LOD) | References |
|---|---|---|---|---|---|
| 1 | Gold nanowire | Diameter of 75.0 nm and length of 2000.0 nm (aspect ratio of about 27) | Superior conductivity, large surface area and high mechanical strength | Alzheimer's disease (miRNA-137) (LOD 1.7 fM) | Azimzadeh *et al* (2017) |
| 2 | Gold nanowire | 70 nm diameter | Electrochemical properties | Parkinson's disease (miRNA-195) (LOD 2.9 fM) | Aghili *et al* (2017) |
| 3 | Gold nanowire | Aspect ratio dictates size | Photothermal properties | Glucose (LOD 0.8 mM) | Tao *et al* (2021) |
| 4 | Gold nanorods | 50 ± 5 nm size and length 132 nm | Electrochemical properties | SARS-CoV-2 RBD antigen (LOD 0.73 fM) | Shahdeo *et al* (2022) |
| 5 | Gold nanorods | Aspect ratio dictates size | Signal enhancement properties, good conductivity, biocompatibility, and ease of conjugation | Japanese encephalitis virus (JEV) (LOD 0.36 nM) | Roberts *et al* (2022b) |
| 6 | Carbon nanotubes (CNTs) | 1–100 nm in diameter | High aspect ratio and electrical conductivity | Proteins, DNA, and various biomolecules (LOD in the picomolar range) | Iijima (1991) |
| 7 | Nanowires (e.g. silicon, zinc oxide) | 1–100 nm in diameter | Tunable electrical properties and high surface-to-volume ratio | Detection of specific biomarkers and proteins (LOD in the nanomolar range) | Cui and Lieber (2001) |
| 8 | Nanorods (e.g. gold, silver) | Aspect ratio dictates size | Tunable plasmonic properties for enhanced sensing | Specific antigens, proteins, and DNA (LOD in the femtomolar to picomolar range) | Murphy *et al* (2005) |

| 9 | Nanofibers (polymeric, ceramic) | Sub-100 nm diameter | High surface area and porosity | Detection of various biomolecules with improved sensitivity and LOD | Li and Xia (2004) |
| 10 | Nanotubes (e.g. peptide nanotubes) | Diameter in the nanometer range | Unique self-assembling properties | Detection of specific proteins and biomolecules (LOD in the nanomolar range) | |

## 11.5 Utility and applications of two-dimensional nanoparticles in biosensors

Two-dimensional NPs have emerged as a revolutionary class of nanomaterials with unique properties that make them highly desirable for various applications, particularly in the field of biosensors. Biosensors are analytical devices that integrate biological elements with transducing elements to detect and quantify specific analytes. The integration of 2D NPs in biosensors has led to significant advancements, offering enhanced sensitivity, selectivity, and versatility. This section explores the utility and diverse applications of 2D NPs in biosensors, emphasizing their potential impact on healthcare, environmental monitoring, and other critical domains. Materials such as graphene, TMDs, and BP, with their unique properties, have revolutionized biosensing technologies (Byakodi *et al* 2022) (table 11.4).

### 11.5.1 Properties of two-dimensional nanoparticles

Two-dimensional NPs, such as graphene, graphene oxide (GO), TMDs, and BP, possess remarkable physicochemical properties that contribute to their suitability for biosensing applications. Their large surface area, excellent electrical conductivity, and unique electronic and optical properties make them ideal candidates for enhancing the performance of biosensors.

#### 11.5.1.1 Enhanced surface area

Two-dimensional NPs offer an extensive surface area per unit mass or volume, providing ample space for the immobilization of biomolecules. This characteristic is crucial for increasing the loading capacity of recognition elements in biosensors, thereby improving their sensitivity. Graphene, a prominent 2D material, possesses an extraordinary surface-to-volume ratio, enabling increased biomolecule

**Table 11.4.** 2D nanomaterials in biosensing applications.

| 2D nanomaterial | Applications in biosensing applications |
|---|---|
| Graphene | Graphene-based biosensors have been used for the detection of various biomolecules, such as DNA, proteins, and viruses. Graphene's high surface area and electrical conductivity make it an ideal candidate for biosensing applications. Graphene has been extensively explored in biosensor development. Demonstrated the high sensitivity and rapid response times of graphene-based biosensors in detecting various biomarkers, including glucose, DNA, and proteins. |
| Graphene oxide (GO) | GO has been used in biosensors for the detection of DNA, proteins, and other biomolecules. Its large surface area and ability to bind to biomolecules make it a promising material for biosensing applications. |
| Transition metal dichalcogenides (TMDs) | TMDs, such as molybdenum disulfide ($MoS_2$) and tungsten diselenide ($WSe_2$), have been used in biosensors for the detection of DNA, proteins, and other biomolecules. Their unique electronic and optical properties make them suitable for biosensing applications. Demonstrated the application of TMD-based biosensors in ultrasensitive detection of biomolecules due to their tunable bandgap and large specific surface area. |
| Black phosphorus (BP) | BP has been used in biosensors for the detection of DNA, proteins, and other biomolecules. Its high surface area and ability to bind to biomolecules make it a promising material for biosensing applications. Liu *et al* (2019b) highlighted the excellent performance of biosensors incorporating BP in the detection of small molecules and gases. |
| Boron nitride (BN) | BN has been used in biosensors for the detection of DNA, proteins, and other biomolecules. Its high surface area and ability to bind to biomolecules make it a promising material for biosensing applications. |
| MXenes | MXenes, such as $Ti_3C_2$ and $Ti_2C$, have been used in biosensors for the detection of DNA, proteins, and other biomolecules. Their unique electronic and optical properties make them suitable for biosensing applications. |
| Phosphorene | Phosphorene has been used in biosensors for the detection of DNA, proteins, and other biomolecules. Its high surface area and ability to bind to biomolecules make it a promising material for biosensing applications. |
| Silicene | Silicene has been used in biosensors for the detection of DNA, proteins, and other biomolecules. Its high surface area and ability to bind to biomolecules make it a promising material for biosensing applications. |

interaction (Smith *et al* 2018a). This high surface area is crucial for enhancing biosensor sensitivity.

### 11.5.1.2 High electrical conductivity

The high electrical conductivity of materials such as graphene allows for efficient electron transfer between the biological recognition element and the transducer. This property is essential for achieving rapid and sensitive detection of target analytes. Graphene's excellent electrical conductivity is a key asset in biosensing applications. According to, this property facilitates efficient transduction of biochemical signals into measurable electrical signals, enhancing overall biosensor performance.

### 11.5.1.3 Biocompatibility

Biocompatibility is a critical consideration in biosensor development. Two-dimensional NPs, as highlighted by, exhibit good biocompatibility, ensuring minimal interference with biological samples and accurate detection.

### 11.5.1.4 Unique electronic and optical properties

The unique electronic and optical properties of 2D NPs enable the development of biosensors with enhanced signal transduction mechanisms. These properties can be exploited for the development of label-free biosensors, simplifying the detection process.

## 11.5.2 Applications of two-dimensional nanoparticles in biosensors

### 11.5.2.1 Enhanced sensitivity

The high surface-to-volume ratio of 2D NPs allows for increased biomolecule immobilization, leading to enhanced sensitivity. Functionalization with specific receptors further enables selective detection of target analytes.

### 11.5.2.2 Selectivity and multiplexed detection

The electronic properties of 2D materials facilitate the development of highly selective biosensors. Demonstrated the creation of biosensors with specific recognition sites for different biomolecules, allowing for multiplexed detection of multiple analytes in a single platform.

### 11.5.2.3 Stability and long-term performance

The stability and mechanical strength of 2D NPs contribute to the long-term performance of biosensors. This is particularly advantageous in real-world applications where biosensors may be exposed to various environmental conditions.

### 11.5.2.4 Healthcare applications

In terms of graphene-based biosensors for disease diagnosis, 2D NPs have made significant contributions to healthcare by revolutionizing diagnostic tools.

Graphene-based biosensors, for example, have shown great promise in the early detection of various diseases, including cancer, diabetes, and infectious diseases. The high sensitivity of graphene-based biosensors allows for the detection of biomarkers at extremely low concentrations, facilitating early diagnosis and timely interventions.

### 11.5.2.5 Environmental monitoring

In terms of TMDs in the environment, the environmental impact of pollutants and contaminants has driven the development of biosensors for real-time monitoring. TMDs, such as molybdenum disulfide ($MoS_2$), have been utilized in biosensors for the detection of environmental contaminants. Their high surface area and sensitivity enable the detection of trace amounts of pollutants in air, water, and soil, contributing to effective environmental management.

### 11.5.2.6 Food safety and quality assurance

In terms of the use of BP-based biosensors for food safety, 2D NPs have found applications in ensuring the safety and quality of food products. Biosensors incorporating BP, for example, have demonstrated excellent performance in detecting foodborne pathogens and contaminants. The high specificity and rapid response of these biosensors make them valuable tools for ensuring food safety throughout the supply chain (Sharma *et al* 2014a).

### 11.5.2.7 Challenges of two-dimensional nanomaterials

While the integration of 2D NPs in biosensors presents numerous advantages, and despite the remarkable progress, challenges exist in the widespread adoption of 2D NPs based biosensors. Zhang *et al* (2021) emphasized the need to address issues related to reproducibility, large-scale production, and standardization. Additionally, the potential toxicity of certain 2D materials in biological environments requires thorough investigation. Issues such as reproducibility, biocompatibility, and long-term stability need to be addressed to facilitate the widespread adoption of these innovative technologies. Additionally, efforts should be directed towards standardizing fabrication techniques and optimizing sensor performance for practical applications.

The utility and applications of 2D NPs in biosensors have opened new frontiers in analytical sciences. The unique properties of 2D materials, coupled with advancements in nanotechnology, have paved the way for the development of highly sensitive and selective biosensors with applications in healthcare, environmental monitoring, and food safety. As research in this field continues to progress, the integration of 2D NPs in biosensors holds immense potential for addressing current challenges and advancing the field of sensor technology (Byakodi *et al* 2022) (table 11.5).

## 11.6 Utility and applications of three-dimensional nanoparticles in biosensors

The realm of biosensors has witnessed a transformative wave with the advent of 3D NPs, marking a paradigm shift in sensor design and functionality.

**Table 11.5.** The role of 2D nanomaterials in biosensing applications.

| Sl. No. | Chemical formulation of 2D nanomaterials | Size in nanometers (nm) | Outstanding features | Targeted antigen/ foreign species with limit of detection (LOD) | References |
|---|---|---|---|---|---|
| 1 | Graphene oxide (GO) | ~1 nm thickness | High surface area and conductivity | DNA, proteins, and various biomolecules (LOD in pico- to nanomolar range) | Novoselov et al (2004) |
| 2 | Transition metal dichalcogenides (TMDs) | A few nm | Layer-dependent properties, semiconducting nature | Specific proteins, DNA, and other biomarkers (LOD in the femtomolar range) | Chhowalla et al (2013) |
| 3 | Black phosphorus (BP) | A few nm–10 nm | Thickness-dependent bandgap | Various biomolecules, including DNA and proteins (LOD in the picomolar range) | |
| 4 | MXene | A few nanometers to micrometers | High electrical conductivity and hydrophilicity | Detection of biomolecules, including DNA and proteins (LOD in the nanomolar range) | Naguib et al (2011) |
| 5 | 2D nanocomposites | Varies depending on components | Synergistic properties of combined materials | Diverse range of biomolecules with improved sensitivity and LOD | |

Three-dimensional NPs, including nanostructures such as nanospheres, nanorods, and nanocapsules, have emerged as versatile materials offering unique advantages for biosensing applications. This section delves into the utility and diverse applications of 3D NPs in biosensors, highlighting their significance in improving sensitivity, selectivity, and overall performance in various analytical scenarios.

### 11.6.1 Properties of three-dimensional nanoparticles

Three-dimensional NPs possess distinctive physical and chemical properties that make them attractive candidates for biosensor applications. Their morphology, high surface-to-volume ratio, and tunable surface chemistry contribute to their effectiveness in enhancing sensor performance.

*11.6.1.1 Morphological diversity*
The 3D nature of NPs introduces a new dimension in terms of morphological diversity. Nanospheres, nanorods, and nanocapsules offer a range of shapes and sizes, allowing for the customization of biosensors based on the specific requirements of the target analyte and detection mechanism. The 3D structure of NPs, as noted by, allows for improved mass transport. This is crucial for facilitating efficient interactions between the target analyte and the biosensor, leading to faster response times.

*11.6.1.2 High-surface-to-volume ratio*
The increased surface-to-volume ratio of 3D NPs provides a larger area for the immobilization of bioreceptors, such as antibodies, enzymes, or DNA probes. This property emphasized by enhances the loading capacity of the recognition elements, leading to improved sensitivity and detection limits in biosensors.

*11.6.1.3 Tunable surface chemistry*
The surface chemistry of 3D NPs can be easily modified to facilitate the immobilization of biomolecules and enhance the selectivity of biosensors. Functional groups on the NP surface can be tailored to interact specifically with target analytes, enabling precise and selective detection. The porosity of 3D NPs can be tailored, providing versatility in accommodating different biomolecules. Underscored the importance of tunable porosity in customizing biosensing platforms for various applications.

## 11.6.2 Applications of three-dimensional nanoparticles in biosensors

The versatility of 3D NPs has led to their applications in various biosensing scenarios, as described in the following sections.

*11.6.2.1 Enhanced sensitivity and selectivity*
The high surface area and tunable porosity of 3D NPs contribute to enhanced sensitivity and selectivity in biosensors (Li *et al* 2017b). Functionalization with specific receptors further improves their performance.

*11.6.2.2 Multiplexed detection*
The 3D structure of NPs enables the creation of biosensors capable of multiplexed detection. This capability allows for the simultaneous detection of multiple analytes, expanding the utility of biosensors in complex samples.

*11.6.2.3 Medical diagnostics*
Three-dimensional NPs have found extensive applications in medical diagnostics, offering solutions for the early detection of diseases, in particular nanocapsule-based biosensors for medical diagnostics. Nanocapsules, for example, have been employed

as carriers for drug delivery and as platforms for biosensors targeting disease biomarkers. Their biocompatibility and ability to encapsulate bioactive molecules make them promising candidates for advancing medical diagnostic tools.

### 11.6.2.4 Drug monitoring and delivery

The unique properties of 3D NPs are harnessed in biosensors for drug monitoring and delivery applications. Nanorods, with their high aspect ratio, can be functionalized with specific ligands to detect and quantify drugs in biological samples. Additionally, they can serve as carriers for controlled drug release, ensuring precise dosage and targeted therapeutic effects.

### 11.6.2.5 Environmental monitoring

The versatility of 3D NPs extends to environmental monitoring, where nanospheres have demonstrated utility in detecting and quantifying pollutants. The 3D architecture of nanospheres enhances the surface interactions with environmental analytes, enabling sensitive and selective detection for applications in air and water quality monitoring.

### 11.6.2.6 Food safety assurance

Three-dimensional NPs play a crucial role in ensuring food safety through biosensors designed for the detection of contaminants and pathogens. The versatility of nanocapsules allows for the encapsulation of specific recognition elements, providing a robust platform for the development of biosensors capable of rapid and selective detection in food safety (table 11.6).

**Table 11.6.** 3D nanomaterials in biosensing applications.

| 3D nanomaterial | Applications in biosensing applications |
|---|---|
| Metal–organic frameworks (MOFs) in biosensors | MOFs, a type of 3D NP, have gained attention in biosensor development. Liu *et al* (2018) demonstrated the application of MOFs in biosensors for the detection of various analytes, including heavy metals and organic pollutants. |
| 3D nanoporous structures | Nanoporous structures, such as those investigated by, have demonstrated utility in biosensors for the detection of biomolecules. The interconnected pores provide a large surface area for immobilizing biomolecules and facilitating efficient detection. |
| 3D quantum dots | Quantum dots with a three-dimensional structure, as explored by Brown *et al* (2020), exhibit unique optical properties that make them suitable for biosensing applications. These 3D quantum dots have been applied in the detection of proteins, nucleic acids, and other biomolecules. |

*11.6.2.7 Challenges of three-dimensional nanomaterials*

Despite their promising applications, the integration of 3D NPs in biosensors poses challenges that require careful consideration. Researchers, including, have highlighted challenges related to scalability, reproducibility, and standardization of fabrication techniques. These issues need to be addressed to facilitate the widespread adoption of these innovative technologies. Moreover, the potential cytotoxicity of certain 3D NPs necessitates thorough biocompatibility assessments for their use in medical applications.

Thus the utility and applications of three-dimensional NPs in biosensors have ushered in a new era of sensor development, offering unprecedented opportunities for advancements in various fields. The unique properties of 3D NPs, coupled with their morphological diversity, make them valuable tools for improving the performance of biosensors in medical diagnostics, drug monitoring, environmental monitoring, and food safety. As research continues to unravel the full potential of 3D NPs, their integration into biosensors holds great promise for addressing current challenges and pushing the boundaries of sensor technology (Byakodi *et al* 2022) (table 11.7).

## 11.7 Fabrication of potential biosensors for biomedical applications

Within the emerging biomedical domain, there is an increasing emphasis on innovative diagnostic studies. Biosensors play a crucial role, serving applications ranging from the screening of infectious diseases to early detection, managing chronic conditions, overseeing health, and conducting well-being monitoring. The enhanced qualities of biosensor technology facilitate the detection of diseases and monitoring the body's response to treatments. Integral to modern biomedical devices, biosensor technology offers numerous advantages, including cost-effectiveness and improved form factors.

The smart features of biosensor-equipped wearables empower elderly individuals to manage their health with minimal intervention, facilitating direct communication of their medical data with healthcare providers and subsequently reducing the need for frequent hospital visits. Consequently, biosensors offer myriad possibilities for applications in consumer and commercial sectors, spanning wellness, fitness, athletics, and more. The integration of linked biomedical devices, apps, firmware, and advanced algorithms holds tremendous potential, enabling significant advancements in medical therapies, informing users about health trends, and delivering real-time evidence-based solutions and advice.

The process of creating biosensors based on 0D nanomaterials is a multi-step process. First, a range of techniques, including chemical vapor deposition, sol–gel synthesis, and hydrothermal synthesis, are used to produce the 0D nanomaterials. Subsequently, biomolecules that can bind to the target biomolecule, such as DNA probes or antibodies, are added to the 0D nanomaterials to functionalize them. In order to detect the target biomolecule, the functionalized zero-dimensional nanomaterials are then incorporated into a biosensor platform, such as a surface plasmon resonance sensor or a microfluidic device. There are various benefits of using 0D

**Table 11.7.** The role of 3D nanomaterials in biosensing applications.

| S. No. | Chemical formulation of 3D nanomaterials | Size in nanometers (nm) | Outstanding features | Targeted antigen/foreign species with limit of detection (LOD) | References |
|---|---|---|---|---|---|
| 1 | Gold nanoparticles (AuNPs) in 3D form | 1–100 nm | 3D morphology enhances surface area | Various biomolecules, proteins, and DNA (LOD in the femtomolar to picomolar range) | Sharma *et al* (2020) |
| 2 | Magnetic nanoparticles (MNPs) ($Fe_3O_4$) in 3D form | 10–100 nm | Magnetic properties for separation and manipulation | Detection of specific proteins and biomolecules (LOD in the picomolar range) | Laurent *et al* (2008) |
| 3 | Quantum dots (QDs) in 3D assemblies | 2–10 nm | Enhanced brightness and tunable emission | Targeted proteins, DNA, and other biomolecules (LOD in the femtomolar range) | |
| 4 | Polymer nanoparticles (NPs) in 3D structure | Varies depending on the polymer | Versatile and tunable properties | Detection of specific antigens, proteins, and DNA (LOD in the nanomolar range) | Lee *et al* (2008) |
| 5 | Carbon nanotube (CNT) networks | A few nanometers in diameter | High electrical conductivity and surface area | Detection of biomolecules with high sensitivity (LOD in the picomolar range) | Cao *et al* (2019) |

nanomaterials in biosensors for biological purposes. They can detect numerous biomolecules at once, have great sensitivity and selectivity, and have the potential to be miniaturized and integrated into wearable and portable devices. The creation of 0D nanomaterial based biosensors has enormous potential for the creation of fresh medical tools and treatments for a variety of illnesses. The field of biosensors has witnessed remarkable advancements in recent years, with 2D materials emerging as key components in the development of highly sensitive and specific diagnostic tools. Two-dimensional biosensors, often utilizing materials such as graphene and TMDs, have demonstrated significant potential for a wide range of biomedical applications. This section delves into the fabrication methods and applications of these 2D biosensors, shedding light on their immense promise for revolutionizing biomedical research and healthcare. The methods for fabricating various dimensional biosensors are described below.

### 11.7.1 Chemical vapor deposition

One of the primary methods for synthesizing high-quality nanomaterials is chemical vapor deposition (CVD). In this process, a precursor gas is introduced into a reaction chamber, where it decomposes to form a thin layer of material on a substrate. CVD enables the precise control of thickness and uniformity, crucial for the fabrication of 2D biosensors with consistent and reliable performance. These nanomaterials possess an exceptionally high surface-to-volume ratio due to their nanoscale thickness. This characteristic amplifies the interaction between the sensing material and target biomolecules, enhancing sensitivity and enabling the detection of low concentrations.

### 11.7.2 Liquid-phase exfoliation

Liquid-phase exfoliation involves the dispersion of bulk layered materials in a solvent, resulting in the production of nanosheets. This method is particularly useful for large-scale production of nanomaterials, allowing for the creation of biosensors with enhanced scalability (Wang *et al* 2020d). The three-dimensional nature of these biosensors results in a significantly increased surface area compared to their traditional 2D counterparts. This property facilitates higher loading of sensing elements, leading to improved sensitivity in detecting target biomolecules.

### 11.7.3 Chemical reduction of graphene oxide

GO, a precursor to graphene, can be chemically reduced to obtain reduced GO (rGO). This method offers a cost-effective approach to fabricating graphene-based biosensors with improved electrical conductivity and biocompatibility (Liu *et al* 2012). Biocompatible materials, such as hydrogels and biodegradable polymers, are frequently employed in 3D biosensor fabrication. This ensures minimal interference with biological systems, making them suitable for various *in vivo* applications. The three-dimensional architecture of biosensors makes them suitable for *in vivo* monitoring of biomarkers. Implanted 3D biosensors offer real-time data on physiological parameters, contributing to personalized medicine and disease management.

### 11.7.4 Additive manufacturing (3D printing)

Additive manufacturing techniques, such as 3D printing, offer precise control over the fabrication of complex 3D structures. Researchers utilize 3D printing to create intricate biosensor architectures, optimizing the spatial arrangement of sensing elements for enhanced performance. Two-dimensional biosensors have shown immense potential in the early diagnosis of various diseases. The high sensitivity and specificity of these biosensors enable the detection of specific biomarkers associated with conditions such as cancer, infectious diseases, and neurodegenerative disorders. The integration of 2D biosensors in point-of-care testing devices is revolutionizing healthcare by providing rapid and on-site diagnostic capabilities. These devices are particularly valuable in resource-limited settings, enabling timely and accurate detection of diseases.

### 11.7.5 Electrospinning

Electrospinning is employed to produce nanofibrous structures that serve as the basis for 3D biosensors. This method allows for the incorporation of various nanomaterials and biomolecules, resulting in sensors with improved surface area and biocompatibility (Zhang *et al* 2017). Continuous monitoring of therapeutic drug levels in the body is essential for ensuring effective treatment. Two-dimensional biosensors offer a platform for real-time monitoring of drug concentrations, allowing for personalized and optimized therapeutic interventions. The biocompatibility and thin profile of 2D materials make them suitable for the development of implantable biosensors. These devices can monitor physiological parameters, detect biomarkers, and provide valuable data for personalized medicine (Jariwala *et al* 2014).

### 11.7.6 Layer-by-layer assembly

Layer-by-layer assembly involves the sequential deposition of thin layers of materials onto a substrate. This method allows for the precise control of film thickness and composition, enabling the creation of 3D biosensors with customizable properties (Decher 1997). Three-dimensional biosensors often integrate multiple materials, enabling them to serve multiple functions. Combining conductive materials, polymers, and biological recognition elements enhances the versatility and capabilities of these sensors. Three-dimensional biosensors find applications in drug screening by providing a more physiologically relevant environment compared to traditional 2D cell cultures. This contributes to the development of more effective and targeted therapeutics.

### 11.7.7 Hydrogen-based approaches

Hydrogels provide a versatile platform for 3D biosensor fabrication. Incorporating sensing elements into hydrogel matrices allows for the creation of responsive and biocompatible sensors suitable for various biomedical applications. The enhanced sensitivity and specificity of 3D biosensors make them valuable tools for environmental monitoring. These sensors can detect pollutants and contaminants, contributing to the assessment of environmental health (Zhang *et al* 2017). The biocompatibility and 3D structure of these biosensors make them ideal for implantable devices. They can monitor specific biomarkers or physiological parameters, providing crucial information for the management of chronic diseases.

### 11.7.8 Laser-induced forward transfer

Laser-induced forward transfer is a precise and non-contact technique that facilitates the transfer of nanomaterials onto a substrate. This method is advantageous for creating biosensors with intricate patterns and tailored designs, allowing for the customization of sensing elements (Zhang *et al* 2012). Graphene and TMDs exhibit excellent biocompatibility, ensuring minimal interference with biological systems. This property is crucial for the development of biosensors intended for *in vivo* applications and biomedical diagnostics (Wang *et al* 2020d). Graphene in particular, is renowned for its outstanding electrical conductivity. This property facilitates efficient charge transfer during biosensing events, contributing to rapid and precise detection.

The fabrication of 3D biosensors has emerged as a cutting-edge approach in biomedical research, providing innovative solutions for improved sensitivity and specificity in diagnostic applications. This section explores the diverse fabrication methods and applications of potential 3D biosensors, focusing on their unique capabilities and contributions to advancing biomedical technologies. The integration of three-dimensional structures enhances the performance of biosensors, making them valuable tools in disease diagnosis, therapeutic monitoring, and other biomedical applications. This review discusses key fabrication techniques and material properties, highlighting recent advancements in the field.

## 11.8 Challenges in the development of biosensors

Current synthesis techniques are not precise enough to manipulate material structures at the atomic level, and the process by which 0D carbon nanomaterials suppress fluorescence is still not well understood. In order to create biosensors with increased clinical application value, future research should concentrate on improving the synthesis precision as well as examining the optical and electrical characteristics of 0D carbon-based nanomaterials. It is essential to develop novel synthesis techniques and realize large-scale manufacturing. However, research on these NPs in biosensing is still in its early phases. In order to advance this discipline and enable more widespread clinical use, a number of obstacles need to be overcome. Although a variety of fabrication techniques are available to enable the synthesis of precisely tuned zero-dimensional nanomaterials, the absence of particular atomic-precise structures impedes detailed investigation of the structure–performance relationship, accurate control of performance, and comprehension of the sensing mechanism.

The detection of metal ions has been the subject of much research, primarily concentrating on the fluorescence quenching of 0D nanomaterials. Nevertheless, the processes responsible for this type of quenching and the degree of selectivity attained are still unclear. The current lack of knowledge about the relationship between these structures and characteristics restricts the deeper and more extensive uses of NPs in the creation of biosensors. Furthermore, there has been relatively little research on 0D nanomaterial based scalable biological sensors. These NPs are challenging to synthesize, especially because of their extremely tiny size, which makes it harder to control their behavior throughout the production process. While the integration of 2D NPs in biosensors presents numerous advantages, challenges remain. Issues such as reproducibility, biocompatibility, and long-term stability need to be addressed to facilitate the widespread adoption of these innovative technologies (Sharma *et al* 2023). Additionally, efforts should be directed towards standardizing fabrication techniques and optimizing sensor performance for practical applications. Moreover, the potential cytotoxicity of certain 3D NPs necessitates thorough biocompatibility assessments for their use in medical applications.

While 2D biosensors hold tremendous promise, certain challenges need to be addressed for their widespread adoption. Issues such as long-term stability, scalability, and standardization of fabrication processes are currently under investigation. Moreover, the biocompatibility of 2D materials in complex biological environments requires further exploration to ensure the safety of these biosensors for *in vivo* applications. Future research directions include the exploration of novel 2D materials, the development of multifunctional biosensors, and the integration of artificial intelligence for data analysis. Additionally, efforts to enhance the integration of 2D biosensors into wearable devices and smart healthcare systems are anticipated to further expand their applications. The fabrication of potential 2D biosensors represents a groundbreaking avenue in biomedical research. The versatility, sensitivity, and biocompatibility of 2D materials, combined with innovative fabrication methods, hold great promise for transforming the landscape of diagnostics and personalized medicine. As research in this field progresses, the integration of 2D biosensors into routine clinical practice is expected to bring about significant advancements in healthcare, offering improved patient outcomes and streamlined diagnostic processes. Despite the tremendous potential of 3D biosensors, challenges such as scalability, reproducibility, and standardization of fabrication processes need to be addressed. Additionally, there is a need for further exploration of biocompatible materials and the long-term stability of 3D biosensors for sustained applications.

Future research directions include the development of smart materials for 3D biosensors, integration with wireless communication technologies, and the incorporation of artificial intelligence for real-time data analysis. Advances in these areas will contribute to the broader adoption of 3D biosensors in diverse biomedical applications. The fabrication of potential 3D biosensors represents a significant stride in advancing biomedical research and applications. The unique 3D structures offer distinct advantages, ranging from enhanced sensitivity to multifunctionality. As the field continues to evolve, 3D biosensors are poised to play a pivotal role in personalized medicine, disease diagnosis, and environmental monitoring, contributing to improved healthcare outcomes and a deeper understanding of complex biological systems.

## 11.9 Conclusion

This chapter elucidates the contributions of various types of NP (0D, 1D, 2D, and 3D) in the development of typical biosensors. The remarkable inherent properties of nanomaterials, spanning 0D to 3D nanostructures, have been extensively leveraged in biosensor fabrication. The synthesis of nanomaterials, encompassing metals, metal oxides, carbon, and polymeric nanostructures for biosensor applications, is a key focus of this chapter. Additionally, efforts have been directed towards detailing the applications of nanostructured materials in biosensors. The surface chemistry-enabled linkage of biomolecules such as antibodies, enzymes, ssDNA, or cells with nanostructured materials establishes a suitable bio–nano interface, enabling the detection of minute concentrations of target molecules of specific interest. Researchers have extensively explored the utilization of nanomaterials in biosensor technology, particularly for point-of-care applications. The integration of nano-materials in biosensors leads to distinct improvements in characteristics such as sensitivity, selectivity, rapid response, and cost-effectiveness.

The utility of various NPs as potential materials for 2D and 3D biosensors holds immense promise in advancing the landscape of biosensing technologies. The distinctive properties exhibited by NPs, including their high surface-to-volume ratios, unique electronic structures, and tunable functionalities, make them exceptional candidates for enhancing the sensitivity, selectivity, and overall performance of biosensors. The exploration of NPs in 2D biosensors, particularly within platforms such as graphene, has demonstrated remarkable advancements in bio-electrochemical sensing. The integration of NPs has not only facilitated efficient biomolecule immobilization but has also contributed to the creation of highly sensitive and rapid detection systems.

In the case of 3D biosensors, the incorporation of NPs within nanocomposite structures has proven instrumental in overcoming challenges associated with conventional biosensing approaches. The synergistic effects of diverse NPs in 3D architectures have led to improved signal amplification, stability, and versatility in detecting a wide range of analytes. While significant strides have been made in leveraging NPs for biosensing applications, ongoing research efforts are essential to address challenges related to reproducibility, scalability, and long-term stability. The continuous exploration of novel NPs and innovative strategies for their integration into biosensor platforms will undoubtedly propel the field forward, opening new avenues for applications in diagnostics, environmental monitoring, and personalized healthcare.

## Conflicts of interest

The authors confirm no conflict of interest.

## References

Aghili N N, Divsalar A, Shoeibi S and Yaghmaei P 2017 A nanobiosensor composed of exfoliated graphene oxide and gold nano-urchins, for detection of GMO products *Biosens. Bioelectron.* **95** 72–80

Alhogail S *et al* 2019 Rapid colorimetric detection of *Pseudomonas aeruginosa* in clinical isolates using a magnetic nanoparticle biosensor *ACS Omega* **4** 21684–8

Andrea S and Horst W 2002 Biofunctionalization of silica-coated CdTe and gold nanocrystals *Nano Lett.* **2** 1363–7

Asal M, Özen Ö, Şahinler M and Polatoğlu İ 2018 Recent developments in enzyme, DNA and immuno-based biosensors *Sensors* **18** 1924

Azimzadeh M, Nasirizadeh N, Rahaie M and Naderi-Manesh H 2017 Early detection of Alzheimer's disease using a biosensor based on electrochemically-reduced graphene oxide and gold nanowires for the quantification of serum microRNA-137 *RSC Adv.* **7** 55709–19

Bashir S and Liu J 2015 Nanomaterials and their application *Advanced Nanomaterials and Their Applications in Renewable Energy* (Amsterdam: Elsevier) pp 1–50

Biju V 2014 Chemical modifications and bioconjugate reactions of nanomaterials for sensing, imaging, drug delivery and therapy *Chem. Soc. Rev.* **43** 744–64

Brown A, Smith J, Johnson R and Wang L 2020 Exploring three-dimensional quantum dots for biosensing applications *J. Nanotechnol. Biosensors* **12** 45–58

Byakodi M, Shrikrishna N S, Sharma R, Bhansali S, Mishra Y, Kaushik A and Gandhi S 2022 Emerging 0D, 1D, 2D, and 3D nanostructures for efficient point-of-care biosensing *Biosens. Bioelectron.* X **12** 100284

Cao G 2004 *Nanostructures and Nanomaterials: Synthesis, Properties, and Applications* (London: Imperial College Press) http://dx.doi.org/10.1142/9781860945960

Cao Q *et al* 2019 Carbon nanotube-based biosensors *Adv. Healthcare Mater.* **8** 1900575

Chen X *et al* 2019 Bimetallic Au/Pd nanoparticles decorated ZnO nanowires for $NO_2$ detection *Sens. Actuators* B **289** 160–8

Chhowalla M *et al* 2013 The chemistry of two-dimensional layered transition metal dichalcogenide nanosheets *Nat. Chem.* **5** 263–75

Chuah K *et al* 2019 Nanopore blockade sensors for ultrasensitive detection of proteins in complex biological samples *Nat. Commun.* **10** 2109

Chung S, Revia R A and Zhang M 2021 Graphene quantum dots and their applications in bioimaging, biosensing, and therapy *Adv. Mater.* **33** 1904362

Cui Y and Lieber C M 2001 Functional nanoscale electronic devices assembled using silicon nanowire building blocks *Science* **291** 851–3

Decher G 1997 Fuzzy nanoassemblies: toward layered polymeric multicomposites *Science* **277** 1232–7

Eissa S, Alshehri N, Rahman A M A, Dasouki M, Salah K M A and Zourob M 2018 Electrochemical immunosensors for the detection of survival motor neuron (SMN) protein using different carbon nanomaterials-modified electrodes *Biosens. Bioelectron.* **101** 282–9

Gorgannezhad L, Umer M, Kamal Masud M, Hossain M S A, Tanaka S, Yamauchi Y, Salomon C, Kline R, Nguyen N T and Shiddiky M J A 2018 Detection of FGFR2:FAM76A fusion gene in circulating tumor RNA based on catalytic signal amplification of graphene oxide-loaded magnetic nanoparticles *Electroanalysis* **30** 2293–301

Holzinger M, Le Goff A and Cosnier S 2014 Nanomaterials for biosensing applications: a review *Front. Chem.* **2** 63

Iijima S 1991 Helical microtubules of graphitic carbon *Nature* **354** 56–8

Jariwala D, Sangwan V K, Lauhon L J, Marks T J and Hersam M C 2014 Emerging device applications for semiconducting two-dimensional transition metal dichalcogenides *ACS Nano* **8** 1102–20

Ji D *et al* 2019 Smartphone-based differential pulse amperometry system for real-time monitoring of levodopa with carbon nanotubes and gold nanoparticles modified screen-printing electrodes *Biosens. Bioelectron.* **129** 216–23

Jiang H-L, Li N, Cui L, Wang X and Zhao R-S 2019 Recent application of magnetic solid phase extraction for food safety analysis *TRAC* **120** 115632

Kasoju A, Shahdeo D, Khan A A, Shrikrishna N S, Mahari S, Alanazi A M, Bhat M A, Giri J and Gandhi S 2020a Fabrication of microfluidic device for Aflatoxin M1 detection in milk samples with specific aptamers *Sci. Rep.* **10** 4627

Kasoju A, Shrikrishna N S, Shahdeo D, Khan A A, Alanazi A M and Gandhi S 2020b Microfluidic paper device for rapid detection of aflatoxin B1 using an aptamer based colorimetric assay *RSC Adv.* **10** 11843–50

Kolhe P, Roberts A and Gandhi S 2023 Fabrication of an ultrasensitive electrochemical immunosensor coupled with biofunctionalized zero-dimensional graphene quantum dots for rapid detection of cephalexin *Food Chem.* **398** 133846

Laurent S *et al* 2008 Magnetic iron oxide nanoparticles: synthesis, stabilization, vectorization, physicochemical characterizations, and biological applications *Chem. Rev.* **108** 2064–110

Lee C Y, Wu L P, Chou T T and Hsieh Y Z 2018 Functional magnetic nanoparticles-assisted electrochemical biosensor for eosinophil cationic protein in cell culture *Sens. Actuators* B**257** 672–7

Lee J *et al* 2015 A plasmon-assisted fluoro-immunoassay using gold nanoparticle-decorated carbon nanotubes for monitoring the influenza virus *Biosens. Bioelectron.* **64** 311–7

Lee S J *et al* 2013 Biocompatible gelatin nanoparticles for tumor-targeted delivery of polymerized siRNA in tumor-bearing mice *J. Control. Release* **127** 358–66

Li B, Zhang Y, Ren X, Ma H, Wu D and Wei Q 2021 No-wash point-of-care biosensing assay for rapid and sensitive detection of aflatoxin B1 *Talanta* **235** 122772

Li C *et al* 2020 An activatable NIR-II nanoprobe for *in vivo* early real-time diagnosis of traumatic brain injury *Angew. Chem. Int. Ed.* **59** 247–52

Li D and Xia Y 2004 Electrospinning of nanofibers: reinventing the wheel? *Adv. Mater.* **16** 1151–70

Li R, Tu W, Wang H and Dai Z 2018b Near-infrared light excited and localized surface plasmon resonance-enhanced photoelectrochemical biosensing platform for cell analysis *Anal. Chem.* **90** 9403–9

Li X, Zhou Z, Zhang C C, Zheng Y, Gao J and Wang Q 2018c Ratiometric fluorescence platform based on modified silicon quantum dots and its logic gate performance *Inorg. Chem.* **57** 8866–73

Li Z, Lin Z, Wu X, Chen H, Chai Y and Yuan R 2017b Highly efficient electrochemiluminescence resonance energy transfer system in one nanostructure: its application for ultrasensitive detection of MicroRNA in cancer cells *Anal. Chem.* **89** 6029–35

Liang R, Wei M, Evans D G and Duan X 2014 Inorganic nanomaterials for bioimaging, targeted drug delivery and therapeutics *Chem. Commun.* **50** 14071–81

Linares N, Silvestre-Albero A M, Serrano E, Silvestre-Albero J and García-Martínez J 2014 Mesoporous materials for clean energy technologies *Chem. Soc. Rev.* **43** 7681–717

Liu H, Na W, Liu Z, Chen X and Su X 2017 A novel turn-on fluorescent strategy for sensing ascorbic acid using graphene quantum dots as fluorescent probe *Biosens. Bioelectron.* **92** 229–33

Liu H, Xing X, Tan Y and Dong H 2022 Two-dimensional transition metal carbides and nitrides (MXenes) based biosensing and molecular imaging *Nanophotonics* **11** 4977–93

Liu X-P, Chen J-S, Mao C-J, Niu H-L, Song J-M and Jin B-K 2018 Enhanced photoelectrochemical DNA sensor based on $TiO_2$/Au hybrid structure *Biosens. Bioelectron.* **116** 23–9

Liu Y, Dong X and Chen P 2012 Biological and chemical sensors based on graphene materials *Chem. Soc. Rev.* **41** 2283–307

Lu S *et al* 2016 Facile and ultrasensitive fluorescence sensor platform for tumor invasive biomaker $\beta$-glucuronidase detection and inhibitor evaluation with carbon quantum dots based on inner-filter effect *Biosens. Bioelectron.* **85** 358–62

Luo J H, Li Q, Chen S H and Yuan R 2019 Coreactant-free dual amplified electrochemiluminescent biosensor based on conjugated polymer dots for the ultrasensitive detection of microRNA *ACS Appl. Mater. Interfaces* **11** 27363–70

Malhotra B D and Ali M A 2018 Nanomaterials in biosensors: fundamentals and applications *Nanomaterials for Biosensors* (Norwich, NY: William Andrew) pp 1–74

Mao K *et al* 2018 A novel biosensor based on Au@Ag core–shell nanoparticles for sensitive detection of methylamphetamine with surface enhanced Raman scattering *Talanta* **190** 263–8

Markwalter C F, Kantor A G, Moore C P, Richardson K A and Wright D W 2019 Inorganic complexes and metal-based nanomaterials for infectious disease diagnostics *Chemical Reviews* **119** 1456–1518

Mekuye B and Abera B 2023 Nanomaterials: an overview of synthesis, classification, characterization, and applications *Nano Select* **4** 486–501

Murphy C J, Gole A M, Stone J W, Sisco P N, Alkilany A M, Goldsmith E C and Baxter S C 2008 Gold nanoparticles in biology: beyond toxicity to cellular imaging *Acc. Chem. Res.* **41** 1721–30

Naguib M *et al* 2011 Two-dimensional nanocrystals produced by exfoliation of $Ti_3AlC_2$ *Adv. Mater.* **23** 4248–53

Novoselov K S *et al* 2004 Electric field effect in atomically thin carbon films *Science* **306** 666–9

Pal M K, Rashid M and Bisht M 2015 Multiplexed magnetic nanoparticle-antibody conjugates (MNPs-ABS) based prognostic detection of ovarian cancer biomarkers, CA-125, $\beta$-2M and ApoA1 using fluorescence spectroscopy with comparison of surface plasmon resonance (SPR) analysis *Biosens. Bioelectron.* **73** 146–52

Pathan S, Jalal M, Prasad S and Bose S 2019 Aggregation-induced enhanced photoluminescence in magnetic graphene oxide quantum dots as a fluorescence probe for As (III) sensing *J. Mater. Chem.* A **7** 8510–20

Qian Z S, Shan X Y, Chai L J, Chen J R and Feng H 2015 A fluorescent nanosensor based on graphene quantum dots–aptamer probe and graphene oxide platform for detection of lead (II) ion *Biosens. Bioelectron.* **68** 225–31

Rabie H, Zhang Y, Pasquale N, Lagos M J, Batson P E and Lee K B 2019 NIR biosensing of neurotransmitters in stem cell-derived neural interface using advanced core–shell upconversion nanoparticles *Adv. Mater.* **31** 1806991

Raj M and Goyal R N 2019 Silver nanoparticles and electrochemically reduced graphene oxide nanocomposite based biosensor for determining the effect of caffeine on Estradiol release in women of child-bearing age *Sens. Actuators* B **284** 759–67

Roberts A, Mahari S and Gandhi S 2022 Signal enhancing gold nanorods (GNR) and antibody modified electrochemical nanosensor for ultrasensitive detection of Japanese encephalitis virus (JEV) secretory non-structural 1 (NS1) biomarker *J. Electroanal. Chem.* **919** 116563

Sabouri S, Ghourchian H, Shourian M and Boutorabi M 2014 A gold nanoparticle-based immunosensor for the chemiluminescence detection of the hepatitis B surface antigen *Anal. Methods* **6** 5059–66

Shahdeo D, Roberts A, Archana G J, Shrikrishna N S, Mahari S, Nagamani K and Gandhi S 2022 Label free detection of SARS CoV-2 receptor binding domain (RBD) protein by fabrication of gold nanorods deposited on electrochemical immunosensor (GDEI) *Biosens. Bioelectron.* **212** 114406

Sharma A, Kashyap B K and Puranik N 2023 *State-of-the-Art of Paper-based Technology and Challenges in its Commercialization* (Bristol: IOP Publishing)

Sharma A, Rao V K and Kamboj D V 2020 Electrochemical immunosensor for the detection of Staphylococcal enterotoxin B using screen-printed electrodes *Indian J. Chem.* **59** 174–80

Sharma A, Rao V K, Kamboj D V, Gaur R, Shaik M and Shrivastava A R 2016a Enzyme free detection of Staphylococcal enterotoxin B (SEB) using ferrocene carboxylic acid labeled monoclonal antibodies: an electrochemical approach *New J. Chem.* **40** 8334–41

Sharma A, Rao V K, Kamboj D V, Gaur R, Upadhyay S and Shaik M 2015 Relative efficiency of zinc sulfide (ZnS) quantum dots (QDs) based electrochemical and fluorescence immunoassay for the detection of Staphylococcal enterotoxin B (SEB) *Biotechnol. Rep.* **6** 129–36

Sharma A, Rao V K, Kamboj D V and Jain R 2014a Electrochemical immunosensor for Staphylococcal enterotoxin B (SEB) based on platinum nanoparticles-modified electrode using hydrogen evolution inhibition approach *Electroanalysis* **26** 2320–7

Sharma A, Rao V K, Kamboj D V, Upadhyay S, Shaik M, Shrivastava A R and Jain R 2014b Sensitive detection of Staphylococcal enterotoxin B (SEB) using quantum dots by various methods with special emphasis on an electrochemical immunoassay approach *RSC Adv.* **4** 34089–95

Sharma A, Rao V K, Roy A, Shrivastava A R, Upadhyay S and Jindal D 2016b Controlled synthesis of water soluble micrometer sized highly luminescent zinc sulfide flowers using green chemistry approach and their characterization *ChemXpress* **9** 108

Shevchenko V Y, Madison A E and Shudegov V E 2003 The structural diversity of the nanoworld *Glass Phys. Chem.* **29** 577

Smith A M, Duan H, Rhyner M N and Ruan G 2018a Synthesis of nanoparticles in microreactors *Chem. Rev.* **118** 11052–121

Sondhi P, Maruf M H U and Stine K J 2020 Nanomaterials for biosensing lipopolysaccharide *Biosensors* **10** 2

Steinmetz M *et al* 2019 A sensitive label-free impedimetric DNA biosensor based on silsesquioxane-functionalized gold nanoparticles for Zika virus detection *Biosens. Bioelectron.* **141** 111351

Takemura K, Lee J, Suzuki T, Hara T, Abe F and Park E Y 2019 Ultrasensitive detection of norovirus using a magnetofluoroimmunoassay based on synergic properties of gold/magnetic nanoparticle hybrid nanocomposites and quantum dots *Sens. Actuators* B **296** 126672

Tao Y, Luo F, Lin Y, Dong N, Li C and Lin Z 2021 Quantitative gold nanorods based photothermal biosensor for glucose using a thermometer as readout *Talanta* **230** 122364

Tavallaie R *et al* 2018 Nucleic acid hybridization on an electrically reconfigurable network of gold-coated magnetic nanoparticles enables microRNA detection in blood *Nat. Nanotech.* **13** 1066–71

Tran D T, Hoa V H, Tuan L H, Kim N H and Lee J H 2018 Cu–Au nanocrystals functionalized carbon nanotube arrays vertically grown on carbon spheres for highly sensitive detecting cancer biomarker *Biosens. Bioelectron.* **119** 134–40

Wang Q, Zhang S, Zhong Y, Yang X F, Li Z and Li H 2017 Preparation of yellow-green-emissive carbon dots and their application in constructing a fluorescent turn-on nanoprobe for imaging of selenol in living cells *Anal. Chem.* **89** 1734–41

Wang Z, Hu T, Liang R and Wei M 2020d Application of zero-dimensional nanomaterials in biosensing *Front. Chem.* **8** 320

Yang Z, Wang Y and Zhang D 2017 A novel multifunctional electrochemical platform for simultaneous detection, elimination, and inactivation of pathogenic bacteria based on the vancomycin-functionalised AgNPs/3D-ZnO nanorod arrays *Biosens. Bioelectron.* **98** 248–53

Yao J, Li P, Li L and Yang M 2018 Biochemistry and biomedicine of quantum dots: From biodetection to bioimaging, drug discovery, diagnostics, and therapy *Acta Biomater.* **74** 36–55

Yuan Q *et al* 2018 Sandwich-type biosensor for the detection of α2,3-sialylated glycans based on fullerene-palladium-platinum alloy and 4-mercaptophenylboronic acid nanoparticle hybrids coupled with Au-methylene blue-MAL signal amplification *Biosens. Bioelectron.* **102** 321–7

Zhang M, Wang M, Chen P, X and Liu Y 2021 Two-dimensional nanoparticles in biosensors: recent developments and future directions *Biosens. Bioelectron.* **178** 113008

Zhang R Q, Hong S L, Wen C Y, Pang D W and Zhang Z L 2018 Rapid detection and subtyping of multiple influenza viruses on a microfluidic chip integrated with controllable micro-magnetic field *Biosens. Bioelectron.* **100** 348–54

Zhang Y, Nayak T R, Hong H and Cai W 2012 Graphene: a versatile nanoplatform for biomedical applications *Nanoscale* **4** 3833–42

Zhang Y S *et al* 2017 Multisensor-integrated organs-on-chips platform for automated and continual *in situ* monitoring of organoid behaviors *Proc. Natl Acad. Sci.* **114** E2293–302

Zhao H *et al* 2021 Ultrasensitive supersandwich-type electrochemical sensor for SARS-CoV-2 from the infected COVID-19 patients using a smartphone *Sensors Actuators* B **327** 128899

Zhou P, Liu H, Gong L, Tang B, Shi Y, Yang C and Han Z 2019 A faster detection method for high-sensitivity cardiac troponin—POCT quantum dot fluorescence immunoassay *J. Thorac. Dis.* **11** 1506–13

Zhu X, Radovic-Moreno A F, Wu J, Langer R and Shi J 2014 Nanomedicine in the management of microbial infection—overview and perspectives *Nano Today* **9** 478–98

# Chapter 12

# Nanobiosensor based rapid detection of circulating biomarkers of cancer

**Nidhi Puranik, Prince Kumar, Priya Paliwal, Shiv Kumar Yadav and Minseok Song**

The treatment and management of patients with cancer are improved by early detection, which is essential for effective therapy. The most common diagnostic method, tissue biopsy, takes a long time and hurts the patient. It has been consistently demonstrated that liquid biopsies, a minimally invasive technique for detecting cancer, may effectively target circulating cancer biomarkers. Circulating tumor cells (CTCs), extracellular vesicles (EVs), tumor proteins, microRNA (miRNA), and circulating tumor DNA are examples of these biomarkers. Nonetheless, certain obstacles persist in attaining elevated sensitivity of detection, such as the remarkably low concentration of biomarkers in fluid specimens. The most recent advancements in nanoparticle-based biosensors have the potential to overcome these practical complications. Recent developments in the nanobiosensors field offer enormous advantages, such as high sensitivity, reproducibility, and fast analysis of biomolecules making this analytical tool very promising for this purpose. This chapter aims to provide a summary of circulatory biomarkers of cancer and current biosensor based approaches for early detection and diagnosis of cancer.

## 12.1 Cancer

According to the World Health Organization's (WHO) 2020 report on cancer, 18.1 million people worldwide had cancer in 2018, and 9.6 million of those people lost their lives to the illness. Furthermore, it was predicted that by 2040, there will be almost twice as many cancer patients worldwide, with the largest increase occurring in low- and middle-income countries (LMIC), home to more than two-thirds of all cancer cases. About 30% of all adult 30- to 69-year-olds' premature deaths from non-communicable diseases are caused by cancer (WHO 2022).

Utilizing central cancer registries (CCR) data for incidence and National Center for Health Statistics (NCHS) data for mortality, the American Cancer Society assessed the latest data on population-based cancer occurrence as well as outcomes and predicted the number of new cancer cases and deaths in the US each year. In the United States, 609 820 cancer deaths and 1 958 310 new cases were expected in 2023 (Siegel *et al* 2023).

'Metastasis' refers to the emergence of secondary tumors in an area of the body distant from the original primary cancer. Even though metastasis is the primary factor contributing to cancer therapy failure and mortality, little is known about it (Seyfried and Huysentruyt 2013). Numerous cancer cells are released into the bloodstream daily in cancer patients; however, studies on melanoma in animal models indicate that less than 0.1% of tumor cells spread to other organs. Cancer cells must travel from their original site, circulate through the bloodstream, withstand blood vessel pressure, adapt to new cellular conditions in a secondary site, and avoid lethal interactions with immune cells for metastases to develop (Fares *et al* 2020).

According to Hanahan and Weinberg, one of the characteristics of cancer is 'activating invasion and metastasis'. (Hanahan and Weinberg 2011). The invasion of nearby tissue and the seeding of distant areas to create metastases remain important aspects of cancer malignancy. After all, for over 90% of cancer patients, metastasis is the main cause of death (Dillekås *et al* 2019). Comprehending the intricacies of this procedure will aid in pinpointing targets for molecular treatments that have the potential to prevent or even reverse the progression and spread of cancer (Fares *et al* 2020).

A markedly higher chance of survival and more efficient treatment are the results of early cancer identification. However, over 50% of malignancies are discovered after they have progressed. Improving early identification of cancer has the potential to greatly increase survival rates. The requirement of several million cells for a precise clinical diagnosis with conventional instruments stands in the way of any early cancer diagnosis. To detect cancer early and treat it effectively, a sensor that is highly selective and sensitive to small amounts of samples is needed. More research and development of early cancer detection techniques are needed, even if recent developments in this field have saved lives.

Particle sizes ranging from 1 to 100 nm are known to exhibit unique physiochemical characteristics, making them viable options for early cancer detection and treatment. The field is changing quickly as a result of growing technological advancements and advances in our understanding of biology (Crosby *et al* 2022). The development of nanotechnology is one of the most significant advances in the field of healthcare for the eradication of emerging health problems. The results of nanotechnology research offer new techniques or tools for the early detection and treatment of cancer. Biosensors are cutting-edge technology that can help treat and prevent a variety of chronic illnesses, including cancer (Chauhan *et al* 2017). These biosensors allow for the early diagnosis of cancer and the tracking of the prognosis of the illness. These devices directly measure physiological fluids such as saliva, milk, blood, urine, and serum, making them affordable, non-invasive, specific, sensitive, and quick to react (Asci Erkocyigit *et al* 2023). Because of their potential uses in drug delivery, magnetic recording media, nanoelectronics, nanosensors, optoelectronics, nanoelectronics, and catalysts, nanoparticles have been the subject of extensive research in recent years (Hossain *et al* 2023). The application of nanoscopic properties of nanomaterials, such as graphene, carbon nanotubes (CNTs), and gold nanoparticles (AuNPs), in electrical biosensors for the early detection of high-risk cancers, such as those of the colon, prostate, lung, and bronchus, and breast, has garnered significant attention (Sharifianjazi *et al* 2021).

## 12.2 Liquid biopsy and circulatory biomarkers

Based on the examination of bodily fluids such as blood, urine, tears, sweat, nipple aspirate fluid, and volatile organic compounds in the breath, liquid biopsy has become a promising non-invasive diagnostic biomarker to enhance existing clinical methods for early detection of breast cancer (Li *et al* 2020). The discovery of numerous highly sensitive and selective tumor markers would be necessary for the widespread application of tumor markers in healthcare (Sharma 2009). Biomarkers present in biological fluids, specifically blood, seem to have the greatest potential for expediting the development of screening assays. Circulating carcinoma antigens (Coronell *et al* 2012), autoantibodies (de Jonge *et al* 2021), circulating tumor cells (Lin *et al* 2021), circulating cell-free tumor nucleic acids (DNA or RNA) (Chaddha *et al* 2023, Stejskal *et al* 2023), and circulating extracellular vesicles in the peripheral blood are the common biomarkers for cancer. Both circulating DNA and RNAs are examples of circulating cell-free tumor nucleic acids. Circulating RNA, also known as extracellular RNA (exRNA), is a signaling molecule that moves between cells in the body's fluids, transmitting data. Longer messenger RNA (mRNA) and non-coding RNA (ncRNA), such as small ncRNA and long ncRNA (lncRNA), are examples of exRNA types.

ncRNAs are classified into two groups: regulatory ncRNAs and housekeeping ncRNAs. Regulatory ncRNAs include lncRNA, microRNA (miRNA), piwi-inter-acting RNA (piRNA), small interfering RNA (siRNA), and transfer RNA (tRNA) derived fragments while housekeeping ncRNAs include ribosomal RNA (rRNA), tRNA, small nucleolar RNA (snoRNA), and small nuclear RNA (snRNA), and ncRNAs have become essential biomolecules for a wide range of biological functions. Their primary function is to regulate the expression of genes at the post-transcriptional level. Housekeeping ncRNAs are very prevalent and necessary for many cellular processes, including transcriptional splicing and the translation of RNA into proteins (Happel *et al* 2020). Among all the circulating RNAs, miRNA expression is recurrently dysregulated in cancer, has tissue-specific expression patterns, and is involved in oncogenesis, disease progression, invasion, and meta-stasis, making miRNA a promising biomarker of human cancer (Condrat *et al* 2020).

### 12.2.1 Circulating tumor cells

Cancer cells known as circulating tumor cells (CTCs) can cause a new, deadly metastasis when they naturally shed from primary or metastatic tumors and circulate in the bloodstream. Over the past ten years, CTC research has gained significant traction. Finding CTCs in a liquid biopsy of a tumor can help with early cancer diagnosis, early assessment of the effectiveness of chemotherapy in preventing cancer recurrence, and selection of specific, sensitive anti-cancer medications. As a result, CTC detection is an essential weapon in the battle against cancer (Shen *et al* 2017). One of the main characteristics of 'invasive behavior' in some cancer cells is the spontaneous circulation of tumor cells and/or tumor microemboli. It is anticipated that their identification will yield a potent instrument for determining the prognosis of cancer, diagnosing minimal residual disease, evaluating tumor sensitivity to anti-cancer medications, and customizing anti-cancer treatment (Paterlini-Brechot and Benali 2007). Although CTCs have the potential to be cancer markers, their low blood concentration necessitates the use of a very sensitive instrument to detect them (Zhang *et al* 2021, Ju *et al* 2022).

### 12.2.2 Blood circulating protein markers

Along with the development of cancer, protein markers may accumulate in tissue(s) and body fluids such as blood. Proteomics analysis can be used for the investigation of variations at a qualitative as well as quantitative level of the protein profiles/ distribution in tissues and blood. Most blood proteins can have abundances that drop to extremely low concentrations, so using extremely sensitive techniques is necessary for quantification (Repetto *et al* 2023). Over time, several blood antigens have been evaluated as possible cancer biomarkers. CYFRA 21-1, neuron-specific enolase (NSE), carcinoembriogenic antigen (CEA), and squamous cell carcinoma antigen (SCC-Ag) are among the most researched biomarkers (Nooreldeen and Bach 2021). A list of a few major protein biomarkers in the early detection of cancers is listed in table 12.1.

### 12.2.3 Exosomes

Tumoral and nontumoral cells release exosomes, a type of microscopic membranous vesicle, into bodily fluids and the surrounding environment. The primary role of these vesicles in cellular communication is to shuttle between donor and destination cells. The various components of an exosome's lumen, which correspond to bioactive chemicals in donor cells, are proteins, lipids, DNA, and RNA. One of the cargos carried by exosomes is miRNA. They are involved in many biological processes, such as metastasis of cancer and angiogenesis. Exosomes are blood-stream-circulating nanovesicles (Zhang *et al* 2019). All types of naturally occurring particles that are confined by a lipid bilayer and incapable of replicating are referred to as EVs. The molecular makeup, size and physical characteristics, biogenesis, and physiological roles of the different subtypes of EVs vary. The release of multi-vesicular endosome intraluminal vesicles into the extracellular space and direct budding from the cell surface are the two primary pathways for EV biogenesis in living cells. Endosomal EVs are known as exosomes, and most of them have a diameter of 30–150 nm. On the other hand, vesicles resulting from plasma membrane budding can have a diameter of up to 1000 nm and are known by

**Table 12.1.** A list of major protein biomarkers in cancer detection and diagnosis.

| Cancer | Fluid | Protein marker | References |
|---|---|---|---|
| Breast cancer | Serum | Epidermal growth factor receptor 2, cancer antigen 15-3, carcinoembryonic antigen, mucin 1, cell biomarkers such as Michigan Cancer foundation-7, MDA-MB-231 | Veyssière *et al* (2022), Mohammadpour-Haratbar *et al* (2023) |
| Lung cancer | Serum | Lactate dehydrogenase, C-reactive protein, prolactin, transthyretin, thrombospondin 1, selectin E, macrophage migration inhibitory factor, plasminogen activator, tissue type, erb-B2 receptor tyrosine kinase 2, epidermal growth factor receptor | Zamay *et al* (2017) |
| Gastric cancer | Serum | Carbohydrate antigen 19-9, carcinoembryonic antigen, carbohydrate antigen 125, and leptin | Repetto *et al* (2023) |
| Liver cancer | Serum | Alpha-fetoprotein, glypican-3, aldo-keto reductase family 1 member B10, des-gamma-carboxyprothrombin | Debes *et al* (2021) |
| Ovary cancer | Serum | Transthyretin, beta-hemoglobin, apolipoprotein AI, and transferrin, leptin, prolactin, osteopontin, and insulin-like growth factor-II | Kozak *et al* (2005), Mor *et al* (2005) |
| Kidney cancer | Urine | Carbonic anhydrase-9, aquaporin-1, perilipin-2, nuclear matrix protein-22, 14-3-3 protein, $\beta/\alpha$ Raf-kinase inhibitory protein, and neutrophil gelatinase-associated lipocalin | Flitcroft *et al* (2022) |
| Prostate cancer | Serum | Prostate-specific antigen, kallikrein 3/PSA, folate hydrolase 1/prostate-specific membrane antigen, and transmembrane protease, serine 2 | Duffy (2020) |
| | Urine | Beta 2-microglobulin protein, pepsinogen A3, mucin | Jedinak *et al* (2015) |

various names, including microvesicles, ectosomes, shedding vesicles, and microparticles.

It is currently not possible to accurately separate EV subtypes based on size, metabolic characteristics, or surface markers, even though different EV subtypes have different mean sizes. Consequently, unless their origin is established, the International Society for Extracellular Vesicles (ISEV) advises using operational terms for EV subtypes such as size, density, marker profile, etc, instead of terms such as exosomes or microvesicles (Vasconcelos *et al* 2019). Recently, EVs have become known as unique analytes for liquid biopsies.

### 12.2.4 Circulating tumor DNA

Circulating tumor DNA (ctDNA) in the blood provides a minimally invasive method for disease monitoring and therapy response assessment (Magbanua *et al* 2021). The year 1948 saw the first description of circulating cell-free DNA (cfDNA). Due to the additional ctDNA fraction, it can be elevated in patients with cancer, as well as in those with autoimmune diseases, stroke, trauma, and myocardial infarction. Furthermore, because leukocytes and other normal cells can actively secrete or release DNA, it is also present in trace amounts in healthy individuals. cfDNA is found in a variety of bodily fluids and is incredibly variable in size and makeup. The exact process through which cells release cfDNA is still unknown. The majority of fragments, according to electrophoresis assays, are between 180 and 200 base pairs (bp), and they are frequently linked to the histone proteins that make up the nucleosome. This suggests that one of the main sources of cfDNA may be apoptotic cells.

The discovery and characterization of epigenetic ctDNA modifications is also a promising biomarker in early cancer, since the methylation of genes or transcription-regulating regions has been connected to the therapy response and outcome (Buono *et al* 2019).

### 12.2.5 Circular RNAs

Circular RNAs (circRNAs), also known as back-splicing or non-canonical splicing RNAs, are a class of single-stranded noncoding RNAs that form a circular conformation. circRNA is a unique kind of RNA that, in most cases, has a covalently closed continuous loop formed by back-splicing in animals from the 5' to 3' ends. The circRNA biogenesis mechanisms are still mainly unknown. The fact that circRNAs are typically derived from pre-mRNAs and are regulated by the canonical spliceosomal machinery is a widely accepted and common mechanism. Numerous circRNAs have aberrant expressions in a variety of cancers, demonstrating their critical roles in tumorigenesis and tumor development. Numerous circRNAs are implicated in the promotion or suppression of cancers to varying degrees through various molecular mechanisms, according to a number of recent pieces of evidence. Recent research has shown that aberrant circRNA expressions are present in nearly all forms of cancer and are essential for the pathophysiology of the disease, acting as tumor suppressors or oncogenes. Through a variety of mechanisms, it has been discovered that circRNAs regulate the growth, migration, invasion, and apoptosis of cancer cells. Finding and using useful biomarkers is desperately needed, as early detection is especially important for cancer patients. circRNAs have special characteristics such as longer half-lives, resistance to exonucleases and RNase R, and patterns specific to specific tissues, cells, and developmental stages. Because of these special characteristics, circRNAs may be able to be targeted as markers in medical interventions (Chen and Shan 2021).

Tumor-suppressor circRNAs and oncogenic circRNAs are the two main categories of circRNAs that have been linked to the emergence of cancer. circRNAs either promote or inhibit the progression of cancer, but the mechanism generally affects drug resistance, invasion, apoptosis, and cell proliferation (Sarkar and Diermeier 2021). circRNAs are single-stranded, covalently closed circular transcripts without $5'$ caps or $3'$ poly(A) tails. They are classified as noncoding RNAs. These characteristics give circRNAs longer half-lives than linear mRNAs by making them resistant to ribonuclease digestion, including RNase R and exonuclease (Sharma *et al* 2021a).

By using electron microscopy, circRNAs were first identified as viroids in RNA viruses in 1976. In 1979, it was discovered that circRNAs were endogenous RNA splicing products in eukaryotes. However, in the twenty-first century, advances in bioinformatics and RNA sequencing (RNA-seq) technologies have revealed that circRNAs are widely distributed in eukaryotic cells and play a role in the biogenesis and progression of a number of diseases, including cancer. For instance, an exome capture RNA-seq protocol that identified and characterized circRNAs in more than 2000 cancer samples was used to determine the cancer landscape of circRNAs in brain, lung, thyroid, breast, and bladder cancers. circRNAs are essential for the development of cancer, metastasis, and treatment resistance. circRNAs exhibit tissue specificity and stability in exosomes or bodily fluids, indicating their potential utility as therapeutic targets for a range of cancers as well as as accurate tumor biomarkers for diagnosis or prognostication (Zeng *et al* 2022).

### 12.2.6 Long noncoding RNAs

Since they are non-invasive biomarkers for better CRC screening techniques, lncRNAs have drawn a lot of interest. Determining the expression of circulating lncRNA offers a novel and promising early diagnostic technique for CRC screening. Exosomes and microvesicles are two examples of extracellular vesicles that store and protect circulating lncRNAs. Numerous studies have demonstrated distinct lncRNA expression profiles in serum or plasma in patients with different tumors. As a result, peripheral blood contains high concentrations of lncRNA in a very stable, cell-free form (Zabeti Touchaei *et al* 2024). Exosomes and microvesicles are two examples of extracellular vesicles that store and protect circulating lncRNAs. Numerous studies have demonstrated distinct lncRNA expression profiles in serum or plasma in patients with different tumors. As a result, peripheral blood contains high concentrations of lncRNA in a very stable, cell-free form (Xu *et al* 2020). lncRNAs participate in a variety of signaling pathways and act as tumor suppressors or oncogenes. There are presently few therapeutic agents and biomarkers available targeting lncRNAs. Currently, the first and only lncRNA approved for clinical use is prostate cancer antigen 3 (PCA3), an early diagnostic biomarker for prostate cancer (PC) (Lemos *et al* 2019). Some major lncRNAs used as biomarkers are listed in table 12.2.

**Table 12.2.** Some lncRNAs related to cancer and used as biomarkers in detection and diagnosis.

| Cancer | Associed lncRNAs |
| --- | --- |
| Breast | CERS6-AS1 (Bao *et al* 2020), H19 (Si *et al* 2019, Wang *et al* 2019), LINC00673 (Qiao *et al* 2019), LINC00511 (Lu *et al* 2018), TROJAN (Jin *et al* 2020), and PTENP1 (Gao *et al* 2019) |
| Gastric | ABHD11-AS1 (Yang *et al* 2016), HOTAIR (Pan *et al* 2016), BANCR (Li *et al* 2015), MEG3 (Wei and Wang 2017), HCP5 (Qin *et al* 2021) |
| Lung | XLOC_009167 (Jiang *et al* 2018), GAS5 (Li *et al* 2019a), UCA1 (Wang *et al* 2015a), LncRNA16 (Zhu *et al* 2017), CCAT2 (Qiu *et al* 2014), TBILA and AGAP2-AS1 (Tao *et al* 2020) |
| Liver | SNHG1 (Li *et al* 2019b), SNHG4 (Jiao *et al* 2020), CDKN2B-AS1 (Zhuang *et al* 2019), NEAT1 (Ling *et al* 2018), CRNDE and SNHG7 (Zhang *et al* 2020) |
| Ovarian | lncRNA ROR (Shen *et al* 2020), LOXL1-AS1 (Liu *et al* 2020), RUNX1-IT1, MALAT1, H19, HOTAIRM1, LOC100190986 and AL132709.8 (Yang *et al* 2017) |
| Prostate | PCAT14 (Yan *et al* 2021), p21 (Işın *et al* 2015), BRE-AS1 (Chen *et al* 2019), TUG1 (Xu *et al* 2019) and RNCR3 (Tian *et al* 2018) |
| Kidney | SLINKY (Gong *et al* 2017), LINC00887 (Xie *et al* 2020), TapSAKI, XIST, MALAT1, CASC2, and HOXA-AS2 (Ma *et al* 2021) |

### 12.2.7 MicroRNAs

By targeting mRNAs for cleavage or translational repression, endogenous ∼22 nt single-stranded noncoding small RNA molecules known as microRNAs (miRNAs) can be secreted into the circulation and exist steadily. In animals, miRNAs play important regulatory roles. The majority of the time, miRNAs bind to target mRNAs' 3′ untranslated region (3′ UTR) to cause translational repression and mRNA destruction. miRNAs are frequently investigated in body fluids, tissue samples, and cell cultures, all of which are easily processed to obtain a tiny RNA subfraction (usually ∼10% by mass) and total RNAs (usually in microgram scale). miRNAs can attach to proteins, such as Argonautes, or be secreted into extracellular fluids and delivered to target cells via vesicles such as exosomes. miRNAs through their impact on protein translation, have become significant regulators of many biological processes and have demonstrated encouraging promise as useful non-invasive biomarkers for cancer screening; a few of them are listed in table 12.3. Tumor-suppressor miRNAs and oncogenic miRNAs are the two main categories of miRNAs, which are separated based on the expression patterns of miRNA and target mRNA. Research findings indicate that tumor-suppressor miRNA expression is down-regulated during the onset of cancer, whereas oncogenic miRNA expression is up-regulated (Mollaei *et al* 2019). Exosomal miRNAs have special properties that make them potentially useful biomarkers for cancer diagnosis. Because exosomes are abundant in a variety of body fluids and because miRNAs in exosomes are

**Table 12.3.** A list of major miRNAs deregulated in cancer patients that could be possible biomarkers.

| Cancer | miRNA down-regulated | miRNA up-regulated |
|---|---|---|
| Breast | miR-145 (Ng *et al* 2013), miR-339-5p, miR-133a-3p, miR-326, miR-331-3p, miR-369-3p, miR-328-3p, miR-26a-3p, miR-139-3p, miR-493-3p, miR-664a-5p, miR-146a-5p, miR-323b-3p, miR-1307-3p, miR-423-3p (Escuin *et al* 2021) | miR-21, miR155 and miR125 (Canatan *et al* 2021), miR-16, miR-21, miR-451 (Ng *et al* 2013), miR-101-3p, miR-144-3p (Escuin *et al* 2021) |
| Lung | miR-200a, miR-200b, miR-200c, miR-141, miR-429 (Han and Li 2018) | miR-429, miR-205, miR-200b, miR-203, miR-125b, miR-34b (Halvorsen *et al* 2016) |
| Gastric | miR-214 (Saliminejad *et al* 2022), let-7a (Tsujiura *et al* 2010) | miR-18a, miR-21, miR-25, miR-92a, miR-125b, miR-221 (Saliminejad *et al* 2022), miR-17-5p, miR-21, miR-106a, miR-106b (Tsujiura *et al* 2010) |
| Liver | miR-101 (Fu *et al* 2013) | miR-16, miR-122 (Fang *et al* 2022), miR-494, miR-1269 (Elemeery *et al* 2017) |
| Ovary | miR-144-3p, miR-142-3p, miR-150-5p, miR-15a-5p, miR-15b-5p, miR-126-3p, miR-191-5p, miR-106b-5p (Niemira *et al* 2023) | miR-1246, miR-4454 + miR-7975, miR-630, miR-4516 (Niemira *et al* 2023) |
| Kidney | miRNA-455-3p, miRNA-487b, miRNA-29a, miRNA-424, miRNA-199b, miRNA-582-3p, miRNA-375, miRNA-196b, miRNA-200c, miRNA-409-3p (Gilyazova *et al* 2023) | miRNA-210, miRNA-642, miRNA-18a, miRNA-483-5p (Gilyazova *et al* 2023) |
| Prostate | let-7e, let-7c, miR-30c (Chen *et al* 2012) | miR-622, miR-1285 (Chen *et al* 2012) |

stable, exosomal miRNAs may constitute a unique class of biomarkers for early and minimally invasive cancer diagnosis (Preethi *et al* 2022).

## 12.3 Superiority of biomarker-based detection in cancer over conventional methods

The prognosis and course of treatment for cancer depend on an early diagnosis. Imaging methods are the primary diagnosis tools among several platforms that could yield important information about cancer patients (Fass 2008). It has been demonstrated that a variety of imaging modalities, including ultrasound, single-photon emission computed tomography (SPECT), positron emission tomography (PET), computed tomography (CT), magnetic resonance imaging (MRI), and mammography, can be used to diagnose and follow patients with breast cancer at different stages (Hussain *et al* 2022, Pulumati *et al* 2023). Mammography is a gold standard method that is frequently used in cancer screening. It is easy to use, causes little damage, is inexpensive, and has a wide range of applications. In particular, it can be used to diagnose lesions that have sand-like calcification and to display the shape and boundaries of breast masses (Li *et al* 2016). PET is a radionuclide-based imaging technique that can be used to find the tumor, determine its stage, and track how well it is responding to therapy. While axillary metastases and ambiguous palpable masses can be effectively characterized by SPECT and PET, these methods are not sensitive enough to identify sub-centimetric tumor deposits (Zhu *et al* 2011). Since individual operator skills have a significant impact on ultrasound imaging, there is still room for improvement in terms of susceptibility and specificity. The size of the malignancy can be accurately determined by MRI, but it requires complex examination procedures, takes a long time, has low patient compliance, and is insensitive to calcifications (Li *et al* 2016). There are several drawbacks to using different imaging modalities for cancer detection, including high costs, low sensitivity and specificity, and non-use as a point-of-care system. In order to get beyond the associated constraints of imaging techniques, more sensitive point-of-care approaches based on biomarkers must be introduced (Das *et al* 2023).

Biochemical techniques that rely on the identification and measurement of biomarkers may provide an early diagnosis. Biomarkers are defined as naturally occurring compounds that are present in abnormal proportions in individuals with cancer or precancerous conditions. These substances can be detected in the body's cells, tissues, or fluids. Cancer biomarkers may be exclusive to one particular type of cancer or they may be linked to multiple cancer types (Wagner *et al* 2004).

The most widely used, technologically limited methods for biomarker screening now in use include immunohistochemistry (IHC), high-performance liquid chromatography (HPLC), enzyme-linked immunosorbent assay (ELISA), polymerase chain reaction (PCR), immunohistochemistry (IHC), and radioimmunoassay (RIA). Thus, there is a great need for the creation of novel, commercially viable methods for finding cancer biomarkers (Hasan *et al* 2021). Researchers have focused on the creation of biosensors in order to identify several indicators for cancer in recent years. Along with biosensors and biomarkers, microwave imaging techniques have also been thoroughly investigated as a potential diagnostic tool for prompt and economical early-stage cancer diagnosis.

A point-of-care (POC) diagnostic tool should ideally be quick, affordable, functional without requiring a lot of sample preparation beforehand, extremely sensitive to allow for early cancer detection, and specific to avoid overdiagnosing, misdiagnosing, or missing diagnoses. To start therapy as soon as feasible and improve the patient's well-being in the long run, results must be returned swiftly (Wang 2017).

## 12.4 Biosensors

The most cutting-edge nanotechnology research being conducted in the modern period is the creation of nanosensors. Applications for nanobiosensors in the biomedical and healthcare fields include monitoring patient health and managing human health, identifying diseases, preventing them, and rehabilitating patients.

These little gadgets serve as step and activity monitors, encouraging individuals to adopt healthier lifestyles (Haleem *et al* 2021).

'Biosensors' are analytical tools that translate a biological response into an electrochemical signal. Cammann coined the term 'biosensor'. It measured glucose in biological samples by electrochemically detecting hydrogen peroxide or oxygen using an immobilized glucose oxidase electrode. Biosensors should, in general, be very specialized, independent of physical constraints such as pH and temperature, and potentially recyclable. In order to effectively build a biosensor, it is necessary to fabricate, immobilize, and transduce devices. These steps collectively provide engineering for transdisciplinary study in both biology and chemistry (Mehrotra 2016). Based on how they function, the materials required for biosensors are categorized into four groups: (i) biocatalytic, or enzyme-based biosensors; (ii) the bioaffinity group, which includes the involvement of nucleic acids, antigens, and antibodies; (iii) microbes, or microorganism-containing biosensors; and (iv) nano-sensors, or sensors that contain active nanoparticles, which often improve sensitivity and specificity for disease early detection (Cash and Clark 2010, Rocchitta *et al* 2016, Metkar and Girigoswami 2019).

Biosensors are instruments that typically provide signals primarily related to the concentration of an analyte in the chemical reaction, allowing them to assess the amounts of biological markers or any chemical reaction. These biosensors typically assist in the monitoring of diseases, medication discovery, pollution detection, and the identification of bacteria that cause disease as well as markers that typically point to the presence of disease, such as bodily fluids (Alhadrami 2018, Parkhey and Mohan 2019). The main industrial uses of nanosensors are in the fields of healthcare, medicine, and clinical services. The application of biosensors in widely classified disciplines, such as contrast imaging during MRIs, illness diagnosis, and health monitoring, is illustrated in figure 12.1. Following the first oxygen biosensor created Led and Clark. then, the development of biosensors as diagnostic tools has drawn significant attention from researchers in biotechnology and medicine. Recent advances in basic and clinical science have been made possible by the capacity to identify biomarkers at low concentrations, and their predictive value in terms of illness prognosis, diagnosis, and course (Palchetti 2016). Future technological diagnostics will be necessary to identify very precise, precise, quantitative, and multiplexed biomarkers. Electrodes specific to metals are built into biosensors to detect hazardous metal concentrations in water (Sharma *et al* 2021b). They are able to identify dangerous illnesses and identify biomarkers.

Biomarker-based electrochemical biosensors have proven useful in the field of cancer research, enabling quicker and more precise diagnosis. Additionally, bio-sensors equipped with optical transducers are able to detect variations in light resulting from the analysis and interaction of biological elements. The application of these nanosensors in our daily lives can help solve a lot of healthcare issues. The most practical examples of nanosensors that improve our lives are those that monitor food, blood quality, body chemistry, biological anomalies, heart rate, and diet. Point-of-care testing, using these very small testing devices, does not require

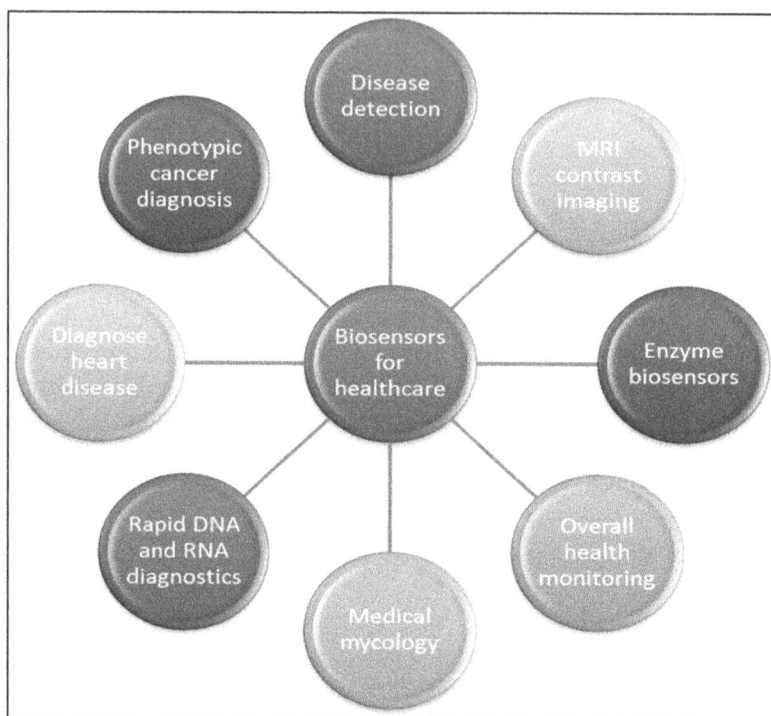

**Figure 12.1.** Different aspects of nanosensors in healthcare services.

additional funding or labor for the diagnosis (Javaid and Haleem 2019, Lin *et al* 2020).

Point-of-care diagnostic tools offer a practical choice for the sensitive and quick identification of cancer indicators. Biosensors can be very helpful in the early identification of cancer, given the rising number of cancer cases being detected globally and the rise in deaths from late illness detection (Tothill 2009).

The use of these biosensors for biomarker-based detection is becoming increasingly important in the diagnosis of various illnesses, including cancer and cardio-vascular disease. The exact diagnosis of cardiac disorders depends on the design and development of highly selective and sensitive biosensors that use nonmaterial and convenient surface chemistries (Tan *et al* 2017). A typical biosensor consists of the components listed below (and shown in figure 12.2.)

**Analyte:** A substance of interest that needs to be detected.

**Bioreceptor:** Molecules such as enzymes that can recognize the analyte are examples of bioreceptors.

**Transducer:** It often transforms a biorecognition event into a quantifiable signal, known as signalization.

**Electronics:** The transduced signal is typically processed and displayed using electronics.

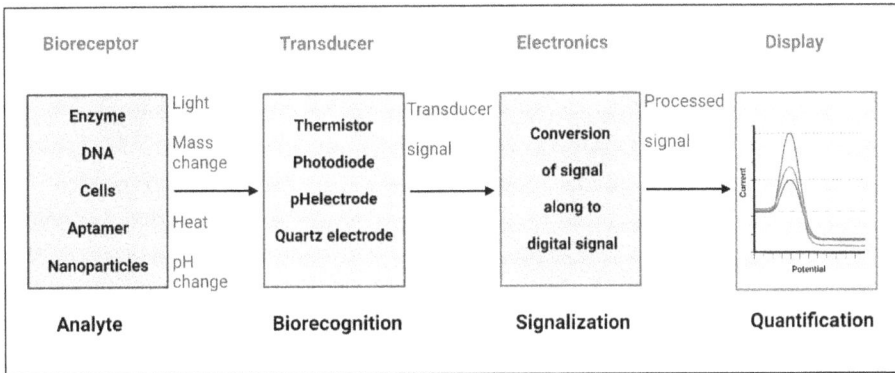

**Figure 12.2.** Schematic representation of biosensors. (Created using Biorender.com.)

**Display:** Typically, a liquid crystal display combined with biosensor production hardware and software produces a user-friendly biosensor.

The two main parts that are combined to create a single device are the transducer and bioreceptor. With this combination, the target analyte can be measured without the need for reagents. Biosensor measurements are straightforward and quick, requiring no specialist laboratory knowledge. Biosensors have been applied in many other domains, including medical science, the marine industry, the food industry, etc. Additionally, these biosensors are designed to have higher linearity and sensitivity than conventional techniques (Sagadevan and Periasamy 2014, Alhadrami 2018). Various biosensors developed for the detection of circulatory biomarkers for the diagnosis of cancer are listed in table 12.4. The application of biosensors in medical science is expanding quickly. The most common use of the glucose biosensor is in medical applications to diagnose diabetes mellitus (Mehrotra 2016).

Many biological molecules (such as DNA and biomarkers) and other physiological markers are helpful for cancer diagnosis and management in the majority of bioresearch domains, particularly for cancer detection. Biological markers are among these molecular analytes that are frequently thought of as a type of quantitative label that denotes particular biological states of human bodies. Consequently, biomarker-based sensors have great promise for early illness diagnosis and individualized treatment. More significantly, biomarkers give us personalized information about underlying medical issues in addition to information about current disorders. This information will quickly offer users biology-related information such as sub-clinical status and morbidity by comparing results between normal samples and patients (Griffiths *et al* 2002, Naylor 2003). Therefore, the detection of biomarkers is of great significance to human health.

### 12.4.1 Characteristics of a nanosensor

A biosensor's design defines its intended purpose, yet performance monitoring of these biosensors still requires additional fundamental components.

**Table 12.4.** Summary of various biosensors developed for the detection of circulatory biomarkers for the diagnosis of cancer.

| Biosensor | Target | Sample | Cancer type | Limit of detection | References |
|---|---|---|---|---|---|
| Ultrasensitive electrochemical biosensor | miRNA-155 | Serum | Breast cancer | 20 zmol | Hakimian and Ghourchian (2020) |
| Electrochemical biosensor | miRNA-155 | Serum | Breast cancer | 5.7 aM | Cardoso et al (2016) |
| Electrochemical biosensor | miRNA-141, miRNA-21 | Plasma | Lung cancer | LODs were 0.89 and 1.24 fM for simultaneous detection of miRNA-141 and miRNA-21 | Khodadoust et al (2023) |
| Electrochemical biosensor | miRNA-21 | Plasma | Breast cancer | 84.3 fM | Rafiee-Pour et al (2016) |
| Field-effect transistor biosensor ($MoS_2$ nanosheets) | miRNA-155 | Serum | Breast cancer | 0.03 fM | Majd et al (2018) |
| Electrochemical nanobiosensor (graphene oxide and gold nanorod) | miRNA-155 | Plasma | Breast cancer | 0.6 fM | Azimzadeh et al (2016) |
| Voltammetric biosensor (reduced graphene oxide (rGO) and modified AuNPs) | miRNA-21 | Serum | Breast cancer | 5 fM | Zouari et al (2020) |
| Silicon nanophotonic biosensor | miRNA-21-5p | Plasma | Lung cancer | 25 pM | Calvo-Lozano et al (2022) |
| Optical biosensor (AuNPs) | miRNA-155 | — | Breast cancer | 100 aM | Hakimian et al (2018) |
| Electrochemical nano-genosensor (AgNPs and graphene) | miRNA-21 | Blood | Breast cancer | 0.2 fM | Salahandish et al (2018) |
| Electrochemical nanosensor | miRNA-21 | Cell lysates | Breast cancer | 6 pmol | Kilic et al (2012) |
| Screen-printed carbon electrode-based electrochemical biosensor | miRNA-141 | Urine | Colorectal and breast cancer | 20 nM | Leung et al (2021) |

| Biosensor | Biomarker | Sample | Cancer type | Detection limit / response | Reference |
|---|---|---|---|---|---|
| Electrochemical biosensor (gold nanorods) | miRNA30e | — | Pancreatic Cancer | 14.9 aM | Sharma and Srivastava (2022) |
| Nanophotonic biosensor | miRNA-21 | Clinical samples | Lung cancer | 25 pM | Calvo-Lozano et al (2022) |
| Plasmonic biosensor | miRNA-21, miRNA-221, miRNA-153 | Clinical samples | Gastric cancer | Optical response of the sample shifted to higher wavelengths of 30 nm | Asl et al (2022) |
| Plasmonic biosensor | miRNA-10b, miRNA-21 | Plasma | Pancreatic cancer | Significantly peak shifted to higher wavelengths for both miRNA | Joshi et al (2014) |
| Amperometric biosensing | miRNA-21 | Serum and cancer cells | Breast cancer | 29 fM | Zouari et al (2018) |
| Electrochemical biosensor | miRNA-222 | Serum | Cancer | 40 pM | Wang et al (2015b) |
| Fluorescence biosensor | Prostate-specific antigen | Serum | Prostate cancer | 0.3 pg ml$^{-1}$ | Yang et al (2018) |
| Electrochemical immunoassay | Carbohydrate antigen 19-9 | Serum | Pancreatic cancer | 0.26 U ml$^{-1}$ | Huang et al (2017) |
| Piezoelectric immunosensor | Carbohydrate antigen 19-9 | Serum | Cancer patients | 12.5–270.0 U ml$^{-1}$ | Ding et al (2008) |
| Electrochemical immunosensor | p53 biomarker | Saliva | Cancer | 5.0 fg ml$^{-1}$ | Ibáñez-Redín et al (2020) |
| Electrochemiluminescence immunosensor | p53 | Human p53 spike sera samples | Cancer | 4 fg ml$^{-1}$ | Heidari et al (2019) |
| SERS immunosensor | Carcinoembryonic antigen | Plasma | Various cancer | 0.033 pg ml$^{-1}$ | Medetalibeyoglu et al (2020) |

(Continued)

**Table 12.4.** (*Continued*)

| Biosensor | Target | Sample | Cancer type | Limit of detection | References |
|---|---|---|---|---|---|
| SPR and quartz crystal microbalance sensor | Prostate-specific antigen | Serum | Prostate cancer | KD of the antibody—$9.46 \times 10^{-10}$ M | Uludag and Tothill (2012) |
| Electrochemical DNA biosensor | DNA (*BRCA1* gene) | Breast cancer cells | Breast cancer | 3.32 $\mu$M | Mansor et al (2014) |
| Electrochemical biosensor | K562 cells | K562 cells | Cancer | 60 cells ml$^{-1}$ | Zheng et al (2019) |
| Piezoelectric biosensor | PSA and $\alpha$-fetoprotein | Commercial | Cancer | 0.25 ng ml$^{-1}$ | Su et al (2017) |
| Piezoelectric biosensor | $\alpha$-fetoprotein | Serum | Liver | Kd-$3.21 \times 10^{-10}$ M | Chen and Shi (2023) |
| Photonic crystal biosensors | Cancer cell | Cancer cell | Cancer | 0.000 236 RIU | Yang et al (2023) |
| Optical biosensor | HER-2 protein | Serum | Breast cancer | 1 fg ml$^{-1}$ | Pourasl et al (2023) |
| Electrochemical cytosensor | Surface protein CD123 | Acute myeloid leukemia cells | Acute myeloid leukemia | 1 cell ml$^{-1}$ | Soleimanian et al (2021) |
| Electrochemical biosensor | Serum | HER-2 protein | Breast cancer | 1 fg ml$^{-1}$ | Nasrollahpour et al (2021) |

### 12.4.1.1 Selectivity

The ability of a nanosensor to separate a particular target analyte from a mixed sample that contains combinations of pollutants or unwanted chemicals. The interaction of a very particular antigen with an immobilized body is the most significant illustration of selectivity.

### 12.4.1.2 Stability

Stability is the capacity of biosensors to elude environmental perturbations that can alter their anticipated response during the test. This is especially important when building biosensors, which may require continuous monitoring and take longer to produce data. A few factors that can impact the stability of the biosensor are temperature, the affinity of the bioreceptor, and membrane fouling.

### 12.4.1.3 Sensitivity and linearity

The two most crucial biosensor characteristics that affect its robustness and potential applications are sensitivity and linearity. The lowest concentration at which a nanosensor can identify an analyte is known as its sensitivity; it can range from femtograms (fg ml$^{-1}$) to nanograms per milliliter (ng ml$^{-1}$). Biosensors intended for use in medical or environmental monitoring applications can have a minimum practicable sensitivity value of ng ml$^{-1}$ or fg ml$^{-1}$. On the other hand, linearity denotes the output's correctness within a working range where the analyte's concentration is directly proportional to the measured signal (Cash and Clark 2010).

### 12.4.1.4 Reproducibility

The yield of obtaining the same results no matter how many times the experiment is done is known as reproducibility (Cash and Clark 2010).

### 12.4.2 Types of nanobiosensors

#### 12.4.2.1 Optical nanobiosensors

Light intensity changes are measured by optical nanobiosensors. An instrument can detect the electric signal produced by measuring and converting the light beam. The components of the system are a detector, an optical fiber sensing material, and a light source (Dey and Goswami 2011). Light used as a sensing material is transmitted via an optical fiber substrate. The detector uses this transmitted light as an output signal. Depending on the light intensity, optical biosensors can be either photometric or colorimetric. Optical biosensors' valuable performance is driving their progress in drug research and clinical diagnostics (Syam *et al* 2012). Surface plasmon resonance, optical waveguides, optical resonators, photonic crystals, and optical fibers are examples of these optical biosensors. Lately, there has been a significant benefit to using fiber grating (FBG) sensors to measure a variety of parameters, including temperature, strain, magnetic field, and refractive index (Kazemi-Darsanaki *et al* 2013). Optical biosensors possess a low detection limit and high sensitivity, making them highly promising for the diagnosis of multiple cancer types. They are also fast, real-time, and portable. Compared to standard detection methods that employ 1 billion cells in tumor tissue with a diameter of 7–10 nm, optical biosensors can detect cancer in a few million malignant cells (Kaur *et al* 2022).

Colorimetric biosensing techniques have been widely used to identify a wide range of targets, including proteins, nucleic acids, metal ions, and tiny particles. This is especially true for identifying target indicators associated with certain diseases. Among the many biomolecule detection methods, calorimetric detection attracted a lot of attention due to its benefits, which included visible radiation, ease of use, quick reading, affordability, and ease of measurement. It has also been extensively used to identify rare levels of cancer target markers (Kal-Koshvandi 2020).

### Surface plasmon resonance (SPR) nanosensors

As illustrated in figure 12.3, this is an evanescent area-based optical sensor that uses a thin gold/metal layer for sensing techniques. The detection of reflection minima on photo-detector array sensors allows one to examine the interaction between analytes flowing over immobilized gold surfaces. SPR has been effectively used to identify disease microorganisms through immunoreactions (Homola *et al* 1999, Kazemi-Darsanaki *et al* 2013).

The SPR effect is the result of incident light energy being linked into surface plasmons at the metal–dielectric interface. This weakens the light beam's total internal reflection. At a particular incidence angle and wavelength, the effect manifests. Within the reflection spectrum, there is a minimum (SPR dip). A change in the refractive index, a shift in the minimum, and, if a polarized beam is being employed, a rotation of the angle of incident light occur when the marker is immobilized on the metal surface. Usually, a glass slide with a small layer of gold covering it serves as the biosensor basis. An alternative is to use a glass prism that has been lightly coated with gold. Nevertheless, gold or silver nanoparticles

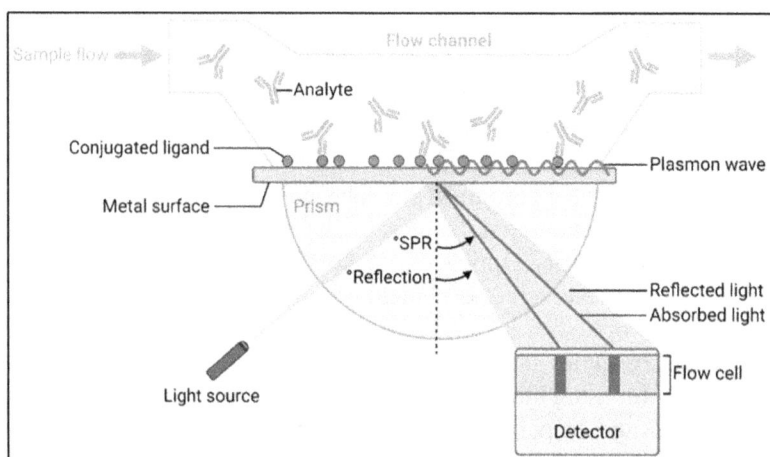

**Figure 12.3.** A schematic representation of the general mechanism of SPR. (Created using Biorender.com.)

dispersed in solution or fixed on a glass slide or optical fiber can also be used for marker identification based on the SPR effect (Falkowski *et al* 2021).

### 12.4.2.2 Piezoelectric nanobiosensors

A class of analytical instruments known as piezoelectric biosensors operates based on recording affinity interactions. A sensor component that operates based on oscillation change as a result of a mass bound on the surface of a piezoelectric crystal is known as a piezoelectric platform or piezoelectric crystal (Pohanka and Skládal 2018). The transduction mechanism in piezoelectric biosensors is based on the ability of piezoelectric crystals to vibrate in response to an electric field and the relationship between changes in resonant frequency and the mass of molecules adsorbed or desorbed from the crystal's surface (Tombelli 2012). Anisotropic crystals such as crystallized topaz, quartz, bones, zinc oxide, aluminum phosphate (berlinite), Rochelle salt, polyvinylidene fluoride, polylactic acids, etc, are utilized in the creation of these biosensors. These biosensors are mass-produced. The fundamental principle of sensing is that a change in voltage induces mechanical stress or oscillation on the surface of piezoelectric materials. When the crystal is inserted into the oscillation circuit, the oscillation frequency is measured. In conclusion, a decline in frequency is directly related to the mass attached to the crystal. Piezoelectric biosensors are frequently employed in applications such as energy harvesting, loudspeakers, electric cigarette lighters, fire alarms, and nano-balancing. Moreover, one of the most often used instruments in the electronic sector is the quartz crystal microbalance (Sappati and Bhadra 2018, Sekhar *et al* 2023).

### 12.4.2.3 Thermal nanobiosensors

This kind of biosensor makes use of one of the fundamental properties of biological processes: heat is absorbed or emitted, changing the reaction medium's temperature. Temperature sensors and immobilized enzyme molecules are coupled to create them. When the analyte and enzyme come into contact, the heat reaction of the enzyme is detected and calibrated against the analyte concentration. This type of biosensor is widely employed in the identification of hazardous substances and germs (Kazemi-Darsanaki *et al* 2013).

### 12.4.2.4 Electrochemical nanobiosensors

Electrochemical nanosensors based on the electrophoretic light scattering approach have three components that make up electrochemical biosensors: the biorecognition element, signal transducer, and three-electrode based systems, as shown in figure 12.4. Such biosensors detect and record electrochemical interactions between target components at the electrode surface triggered by changes in electrical signal. A collection of biorecognition components, including enzymes, antibodies, and synthetic molecules (aptamers, DNA fragments, peptides, etc), are used to identify cancer biomarkers.

As a surface approach, electrochemistry has some benefits for biosensor detection. It is not highly dependent on the reaction volume, and measurements can be made with incredibly small sample quantities (Hammond *et al* 2016). Because

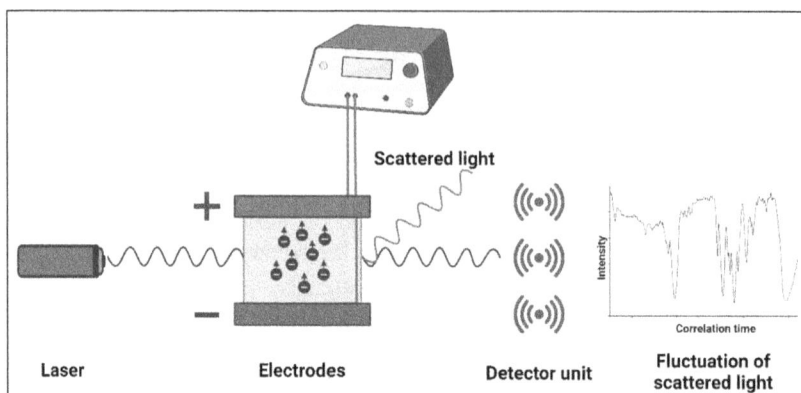

**Figure 12.4.** A mechanistic representation of the electrophoretic light scattering method. (Created using Biorender.com.)

electrochemical detection is inexpensive, user-friendly, portable, and has a straight-forward structure, it is commonly used as a transducer in biosensors. Typically, an electrochemical reaction under observation produces a detectable current (amper-ometry), a measurable charge buildup or potential (potentiometry), or a change in the medium's conductive characteristics between electrodes (conductometry). It is also becoming more usual to utilize electrochemical impedance spectroscopy to assess the biosensor's resistance and reactance (Grieshaber *et al* 2008, Pohanka and Skládal 2008).

Because they are inexpensive to produce and easily miniaturized, electrochemical biosensors are of interest. Furthermore, compelling outcomes using flexible method-ologies based on recently created materials and nanomaterials, naturally occurring organic and bioorganic polymers, electroactive compounds, catalysts, and biocatal-ysis, among other things (El Aamri *et al* 2020).

*Voltammetry/amperometry nanosensors*
Applying a potential to a working (or indicator) electrode in comparison to a reference electrode and measuring the current are the characteristics of both amperometric and voltage-metering approaches. By employing an electrochemical reduction or oxidation at the working electrode, electrolysis produces the current (Pohanka and Skládal 2008). The mass transport rate of molecules to the electrode sets a limit on the electrolysis current. Techniques that scan the potential over a predetermined potential range are referred to as voltammetry. Usually, the current response peaks or plateaus in proportion to the analyte's concentration as shown in figure 12.5. In amperometry, a constant potential is maintained at the working electrode concerning a reference electrode, and variations in the current produced by the electrochemical oxidation or reduction are directly monitored over time. What separates voltammetry and amperometry is the lack of a scanning potential (Kimmel *et al* 2012, Meirinho *et al* 2016).

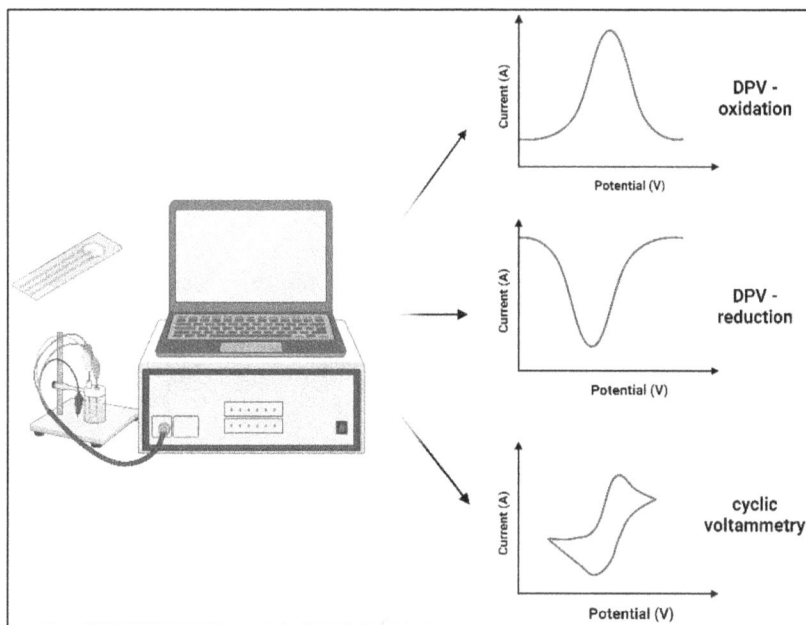

**Figure 12.5.** A schematic representation of the voltammetry technique. (Created with Biorender.com.)

### *Conductimetric nanosensors*

This electrochemical method can be used to measure a solution's electrical conductivity or resistance. The overall conductivity/resistivity has changed and is now an electrochemical signal as a result of the electrochemical reactions producing electrons or ions. Relatively speaking, this type of electrochemical measurement is less sensitive (Lazcka *et al* 2007).

### *Electrochemical impedance spectroscopy (EIS)*

EIS uses a small amplitude sinusoidal ac excitation pulse, usually between 2 and 10 mV, to disturb a system to assess the resistive and capacitive properties of materials. The impedance spectrum is obtained by varying the frequency over a large range. The resistive and capacitive components of impedance are then obtained, respectively, by determining the in-phase and out-of-phase current responses. Because they can sample mass transfer at low frequencies and electron transfer at high frequencies, impedance approaches are quite effective (Lisdat and Schäfer 2008, Chang and Park 2010).

## 12.5 Nanobiosensors and cancer detection and diagnosis

Tumor-specific signature markers expressed on the cell surface, or cancer biomarkers, can be used to identify and diagnose the illness early. According to preliminary data, these cancer marker signals can be used with different biosensing technologies to enable early cancer diagnosis (Cheng *et al* 2019).

The greatest opportunity to improve treatment outcomes and lower the number of cancer deaths is through early cancer diagnosis. Because of their distinct chemical and physical characteristics, large surface area, and ease of functionalization with various biomolecules that can recognize pertinent cancer biomarkers, nanomaterial based biosensors that use graphene quantum dots (GQDs) as a sensing platform show great promise in the early and sensitive detection of cancer biomarkers. It has been demonstrated that the developed optical, electrochemical, and chemiluminescent biosensors based on GQDs guarantee the accurate detection of several cancer disorders as well as the ability to assess the efficacy of anti-cancer therapy. It has been reported that ferrosoferric oxide, GQDs, and molybdenum disulfide-based magnetic fluorescence biosensors can be utilized to identify and separate CTCs (Cui et al 2019). The majority of the biosensors that have been reported have low detection limits and a wide linear range of detection, which indicates their tremendous potential for use in cancer clinics for cancer diagnosis and treatment (Iannazzo et al 2021).

Sequence-specific DNA serves as the recognition element of amperometric-based biosensors for cancer detection, which show great promise for cancer diagnosis. These sensors recognize and hybridize to specific DNA sequences found in the genomes of malignant cells, allowing them to identify the presence of gene mutations linked to cancer (Bohunicky and Mousa 2010).

Effective biosensors for quick examination of cellular changes to find associated biomarkers are highly sought after to ultimately improve the prognosis and treatment approaches for malignancies. However, to create low-cost lab-on-chips and next-generation innovative biosensors, new strategies including nanofabrication and clinical applications are required. It is interesting to note that the most frequently reported sensing technique for finding cancer biomarkers is electrochemical biosensors. Future research is anticipated to make more use of nanostructured materials and nanocomposites, which are crucial to the creation and design of a variety of electrochemical biosensors. To improve the stability and repeatability of the sensor, more research is needed in the manufacture of electrochemical transducers. Biomarker biosensors are still in their early stages of commercialization due to difficulties in downsizing the apparatus and incorporating microfluidics technology for the creation of a clinical justification (Hasan et al 2021). Various reported biosensors for the detection of biomarkers in cancer patients are listed in table 12.4.

Affinity-based electrochemical biosensors are typically used in cancer biomarker analysis to find gene alterations in biomarkers and protein biomarkers. However, a lot of the technology is still in its research and development phase. One of the most successful methods for identifying cancer biomarkers early on is the use of DNA-based electrochemical biosensors (Tothill 2009). Based on the hybridization of ssDNA and the immobilization of complementary DNA/RNA molecules (probe) on the modified electrode surface, DNA-based biosensors collect the sequential information of the target-DNA to further produce an electrical signal of that particular analyte to be evaluated. To achieve quick, precise, and stable detection, various immobilization strategies are introduced based on the characteristics of the transducer. The immobilization and hybridization processes are influenced by the alteration of the electrode surface with various nanoparticles. Because single-base mismatch, low concentration of oligonucleotides, and simple structural assembly are recognized by DNA biosensors, they can quickly identify cancer biomarkers produced by malignant cells (Abu-Salah *et al* 2015).

Typically, piezoelectric immunosensors are made to identify cancer signs by immobilizing a particular antibody on the sensor chip. These technologies have led to the release of more sophisticated gadgets on the market. Human ferritin and hCG may now be detected using piezoelectric immunosensors (Tothill 2009).

The SPR that results from the complete internal reflection of light at a metal film–liquid interface is one of the most widely utilized label-free optical methods for biomolecular interaction detection. To diagnose prostate cancer in human serum samples, Uludag and Tothill (2012) developed a sensitive SPR and quartz crystal microbalance (QCM) point-of-care immunosensor. The assay's high affinity was indicated by the predicted KD of the antibody used against PSA, which was $9.46 \times 10^{-10}$ M. It was discovered that the SPR sensor results were similar to those obtained with a QCM sensor platform, suggesting that disease biomarker screening can be conducted with both systems. It is consequently possible to successfully use the developed immunoassay's clinical applicability with serum samples from patients. This highlights how very promising the proposed sensor devices are as platforms for clinical prostate cancer diagnosis and prognosis (Uludag and Tothill 2012).

The biochemical tests and labeling procedures utilized in traditional cancer screening techniques are costly overall. Cancer cells have been identified by the use of label-free microwave biosensors. In short, these biosensors feature a coplanar waveguide transmission line and a detection window that allow the dielectric characterization of different cancer cells, such as human hepatoma and human LC (A549) cell lines, to be observed. Biosensors have been reported to be employed in the *in vitro* diagnosis of a variety of malignancies because they block the effects of microwave parasites and measure the dielectric characteristics of cancer cells (Iqbal *et al* 2022).

## 12.6 Conclusion

Worldwide, cancer is the primary cause of illness. Exposure to variable environmental, lifestyle, and cultural factors is the primary cause of the majority of malignancies. Of all cancers, lung cancer in men and breast cancer in women are the most prevalent and pose a global public health threat. Therefore, early cancer detection is crucial for the effective therapy of patients. Based on the examination of bodily fluids, liquid biopsy has become a promising non-invasive diagnostic biomarker for early cancer identification. DNA and RNA in circulation are promising non-invasive biomarkers for early cancer detection. The pico-to-femtomolar concentration of circulating RNA in serum can be difficult to detect accurately and sensitively, especially when there are other analogs present that produce strong background signals. Recent advancements in the field of nanosensors could result in the creation of point-of-care cancer diagnostic techniques that are rapid, accurate, and reasonably priced.

# References

Abu-Salah K M, Zourob M M, Mouffouk F, Alrokayan S A, Alaamery M A and Ansari A A 2015 DNA-based nanobiosensors as an emerging platform for detection of disease *Sensors* **15** 14539–68

Alhadrami H A 2018 Biosensors: classifications, medical applications, and future prospective *Biotechnol. Appl. Biochem.* **65** 497–508

Asci Erkocyigit B, Ozufuklar O, Yardim A, Guler Celik E and Timur S 2023 Biomarker detection in early diagnosis of cancer: recent achievements in point-of-care devices based on paper microfluidics *Biosensors* **13** 387

Asl M B, Karamdel J, Khoshbaten M and Rostami A 2022 Plasmonic biosensor for early gastric cancer detection *Opt. Contin.* **9** 2043–61

Azimzadeh M, Rahaie M, Nasirizadeh N, Ashtari K and Naderi-Manesh H 2016 An electro-chemical nanobiosensor for plasma miRNA-155, based on graphene oxide and gold nano-rod, for early detection of breast cancer *Biosens. Bioelectron.* **77** 99–106

Bao G, Huang J, Pan W, Li X and Zhou T 2020 Long noncoding RNA CERS6-AS1 functions as a malignancy promoter in breast cancer by binding to IGF2BP3 to enhance the stability of CERS6 mRNA *Cancer Med.* **9** 278–89

Bohunicky B and Mousa S A 2010 Biosensors: the new wave in cancer diagnosis *Nanotechnol. Sci. Appl.* **4** 1–10

Buono G *et al* 2019 Circulating tumor DNA analysis in breast cancer: is it ready for prime-time? *Cancer Treat. Rev.* **73** 73–83

Calvo-Lozano O, Garcia-Aparicio P, Raduly L Z, Estévez M C, Berindan-Neagoe I, Ferracin M and Lechuga L M 2022 One-step and real-time detection of microRNA-21 in human samples for lung cancer biosensing diagnosis *Anal. Chem.* **94** 14659–65

Canatan D, Yılmaz Ö, Sönmez Y, Çim A, Coşkun H, Göksu S S, Ucar S and Aktekin M R 2021 Circulating microRNAs as potential non-invasive biomarkers for breast cancer detection *Acta Biomed.* **92** e2021028

Cardoso A R, Moreira F T, Fernandes R and Sales M G 2016 Novel and simple electrochemical biosensor monitoring attomolar levels of miRNA-155 in breast cancer *Biosens. Bioelectron.* **80** 621–30

Cash K J and Clark H A 2010 Nanosensors and nanomaterials for monitoring glucose in diabetes *Trends Mol. Med.* **16** 584–93

Chaddha M, Rai H, Gupta R and Thakral D 2023 Integrated analysis of circulating cell free nucleic acids for cancer genotyping and immune phenotyping of tumor microenvironment *Front. Genet.* **14** 1138625

Chang B Y and Park S M 2010 Electrochemical impedance spectroscopy *Annu. Rev. Anal. Chem.* **3** 207–29

Chauhan N, Maekawa T and Kumar D N 2017 Graphene based biosensors—accelerating medical diagnostics to new-dimensions *J. Mater. Res.* **32** 2860–82

Chen L and Shan G 2021 CircRNA in cancer: fundamental mechanism and clinical potential *Cancer Lett.* **505** 49–57

Chen Y and Shi H 2023 Rapid and label-free analysis of antigen–antibody dynamic binding of tumor markers using piezoelectric quartz crystal biosensor *Biosensors* **13** 917

Chen Z, Zhen M and Zhou J 2019 LncRNA BRE-AS1 interacts with miR-145-5p to regulate cancer cell proliferation and apoptosis in prostate carcinoma and has early diagnostic values *Biosci. Rep.* **39** BSR20182097

Chen Z H, Zhang G L, Li H R, Luo J D, Li Z X, Chen G M and Yang J 2012 A panel of five circulating microRNAs as potential biomarkers for prostate cancer *Prostate* **72** 1443–52

Cheng N, Du D, Wang X, Liu D, Xu W, Luo Y and Lin Y 2019 Recent advances in biosensors for detecting cancer-derived exosomes *Trends Biotechnol.* **37** 1236–54

Condrat C E, Thompson D C, Barbu M G, Bugnar O L, Boboc A, Cretoiu D, Suciu N, Cretoiu S M and Voinea S C 2020 miRNAs as biomarkers in disease: latest findings regarding their role in diagnosis and prognosis *Cells* **9** 276

Coronell J A, Syed P, Sergelen K, Gyurján I and Weinhäusel A 2012 The current status of cancer biomarker research using tumour-associated antigens for minimal invasive and early cancer diagnostics *J. Proteomics* **76** 102–15

Crosby D *et al* 2022 Early detection of cancer *Science* **375** eaay9040

Cui F, Ji J, Sun J, Wang J, Wang H, Zhang Y, Ding H, Lu Y, Xu D and Sun X 2019 A novel magnetic fluorescent biosensor based on graphene quantum dots for rapid, efficient, and sensitive separation and detection of circulating tumor cells *Anal. Bioanal. Chem.* **411** 985–95

Das S, Dey M K, Devireddy R and Gartia M R 2023 Biomarkers in cancer detection, diagnosis, and prognosis *Sensors* **24** 37

de Jonge H, Iamele L, Maggi M, Pessino G and Scotti C 2021 Anti-cancer auto-antibodies: roles, applications and open issues *Cancers* **13** 813

Debes J D, Romagnoli P A, Prieto J, Arrese M, Mattos A Z and Boonstra A 2021 Escalon consortium. Serum biomarkers for the prediction of hepatocellular carcinoma *Cancers* **13** 1681

Dey D and Goswami T 2011 Optical biosensors: a revolution towards quantum nanoscale electronics device fabrication *BioMed Res. Int.* **2011** 348218

Dillekås H, Rogers M S and Straume O 2019 Are 90% of deaths from cancer caused by metastases? *Cancer Med.* **8** 5574–6

Ding Y, Liu J, Jin X, Lu H, Shen G and Yu R 2008 Poly-L-lysine/hydroxyapatite/carbon nanotube hybrid nanocomposite applied for piezoelectric immunoassay of carbohydrate antigen 19-9 *Analyst* **133** 184–90

Duffy M J 2020 Biomarkers for prostate cancer: prostate-specific antigen and beyond *Clin. Chem. Lab. Med.* **58** 326–39

El Aamri M, Yammouri G, Mohammadi H, Amine A and Korri-Youssoufi H 2020 Electrochemical biosensors for detection of microRNA as a cancer biomarker: pros and cons *Biosensors* **10** 186

Elemeery M N, Badr A N, Mohamed M A and Ghareeb D A 2017 Validation of a serum microRNA panel as biomarkers for early diagnosis of hepatocellular carcinoma post-hepatitis C infection in Egyptian patients *World J. Gastroenterol.* **23** 3864

Escuin D *et al* 2021 Circulating microRNAs in early breast cancer patients and its association with lymph node metastases *Front. Oncol.* **11** 627811

Falkowski P, Lukaszewski Z and Gorodkiewicz E 2021 Potential of surface plasmon resonance biosensors in cancer detection *J. Pharm. Biomed. Anal.* **194** 113802

Fang Y, Yan D, Wang L, Zhang J and He Q 2022 Circulating microRNAs (miR-16, miR-22, miR-122) expression and early diagnosis of hepatocellular carcinoma *J. Clin. Lab. Anal.* **36** e24541

Fares J, Fares M Y, Khachfe H H, Salhab H A and Fares Y 2020 Molecular principles of metastasis: a hallmark of cancer revisited *Signal Transduct. Target. Therapy* **5** 28

Fass L 2008 Imaging and cancer: a review *Mol. Oncol.* **2** 115–52

Flitcroft J G, Verheyen J, Vemulkar T, Welbourne E N, Rossi S H, Welsh S J, Cowburn R P and Stewart G D 2022 Early detection of kidney cancer using urinary proteins: a truly non-invasive strategy *BJU Int.* **129** 290–303

Fu Y, Wei X, Tang C, Li J, Liu R, Shen A and Wu Z 2013 Circulating microRNA-101 as a potential biomarker for hepatitis B virus-related hepatocellular carcinoma *Oncol. Lett.* **6** 1811–5

Gao X, Qin T, Mao J, Zhang J, Fan S, Lu Y, Sun Z, Zhang Q, Song B and Li L 2019 PTENP1/miR-20a/PTEN axis contributes to breast cancer progression by regulating PTEN via PI3K/AKT pathway *J. Exp. Clin. Cancer Res.* **38** 1–4

Gilyazova I *et al* 2023 MicroRNA expression signatures in clear cell renal cell carcinoma: high-throughput searching for key miRNA markers in patients from the volga-ural region of eurasian continent *Int. J. Mol. Sci.* **24** 6909

Gong X *et al* 2017 Novel lincRNA SLINKY is a prognostic biomarker in kidney cancer *Oncotarget* **8** 18657

Grieshaber D, MacKenzie R, Vörös J and Reimhult E 2008 Electrochemical biosensors-sensor principles and architectures *Sensors* **8** 1400–58

Griffiths H R *et al* 2002 Biomarkers *Mol. Asp. Med.* **23** 101–208

Hakimian F and Ghourchian H 2020 Ultrasensitive electrochemical biosensor for detection of microRNA-155 as a breast cancer risk factor *Anal. Chim. Acta* **1136** 1–8

Hakimian F, Ghourchian H, Hashemi A S, Arastoo M R and Behnam Rad M 2018 Ultrasensitive optical biosensor for detection of miRNA-155 using positively charged Au nanoparticles *Sci. Rep.* **8** 2943

Haleem A, Javaid M, Singh R P, Suman R and Rab S 2021 Biosensors applications in medical field: a brief review *Sens. Int.* **2** 100100

Halvorsen A R *et al* 2016 A unique set of 6 circulating microRNAs for early detection of non-small cell lung cancer *Oncotarget* **7** 37250

Hammond J L, Formisano N, Estrela P, Carrara S and Tkac J 2016 Electrochemical biosensors and nanobiosensors *Essays Biochem.* **60** 69–80

Han Y and Li H 2018 miRNAs as biomarkers and for the early detection of non-small cell lung cancer (NSCLC) *J. Thorac. Dis.* **10** 3119

Hanahan D and Weinberg R A 2011 Hallmarks of cancer: the next generation *Cell* **144** 646–74

Happel C, Ganguly A and Tagle D A 2020 Extracellular RNAs as potential biomarkers for cancer *J. Cancer Metastasis Treat.* **6** 32

Hasan M R, Ahommed M S, Daizy M, Bacchu M S, Ali M R, Al-Mamun M R, Aly M A, Khan M Z and Hossain S I 2021 Recent development in electrochemical biosensors for cancer biomarkers detection *Biosens. Bioelectron.* X **8** 100075

Heidari R *et al* 2019 CdS nanocrystals/graphene oxide-AuNPs based electrochemiluminescence immunosensor in sensitive quantification of a cancer biomarker: p53 *Biosens. Bioelectron.* **126** 7–14

Homola J, Yee S S and Gauglitz G 1999 Surface plasmon resonance sensors *Sensors Actuators* B **54** 3–15

Hossain N, Mobarak M H, Mimona M A, Islam M A, Hossain A, Zohur F T and Chowdhury M A 2023 Advances and significances of nanoparticles in semiconductor applications—a review *Res. Eng.* **19** 101347

Huang Z, Jiang Z, Zhao C, Han W, Lin L, Liu A, Weng S and Lin X 2017 Simple and effective label-free electrochemical immunoassay for carbohydrate antigen 19-9 based on polythionine-Au composites as enhanced sensing signals for detecting different clinical samples *Int. J. Nanomed.* **12** 3049–58

Hussain S, Mubeen I, Ullah N, Shah S S, Khan B A, Zahoor M, Ullah R, Khan F A and Sultan M A 2022 Modern diagnostic imaging technique applications and risk factors in the medical field: a review *BioMed Res. Int.* **2022** 5164970

Iannazzo D, Espro C, Celesti C, Ferlazzo A and Neri G 2021 Smart biosensors for cancer diagnosis based on graphene quantum dots *Cancers* **13** 3194

Ibáñez-Redín G, Joshi N, do Nascimento G F, Wilson D, Melendez M E, Carvalho A L, Reis R M, Gonçalves D and Oliveira O N 2020 Determination of p53 biomarker using an electrochemical immunoassay based on layer-by-layer films with NiFe$_2$O$_4$ nanoparticles *Microchim. Acta* **187** 619

Iqbal M J *et al* 2022 Biosensing chips for cancer diagnosis and treatment: a new wave towards clinical innovation *Cancer Cell Int.* **22** 354

Işın M, Uysaler E, Özgür E, Köseoğlu H, Şanlı Ö, Yücel Ö B, Gezer U and Dalay N 2015 Exosomal lncRNA-p21 levels may help to distinguish prostate cancer from benign disease *Front. Genet.* **6** 168

Javaid M and Haleem A 2019 Industry 4.0 applications in medical field: a brief review *Curr. Med. Res. Pract.* **9** 102–9

Jedinak A, Curatolo A, Zurakowski D, Dillon S, Bhasin M K, Libermann T A, Roy R, Sachdev M, Loughlin K R and Moses M A 2015 Novel non-invasive biomarkers that distinguish between benign prostate hyperplasia and prostate cancer *BMC Cancer* **15** 1–9

Jiang N *et al* 2018 Circulating lncRNA XLOC_009167 serves as a diagnostic biomarker to predict lung cancer *Clin. Chim. Acta* **486** 26–33

Jiao Y, Li Y, Jia B, Chen Q, Pan G, Hua F and Liu Y 2020 The prognostic value of lncRNA SNHG4 and its potential mechanism in liver cancer *Biosci. Rep.* **40** BSR20190729

Jin X, Ge L P, Li D Q, Shao Z M, Di G H, Xu X E and Jiang Y Z 2020 LncRNA TROJAN promotes proliferation and resistance to CDK4/6 inhibitor via CDK2 transcriptional activation in ER+ breast cancer. *Mol. Cancer* **19** 1–8

Joshi G K, Deitz-McElyea S, Johnson M, Mali S, Korc M and Sardar R 2014 Highly specific plasmonic biosensors for ultrasensitive microRNA detection in plasma from pancreatic cancer patients *Nano Lett.* **14** 6955–63

Ju S, Chen C, Zhang J, Xu L, Zhang X, Li Z, Chen Y, Zhou J, Ji F and Wang L 2022 Detection of circulating tumor cells: opportunities and challenges *Biomark. Res.* **10** 58

Kal-Koshvandi A T 2020 Recent advances in optical biosensors for the detection of cancer biomarker α-fetoprotein (AFP) *TrAC, Trends Anal. Chem.* **128** 115920

Kaur B, Kumar S and Kaushik B K 2022 Recent advancements in optical biosensors for cancer detection *Biosens. Bioelectron.* **197** 113805

Kazemi-Darsanaki R, Azizzadeh A, Nourbakhsh M, Raeisi G and AzizollahiAliabadi M 2013 Biosensors: functions and applications *J. Biol. Today's World* **2** 53–61

Khodadoust A, Nasirizadeh N, Seyfati S M, Taheri R A, Ghanei M and Bagheri H 2023 High-performance strategy for the construction of electrochemical biosensor for simultaneous detection of miRNA-141 and miRNA-21 as lung cancer biomarkers *Talanta* **252** 123863

Kilic T, Topkaya S N, Ariksoysal D O, Ozsoz M, Ballar P, Erac Y and Gozen O 2012 Electrochemical based detection of microRNA, mir21 in breast cancer cells *Biosens. Bioelectron.* **38** 195–201

Kimmel D W, LeBlanc G, Meschievitz M E and Cliffel D E 2012 Electrochemical sensors and biosensors *Anal. Chem.* **84** 685–707

Kozak K R, Su F, Whitelegge J P, Faull K, Reddy S and Farias-Eisner R 2005 Characterization of serum biomarkers for detection of early stage ovarian cancer *Proteomics* **5** 4589–96

Lazcka O, Del Campo F J and Munoz F X 2007 Pathogen detection: a perspective of traditional methods and biosensors *Biosens. Bioelectron.* **22** 1205–17

Lemos A E, da Rocha Matos A and Ferreira L B 2019 The long non-coding RNA PCA3: an update of its functions and clinical applications as a biomarker in prostate cancer *Oncotarget* **10** 6589

Leung W H, Pang C C, Pang S N, Weng S X, Lin Y L, Chiou Y E, Pang S T and Weng W H 2021 High-sensitivity dual-probe detection of urinary miR-141 in cancer patients via a modified screen-printed carbon electrode-based electrochemical biosensor *Sensors* **21** 3183

Li C, Lv Y, Shao C, Chen C, Zhang T, Wei Y, Fan H, Lv T, Liu H and Song Y 2019a Tumor-derived exosomal lncRNA GAS5 as a biomarker for early-stage non-small-cell lung cancer diagnosis *J. Cell. Physiol.* **234** 20721–7

Li H, Zhang S, Wang Q and Zhu R 2016 Clinical value of mammography in diagnosis and identification of breast mass *Pak. J. Med. Sci.* **32** 1020

Li J, Guan X, Fan Z, Ching L M, Li Y, Wang X, Cao W M and Liu D X 2020 Non-invasive biomarkers for early detection of breast cancer *Cancers* **12** 2767

Li L, Zhang L, Zhang Y and Zhou F 2015 Increased expression of LncRNA BANCR is associated with clinical progression and poor prognosis in gastric cancer *Biomed. Pharmacother.* **72** 109–12

Li S J, Wang L, Sun Z X, Sun S J, Gao J and Ma R L 2019b LncRNA SNHG1 promotes liver cancer development through inhibiting p53 expression via binding to DNMT1 *Eur. Rev. Med. Pharmacol. Sci.* **23** 2768–76

Lin D *et al* 2020 Circulating tumor cells: biology and clinical significance *Signal Transduct. Target. Ther.* **6** 404

Lin Y, Bariya M and Javey A 2021 Wearable biosensors for body computing *Adv. Funct. Mater.* **31** 2008087

Ling Z A, Xiong D D, Meng R M, Cen J M, Zhao N, Chen G, Li R L and Dang Y W 2018 LncRNA NEAT1 promotes deterioration of hepatocellular carcinoma based on *in vitro* experiments, data mining, and RT-qPCR analysis *Cell. Physiol. Biochem.* **48** 540–55

Lisdat F and Schäfer D 2008 The use of electrochemical impedance spectroscopy for biosensing *Anal. Bioanal. Chem.* **391** 1555–67

Liu C N and Zhang H Y 2020 Serum lncRNA LOXL1-AS1 is a diagnostic and prognostic marker for epithelial ovarian cancer *J. Gene Med.* **22** e3233

Lu G *et al* 2018 Long noncoding RNA LINC00511 contributes to breast cancer tumourigenesis and stemness by inducing the miR-185-3p/E2F1/Nanog axis *J. Exp. Clin. Cancer Res.* **37** 1

Ma T, Jia H, Ji P, He Y and Chen L 2021 Identification of the candidate lncRNA biomarkers for acute kidney injury: a systematic review and meta-analysis *Expert Rev. Mol. Diagn.* **21** 77–89

Magbanua M J *et al* 2021 Circulating tumor DNA in neoadjuvant-treated breast cancer reflects response and survival *Ann. Oncol.* **32** 229–39

Majd S M, Salimi A and Ghasemi F 2018 An ultrasensitive detection of miRNA-155 in breast cancer via direct hybridization assay using two-dimensional molybdenum disulfide field-effect transistor biosensor *Biosens. Bioelectron.* **105** 6–13

Mansor N A, Zain Z M, Hamzah H H, Noorden M S, Jaapar S S, Beni V and Ibupoto Z H 2014 Detection of breast cancer 1 (*BRCA1*) gene using an electrochemical DNA biosensor based on immobilized ZnO nanowires *Open J. Appl. Biosensor.* **3** 9

Medetalibeyoglu H, Kotan G, Atar N and Yola M L 2020 A novel sandwich-type SERS immunosensor for selective and sensitive carcinoembryonic antigen (CEA) detection *Anal. Chim. Acta* **1139** 100–10

Mehrotra P 2016 Biosensors and their applications: a review *J. Oral Biol. Craniofac. Res.* **6** 153–9

Meirinho S G, Dias L G, Peres A M and Rodrigues L R 2016 Voltammetric aptasensors for protein disease biomarkers detection: a review *Biotechnol. Adv.* **34** 941–53

Metkar S K and Girigoswami K 2019 Diagnostic biosensors in medicine: a review. *Biocatal. Agric. Biotechnol.* **17** 271–83

Mohammadpour-Haratbar A, Boraei S B, Zare Y, Rhee K Y and Park S J 2023 Graphene-based electrochemical biosensors for breast cancer detection *Biosensors* **13** 80

Mollaei H, Safaralizadeh R and Rostami Z 2019 MicroRNA replacement therapy in cancer *J. Cell. Physiol.* **234** 12369–84

Mor G, Visintin I, Lai Y, Zhao H, Schwartz P, Rutherford T, Yue L, Bray-Ward P and Ward D C 2005 Serum protein markers for early detection of ovarian cancer *Proc. Natl Acad. Sci.* **102** 7677–82

Nasrollahpour H, Naseri A, Rashidi M R and Khalilzadeh B 2021 Application of green synthesized WO$_3$-poly glutamic acid nanobiocomposite for early stage biosensing of breast cancer using electrochemical approach *Sci. Rep.* **11** 23994

Naylor S 2003 Biomarkers: current perspectives and future prospects *Expert Rev. Mol. Diagn.* **3** 525–9

Ng E K *et al* 2013 Circulating microRNAs as specific biomarkers for breast cancer detection *PLoS One* **8** e53141

Niemira M *et al* 2023 Identification of serum miR-1246 and miR-150-5p as novel diagnostic biomarkers for high-grade serous ovarian cancer *Sci. Rep.* **13** 19287

Nooreldeen R and Bach H 2021 Current and future development in lung cancer diagnosis *Int. J. Mol. Sci.* **22** 8661

Palchetti I 2016 New trends in the design of enzyme-based biosensors for medical applications *Mini-Rev. Med. Chem.* **16** 1125–33

Pan W, Liu L, Wei J, Ge Y, Zhang J, Chen H, Zhou L, Yuan Q, Zhou C and Yang M 2016 A functional lncRNA HOTAIR genetic variant contributes to gastric cancer susceptibility *Mol. Carcinogen.* **55** 90–6

Parkhey P and Mohan S V 2019 Biosensing applications of microbial fuel cell: approach toward miniaturization *Microbial Electrochemical Technology* (Amsterdam: Elsevier) pp 977–97

Paterlini-Brechot P and Benali N L 2007 Circulating tumor cells (CTC) detection: clinical impact and future directions *Cancer Lett.* **253** 180–204

Pohanka M and Skládal P 2008 Electrochemical biosensors—principles and applications *J. Appl. Biomed.* **6** 57–64

Pourasl M H, Vahedi A, Tajalli H, Khalilzadeh B and Bayat F 2023 Liquid crystal-assisted optical biosensor for early-stage diagnosis of mammary glands using HER-2 *Sci. Rep.* **13** 6847

Preethi K A, Selvakumar S C, Ross K, Jayaraman S, Tusubira D and Sekar D 2022 Liquid biopsy: exosomal microRNAs as novel diagnostic and prognostic biomarkers in cancer *Mol. Cancer* **21** 54

Pulumati A, Pulumati A, Dwarakanath B S, Verma A and Papineni R V 2023 Technological advancements in cancer diagnostics: improvements and limitations *Cancer Rep.* **6** e1764

Qiao K, Ning S, Wan L, Wu H, Wang Q, Zhang X, Xu S and Pang D 2019 LINC00673 is activated by YY1 and promotes the proliferation of breast cancer cells via the miR-515-5p/MARK4/Hippo signaling pathway *J. Exp. Clin. Cancer Res.* **38** 1–5

Qin S, Yang L, Kong S, Xu Y, Liang B and Ju S 2021 LncRNA HCP5: a potential biomarker for diagnosing gastric cancer *Front. Oncol.* **11** 684531

Qiu M, Xu Y, Yang X, Wang J, Hu J, Xu L and Yin R 2014 CCAT2 is a lung adenocarcinoma-specific long non-coding RNA and promotes invasion of non-small cell lung cancer *Tumor Biol.* **35** 5375–80

Rafiee-Pour H A, Behpour M and Keshavarz M 2016 A novel label-free electrochemical miRNA biosensor using methylene blue as redox indicator: application to breast cancer biomarker miRNA-21 *Biosens. Bioelectron.* **77** 202–7

Repetto O, Vettori R, Steffan A, Cannizzaro R and De Re V 2023 Circulating proteins as diagnostic markers in gastric cancer *Int. J. Mol. Sci.* **24** 16931

Rocchitta G *et al* 2016 Enzyme biosensors for biomedical applications: strategies for safeguarding analytical performances in biological fluids *Sensors* **16** 780

Sagadevan S and Periasamy M 2014 Recent trends in nanobiosensors and their applications—a review *Rev. Adv. Mater. Sci.* **36** 62–9

Salahandish R, Ghaffarinejad A, Omidinia E, Zargartalebi H, Majidzadeh-A K, Naghib S M and Sanati-Nezhad A 2018 Label-free ultrasensitive detection of breast cancer miRNA-21 biomarker employing electrochemical nano-genosensor based on sandwiched AgNPs in PANI and N-doped graphene *Biosens. Bioelectron.* **120** 129–36

Saliminejad K, Mahmoodzadeh H, Fard S S, Yaghmaie M, Khorshid H R, Mousavi S A, Vaezi M and Ghaffari S H 2022 A panel of circulating microRNAs as a potential biomarker for the early detection of gastric cancer *Avicenna J. Med. Biotechnol.* **14** 278

Sappati K K and Bhadra S 2018 Piezoelectric polymer and paper substrates: a review *Sensors* **18** 3605

Sarkar D and Diermeier S D 2021 Circular RNAs: potential applications as therapeutic targets and biomarkers in breast cancer *Non-coding RNA* **7** 2

Sekhar M C, Veena E, Kumar N S, Naidu K C, Mallikarjuna A and Basha D B 2023 A review on piezoelectric materials and their applications *Cryst. Res. Technol.* **58** 2200130

Seyfried T N and Huysentruyt L C 2013 On the origin of cancer metastasis *Crit. Rev. Oncogen.* **18** 43–73

Sharifianjazi F, Rad A J, Bakhtiari A, Niazvand F, Esmaeilkhanian A, Bazli L, Abniki M, Irani M and Moghanian A 2021 Biosensors and nanotechnology for cancer diagnosis (lung and bronchus, breast, prostate, and colon): a systematic review *Biomed. Mater.* **17** 012002

Sharma A R, Bhattacharya M, Bhakta S, Saha A, Lee S S and Chakraborty C 2021a Recent research progress on circular RNAs: biogenesis, properties, functions, and therapeutic potential *Mol. Ther.-Nucl. Acids* **25** 355–71

Sharma A, Badea M, Tiwari S and Marty J L 2021b Wearable biosensors: an alternative and practical approach in healthcare and disease monitoring *Molecules* **26** 748

Sharma N and Srivastava S 2022 Diagnosis of pancreatic cancer using miRNA30e biosensor *Interdiscip. Sci.: Comput. Life Sci.* **14** 804–13

Sharma S 2009 Tumor markers in clinical practice: general principles and guidelines *Indian J. Med. Paediatr. Oncol.* **30** 1–8

Shen W, Xie X, Liu M and Wang L 2020 Diagnostic value of lncRNA ROR in differentiating ovarian cancer patients *Clin. Lab.* **66**

Shen Z, Wu A and Chen X 2017 Current detection technologies for circulating tumor cells *Chem. Soc. Rev.* **46** 2038–56

Si H, Chen P, Li H and Wang X 2019 Long non-coding RNA H19 regulates cell growth and metastasis via miR-138 in breast cancer *Am. J. Transl. Res.* **11** 3213

Siegel R L, Miller K D, Wagle N S and Jemal A 2023 Cancer statistics, 2023 *CA: Cancer J. Clin.* **73** 17–48

Soleimanian A, Khalilzadeh B, Mahdipour M, Aref A R, Kalbasi A, Bazaz S R, Warkiani M E, Rashidi M R and Mahdavi M 2021 An efficient graphene quantum dots-based electrochemical cytosensor for the sensitive recognition of CD123 in acute myeloid leukemia cells *IEEE Sens. J.* **21** 16451–63

Stejskal P, Goodarzi H, Srovnal J, Hajdúch M, van't Veer L J and Magbanua M J 2023 Circulating tumor nucleic acids: biology, release mechanisms, and clinical relevance *Mol. Cancer* **22** 15

Su L, Fong C C, Cheung P Y and Yang M 2017 Development of novel piezoelectric biosensor using PZT ceramic resonator for detection of cancer markers *Biosens. Biodetect.* **1572** 277–91

Syam R, Davis K J, Pratheesh M D, Anoopraj R and Joseph B S 2012 Biosensors: a novel approach for pathogen detection *Vet. Scan* **7** 102

Tan T H, Gochoo M, Chen Y F, Hu J J, Chiang J Y, Chang C S, Lee M H, Hsu Y N and Hsu J C 2017 Ubiquitous emergency medical service system based on wireless biosensors, traffic information, and wireless communication technologies: development and evaluation *Sensors* **17** 202

Tao Y *et al* 2020 Exploration of serum exosomal LncRNA TBILA and AGAP2-AS1 as promising biomarkers for diagnosis of non-small cell lung cancer *Int. J. Biol. Sci.* **16** 471

Tian C, Deng Y, Jin Y, Shi S and Bi H 2018 Long non-coding RNA RNCR3 promotes prostate cancer progression through targeting miR-185-5p *Am. J. Transl. Res.* **10** 1562

Tombelli S 2012 Piezoelectric biosensors for medical applications *Biosensors for Medical Applications* (Cambridge: Woodhead) pp 41–64

Tothill I E 2009 Biosensors for cancer markers diagnosis *Semin. Cell Dev. Biol.* **20** 55–62

Tsujiura M *et al* 2010 Circulating microRNAs in plasma of patients with gastric cancers *Br. J. Cancer* **102** 1174–9

Uludag Y and Tothill I E 2012 Cancer biomarker detection in serum samples using surface plasmon resonance and quartz crystal microbalance sensors with nanoparticle signal amplification *Anal. Chem.* **84** 5898–904

Vasconcelos M H, Caires H R, Ābols A, Xavier C P and Linē A 2019 Extracellular vesicles as a novel source of biomarkers in liquid biopsies for monitoring cancer progression and drug resistance *Drug Resist. Updat.* **47** 100647

Veyssière H, Bidet Y, Penault-Llorca F, Radosevic-Robin N and Durando X 2022 Circulating proteins as predictive and prognostic biomarkers in breast cancer *Clin. Proteom.* **19** 25

Wagner P D, Verma M and Srivastava S 2004 Challenges for biomarkers in cancer detection *Ann. NY Acad. Sci.* **1022** 9–16

Wang H M, Lu J H, Chen W Y and Gu A Q 2015a Upregulated lncRNA-UCA1 contributes to progression of lung cancer and is closely related to clinical diagnosis as a predictive biomarker in plasma *Int. J. Clin. Exp. Med.* **8** 11824

Wang J *et al* 2019 The long noncoding RNA H19 promotes tamoxifen resistance in breast cancer via autophagy *J. Hematol. Oncol.* **12** 1–4

Wang L 2017 Early diagnosis of breast cancer *Sensors* **17** 1572

Wang M, Shen B, Yuan R, Cheng W, Xu H and Ding S 2015b An electrochemical biosensor for highly sensitive determination of microRNA based on enzymatic and molecular beacon mediated strand displacement amplification *J. Electroanal. Chem.* **756** 147–52

Wei G H and Wang X 2017 lncRNA MEG3 inhibit proliferation and metastasis of gastric cancer via p53 signaling pathway *Eur. Rev. Med. Pharmacol. Sci.* **21** 3850–6

WHO 2022 https://www.who.int/news/item/01-02-2024-global-cancer-burden-growing--amidst-mounting-need-for-services

Xie J *et al* 2020 Serum long non-coding RNA LINC00887 as a potential biomarker for diagnosis of renal cell carcinoma *FEBS Open Bio* **10** 1802–9

Xu T, Liu C L, Li T, Zhang Y H and Zhao Y H 2019 LncRNA TUG1 aggravates the progression of prostate cancer and predicts the poor prognosis *Eur. Rev. Med. Pharmacol. Sci.* **23** 4698–4705

Xu W, Zhou G, Wang H, Liu Y, Chen B, Chen W, Lin C, Wu S, Gong A and Xu M 2020 Circulating lncRNA SNHG11 as a novel biomarker for early diagnosis and prognosis of colorectal cancer *Int. J. Cancer* **146** 2901–12

Yan Y, Liu J, Xu Z, Ye M and Li J 2021 lncRNA PCAT14 is a diagnostic marker for prostate cancer and is associated with immune cell infiltration *Dis. Markers* **2021** 9494619

Yang K, Hou Y, Li A, Li Z, Wang W, Xie H, Rong Z, Lou G and Li K 2017 Identification of a six-lncRNA signature associated with recurrence of ovarian cancer *Sci. Rep.* **7** 752

Yang L, Li N, Wang K, Hai X, Liu J and Dang F 2018 A novel peptide/Fe$_3$O$_4$@ SiO$_2$-Au nanocomposite-based fluorescence biosensor for the highly selective and sensitive detection of prostate-specific antigen *Talanta* **179** 531–7

Yang Y, Shao Y, Zhu M, Li Q, Yang F, Lu X, Xu C, Xiao B, Sun Y and Guo J 2016 Using gastric juice lncRNA-ABHD11-AS1 as a novel type of biomarker in the screening of gastric cancer *Tumor Biol.* **37** 1183–8

Yang Y, Xiang Y and Qi X 2023 Design of photonic crystal biosensors for cancer cell detection *Micromachines* **14** 1478

Zabeti Touchaei A, Vahidi S and Samadani A A 2024 Decoding the regulatory landscape of lncRNAs as potential diagnostic and prognostic biomarkers for gastric and colorectal cancers *Clin. Exp. Med.* **24** 29

Zamay T N, Zamay G S, Kolovskaya O S, Zukov R A, Petrova M M, Gargaun A, Berezovski M V and Kichkailo A S 2017 Current and prospective protein biomarkers of lung cancer *Cancers* **9** 155

Zeng Y, Zou Y, Gao G, Zheng S, Wu S, Xie X and Tang H 2022 The biogenesis, function and clinical significance of circular RNAs in breast cancer *Cancer Biol. Med.* **19** 14

Zhang H *et al* 2021 Detection methods and clinical applications of circulating tumor cells in breast cancer *Front. Oncol.* **11** 652253

Zhang P, Shi L, Song L, Long Y, Yuan K, Ding W and Deng L 2020 LncRNA CRNDE and lncRNA SNHG7 are promising biomarkers for prognosis in synchronous colorectal liver metastasis following hepatectomy *Cancer Manag. Res.* **12** 1681–92

Zhang Y, Liu Y, Liu H and Tang W H 2019 Exosomes: biogenesis, biologic function and clinical potential *Cell Biosci.* **9** 1–8

Zheng Y, Wang X, He S, Gao Z, Di Y, Lu K, Li K and Wang J 2019 Aptamer-DNA concatamer-quantum dots based electrochemical biosensing strategy for green and ultrasensitive detection of tumor cells via mercury-free anodic stripping voltammetry *Biosens. Bioelectron.* **126** 261–8

Zhu A, Lee D and Shim H 2011 Metabolic positron emission tomography imaging in cancer detection and therapy response *Semin. Oncol.* **38** 55–69

Zhu H *et al* 2017 LncRNA16 is a potential biomarker for diagnosis of early-stage lung cancer that promotes cell proliferation by regulating the cell cycle *Oncotarget* **8** 7867

Zhuang H, Cao G, Kou C and Li D 2019 Overexpressed lncRNA CDKN2B-AS1 is an independent prognostic factor for liver cancer and promotes its proliferation *J. BUON* **24** 1441–8

Zouari M, Campuzano S, Pingarrón J M and Raouafi N 2018 Amperometric biosensing of miRNA-21 in serum and cancer cells at nanostructured platforms using anti-DNA–RNA hybrid antibodies *ACS Omega* **3** 8923–31

Zouari M, Campuzano S, Pingarrón J M and Raouafi N 2020 Determination of miRNAs in serum of cancer patients with a label-and enzyme-free voltammetric biosensor in a single 30-min step *Microchim. Acta* **187** 444

# Chapter 13

## Challenges in the development of nanobiosensors in the diagnosis of cancer

**Manish S Sengar, Priya Kumari and Neha Sengar**

The integration of nanotechnology and biosensing platforms holds great promise for advancing cancer diagnostics, offering unprecedented sensitivity and specificity. Nanobiosensors, as powerful tools in this domain, exhibit unique capabilities for detecting cancer-related biomarkers with enhanced precision. However, the translation of these promising technologies from bench to bedside faces significant challenges that must be addressed to fully realize their clinical potential. This review explores the multifaceted challenges associated with the development of nanobiosensors for cancer diagnosis. Key issues encompass biocompatibility, scalability, reproducibility, and standardization of fabrication processes. Additionally, concerns related to the stability, functionalization, and integration of nanomaterials into biosensing platforms are discussed. Advances in addressing these challenges are crucial for fostering the successful deployment of nanobiosensors in clinical settings, ultimately contributing to earlier and more accurate cancer detection. The critical analysis presented herein aims to guide researchers, engineers, and clinicians toward overcoming obstacles and unlocking the full capabilities of nanobiosensors for improved cancer diagnostics.

## 13.1 Introduction

Nanobiosensors represent a groundbreaking technology in the field of diagnostics, offering unprecedented sensitivity, specificity, and portability. These miniature devices, capable of detecting biomolecules at the nanoscale, hold immense potential for revolutionizing healthcare by enabling early disease detection, monitoring of treatment efficacy, and personalized medicine [1, 2]. Nanotechnology has ushered in a significant shift, leading to the widespread adoption of biosensors and nanobiosensors across diverse scientific fields such as the biomedical, clinical, and healthcare sciences along with the agricultural environmental and sciences. The

doi:10.1088/978-0-7503-6234-4ch13

features of different nanobiosensors largely stem from the specific nanomaterials/ nanoparticles utilized in their sensing mechanisms. Over recent years, the recognition and detection of biological markers associated with various diseases (both communicable and non-communicable) have been achieved through numerous sensing methods employing nanotechnology alongside nanobiosensors. In the context of cancer diagnosis, nanobiosensors offer a promising avenue for improving early detection, prognosis, and therapeutic monitoring. Research into nanobiosensor technology is exploring its potential medical applications across a spectrum of areas, such as diagnostics, encompassing antibiotics, hormones, DNA, antibodies, disease markers, and more. It is also delving into the investigation of biomolecular interactions and biochemical assays, including nucleic acids, enzyme assays, proteins, antigen–antibodies, and drug carriers [3, 4].

However, despite their promising prospects, the development of nanobiosensors encounters several challenges. Ranging from technical hurdles to regulatory concerns, these challenges must be addressed to realize the full potential of nanobiosensors in cancer diagnosis and management. This chapter explores the key challenges hindering the widespread adoption of nanobiosensors in the diagnosis of cancer and discusses potential strategies to address them. Cancer is a complex and heterogeneous disease characterized by abnormal cell growth and proliferation [5, 6]. Early detection is critical for successful treatment outcomes, as it enables intervention at a stage when the disease is more amenable to therapy. Nanobiosensors offer the potential for detecting cancer biomarkers with high sensitivity and specificity, even at early stages of the disease. By leveraging nanotechnology and advanced sensing mechanisms, nanobiosensors hold the promise of enabling rapid, non-invasive, and accurate cancer diagnosis. Detecting cancer early increases the likelihood of successful treatment, leading to improved survival rates and reduced treatment expenses. Timely identification and treatment of cancer can markedly enhance the quality of life for patients. Despite a wealth of understanding about the causes, prevention, and management of cancer, significant strides in curing the disease remain limited. However, it has been established that early detection is the key to enhancing both quality of life and life expectancy. To achieve this goal, nanosensors and advanced nanomaterial based devices have been created to detect circulating tumor cells (CTCs), biomarkers, or tumor-derived vesicles. These elements are released relatively early from the tumor into the bloodstream, promising a substantial impact on the morbidity and mortality associated with the disease. For example, in pursuit of the early detection of lung cancer, a seed-mediated growth approach was employed to fabricate AuNR, while solution co-blending techniques were utilized to produce MTPP-AuNR nanocomposites. These nanocomposites served as the foundation for constructing an optical chemical sensor aimed at detecting specific biomarkers associated with lung cancer. Among the biomarkers targeted were decane, undecane, hexanal, heptanal, benzene, and TMB. Chen and colleagues utilized a nanoscale-gated biological field-effect transistor to detect the breast cancer serum biomarker protein CA15.3, achieving detection sensitivity down to concentrations of less than 20 units/ml. They employed a 'top-up' technique to fabricate the nanoscale biosensor, ensuring precise control of geometry through lithography and standard semiconductor processing techniques within a complementary metal oxide semiconductor (CMOS)-compatible process. Functionalization of the nanowires with CA15.3 was carried out, and 3-amino-propyl-triethoxysilane (APTES) was utilized for device silanization.

In the realm of cancer detection, electrochemical techniques have the capability to identify distinct cancer biomarkers present in breath or blood samples. This aids in the early detection of cancer and facilitates the monitoring of treatment response. Meanwhile, fluorescence methodologies facilitate the targeted imaging of cancer cells or tumor markers, thereby assisting in accurate localization and staging of the disease [7]. Table 13.1 shows some reported studies on nanobiosensors for cancer detection. Despite their potential, several challenges impede the development and clinical translation of nanobiosensors for cancer diagnosis (figure 13.1). Technical challenges include achieving high sensitivity and specificity while minimizing non-specific binding and signal interference, as well as ensuring the stability and reproducibility of sensor performance. Moreover, issues related to biocompatibility, integration with existing diagnostic platforms, and scalability also pose significant hurdles [8, 9]. In addition to technical challenges, regulatory considerations play a crucial role in the development and commercialization of nanobiosensors for cancer diagnosis. Regulatory agencies require comprehensive validation of sensor perform-ance, safety assessments, and clinical trials to demonstrate efficacy and reliability. Addressing regulatory requirements in a timely and cost-effective manner is essential for accelerating the translation of nanobiosensors from the laboratory to clinical practice [7, 10–12].

Furthermore, ethical considerations surrounding patient privacy, data security, and informed consent must be carefully addressed in the development and deploy-ment of nanobiosensors for cancer diagnosis. Collaborating with regulatory author-ities, stakeholders, and ethicists from the early stages of development can help navigate these complex ethical considerations and ensure the responsible and ethical use of nanobiosensors in healthcare.

Despite the challenges, the potential benefits of nanobiosensors in cancer diagnosis are substantial. Although there has been notable advancement over the past decade, conventional medical diagnostic methods for monitoring disease stages continue to face significant obstacles. These challenges include the absence of point-of-care (POC) diagnostic devices, the requirement for specialized expertise, low sensitivity, and selectivity issues leading to false-positive results. Consequently, there is a pressing demand for the development of POC diagnostic tools tailored for cancer biomarkers. The significance of particular cancer biomarkers and nano-materials, such as metal nanoparticles and graphene derivatives, cannot be over-stated in the development of electrochemical nanobiosensors for POC testing (POCT). Their straightforward operation, reliable performance, and potential for easy miniaturization and portability are key factors driving their utilization in cancer detection. Among these, ultrasensitive affinity-based electrochemical nanobiosen-sors stand out as highly promising candidates due to their distinctive properties. These nanobiosensors hold significant potential for advancing cancer detection and are poised to be the focal point of future research in this field [13].

**Table 13.1.** Nanobiosensor breakthroughs: advancements in cancer detection research.

| Type of cancer | Biomarker | Procedure | Nanoparticles used | LOD | References |
|---|---|---|---|---|---|
| Lung | miRNA-182 | ETC | Molybdenum disulfide $(MoS_2)/Ti_3C_2$ nanohybrids and modified GCE | 0.43 fM | [17] |
| Lung | MAGE A2 | ETC | Graphite/CN-chitosan/Ag (silver)/AB | 5.00 fg ml$^{-1}$ | [18] |
| Breast | HER2 | ETC | Polyaniline (PANI) functonalized with grafted AuNP and NS | 2 cells ml$^{-1}$ | [19] |
| Breast | BRCA1 | Cyclic voltammetry | GCE multiwalled CN modified with polycyclic aromatic nitrogen heterocycles (PANHS) and ssDNA probe targeting BRCA1 | $3.00 \times 10^{-18}$ mol l$^{-1}$ | [20] |
| Colorectal | CXCL5 | EIS and voltammetry | Conducting polymer-AuNP film with attached chemokine receptor 2 (CXCR2) | $0.078 \pm 0.004$ ng ml$^{-1}$ | [21] |
| Gastric | let-7a and miR-106a | ETC | Polyphenol/reduced GPO-modified GCE with AuNP and CdSe@CdS QTD contained magnetic NCs | 0.06 fM, 0.02 fM for miR-106a and let-7a, respectively | [22] |
| TNBC | miR-199a-5p | ETC | GCE modified with Au nanorods and GPO | 4.50 fM | [23] |

ETC—electrochemical; AuNP—gold nanoparticles; GCE—glassy carbon electrode; EIS—ETC impedance spectroscopy; GPO—graphene oxide; CdSe—cadmium selenide; CdS—cadmium sulfide; QTD—quantum dots; NCs—nanocomposites; TNBC—triple-negative breast cancer.

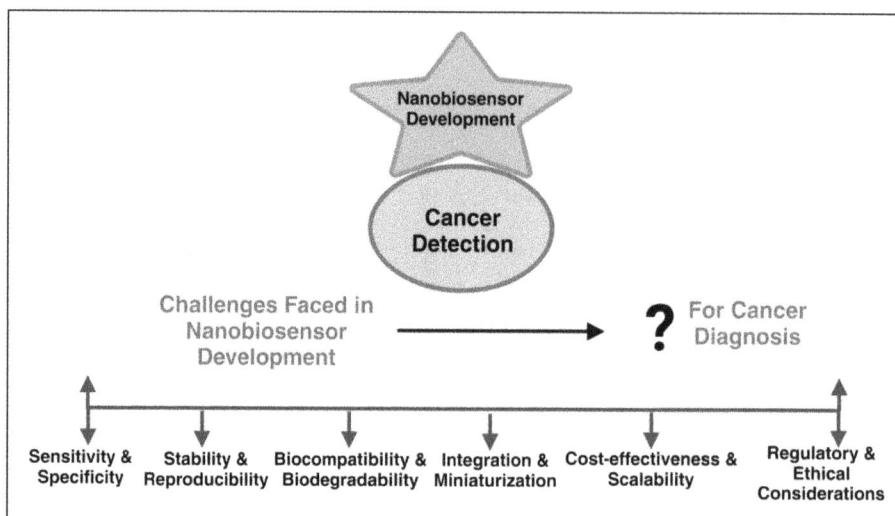

**Figure 13.1.** Diagram depicting different challenges faced in nanobiosensor development for cancer diagnosis.

By overcoming technical hurdles, addressing regulatory concerns, and navigating ethical considerations, nanobiosensors have the potential to revolutionize cancer diagnosis and improve patient outcomes. Continued innovation, interdisciplinary collaboration, and strategic partnerships are essential for overcoming these challenges and unlocking the full potential of nanobiosensors in the fight against cancer [14–16]. This chapter provides a comprehensive exploration of the multifaceted challenges encountered in the development of nanobiosensors for cancer diagnosis. By delving into the intricate complexities and hurdles inherent in this cutting-edge field, the chapter provides invaluable insights for researchers and practitioners striving to overcome obstacles and advance the frontier of early cancer detection. Through a meticulous examination of technological limitations, biological intricacies, and clinical requirements, this chapter offers a holistic understanding of the unique challenges that must be addressed to harness the full potential of nanobiosensors in the fight against cancer.

## 13.2 Sensitivity and specificity

One of the foremost challenges in nanobiosensor development is achieving high sensitivity and specificity while minimizing non-specific binding and signal interference. The nanobiosensor comprises several key components, including the analyte, biological probe, transducer, and data recording unit. The analyte represents the substance under investigation, easily identifiable within the system. The transducer plays a crucial role by converting information derived from the interaction between the biological layer and the analyte. It not only translates biological signals into digital format but also facilitates the conversion of signals. The biological probe employs affinity-based materials to explore interactions between various elements such as antigens and antibodies, digestive enzymes and substrates, nucleic acids, and cells. Lastly, the data recording unit serves to capture, store, and transmit the gathered data effectively [24].

For example, a highly sensitive platform was developed, comprising a nano-composite featuring silver and bovine serum albumin (Ag@BSA) nanoflowers decorated with single-walled carbon nanotubes (SWCNTs) and reduced graphene oxide (rGO), along with adsorbedpoly(3,4-ethylenedioxythiophene (PEDOT). This platform was designed for the detection of carcinoembryonic antigen (CEA), with anti-CEA antibodies immobilized onto its surface. The electrochemical sensor exhibited excellent performance characteristics, including linearity across a concentration range of 0.002–50 ng ml$^{-1}$ and a limit of detection (LOD) of $1 \times 10^{-4}$ ng ml$^{-1}$. Evaluation using cyclic voltammetry (CV) and linear sweep voltammetry (LSV) confirmed the sensor's stability, reproducibility, and high selectivity. Furthermore, the sensor offered the additional advantage of enabling real-time measurement of analytes in patient serum specimens [25].

Table 13.2 provides a summary of the sensitivity and specificity values of certain nanobiosensors utilized in early cancer detection. Nanobiosensors are designed to detect target biomolecules, such as proteins, nucleic acids, or small molecules, with exceptional precision and accuracy. These biomarkers often exist in bodily fluids at extremely low concentrations, making their detection challenging amidst the complex biological milieu [9, 26].

### 13.2.1 The importance of sensitivity and specificity

Sensitivity refers to the ability of a nanobiosensor to detect low concentrations of target biomolecules, while specificity denotes its ability to distinguish between the target molecule and other substances present in the sample. Achieving high sensitivity and specificity is crucial for accurate diagnosis, as it ensures that the sensor can reliably detect the presence of disease markers even at very low levels, while minimizing false positives due to non-specific binding [27, 28].

### 13.2.2 Challenges in sensitivity and specificity

Several factors contribute to the challenges associated with sensitivity and specificity in nanobiosensor development (figure 13.1).

#### 13.2.2.1 Non-specific binding
Nanobiosensors may interact with molecules other than the target biomolecule, leading to non-specific binding and false-positive results. This can arise from surface adsorption, electrostatic interactions, or chemical affinity with other components in the sample.

#### 13.2.2.2 Signal interference
Background signals from the sample matrix or interference from contaminants can interfere with the detection of the target molecule, reducing the sensor's sensitivity and specificity. Signal interference can arise from various sources, including auto-fluorescence, cross-reactivity with similar molecules, or environmental noise.

**Table 13.2.** Early cancer detection: harnessing the power of nanobiosensors.

| Nanomaterials/methods | Type of cancer | Target biomarkers | Sensitivity | Specificity | References |
|---|---|---|---|---|---|
| AuNPs: The sensors comprised layers of GNPs with 13 distinct organic ligands presented in two formats (manual and printed), resulting in 26 unique sensors within each nanosensor system | Lung | Various VOCs | 76%–100% | 75%–100% | [32] |
| AuNPs and SWCNT capped with polycyclic aromatic hydrocarbons | Lung | α-phellandrene, 4-methyl, dodecane and vinyl benzene | 100% | 95% | [33] |
| Chitosan-PDA-AgNPs: Chitosan was electrodeposited onto a GCE surface modified with PDA, followed by deposition of AgNPs onto the chitosan-PDA layer | Lung | Malondialdehyde | 1.45 $\mu$M | ND | [34] |
| CMOS-compatible SiNW: A CMOS-compatible SiNW-FET biosensor utilizing self-limiting anisotropic wet etching for SiNW fabrication | Lung | microRNAs (miRNAs) | 1 | | |
| zeptamole | High | [35] | | | |
| PVP bound iridium (III): The iridium (III) complex conjugated with poly (N-vinylpyrrolidone)-(Ir-PVP) was combined with PCL-PVP to form comicelles, subsequently employed in nanosensor fabrication | Lung | Hypoxia | High | High | [36] |
| WS$_2$ NW/TM was utilized for a biosensor | Breast | HER2 | 0.36 ng ml$^{-1}$ | 1 ng ml$^{-1}$ | [37] |
| Ti$_3$C$_2$:CdS NC: Initially, the surface of FTO electrode was coated with Ti$_3$C$_2$:CdS | Breast | miRNA 159c | 33 fmol l$^{-1}$ | Good | [38] |

(*Continued*)

**Table 13.2.** (*Continued*)

| Nanomaterials/methods | Type of cancer | Target biomarkers | Sensitivity | Specificity | References |
|---|---|---|---|---|---|
| NC. Subsequently, the SH-miRNA were anchored onto the electrode surface through the S–Cd following the removal of chitosan | | | | | |
| SPC-ECL sensor utilizing DNA-mediated Au-Au dimer | Breast | *BRCA1* gene | 0.83 fM | Good | [39] |
| Hairpin DNA strands H1 and H2 attached to AuNPs: The two hairpin DNA strands, H1 and H2, along with PEG, were tethered to the surface of AuNPs to form the photoacoustic nanoprobes (Au-H1/PEG and Au-H2/PEG) | Breast | miRNA 155 | 0.25 nM | Superior | [40] |
| AgNPs-modified MNFs: MNFs were fabricated through the self-assembly of peptide probes, attracting AgNPs to generate electrochemical signals and providing numerous reaction sites to amplify the signals | Breast | CD44 | 6 cells/ml | High | [41] |

GNPs—gold nanoparticles; SWCNT—single-walled carbon nanotubes; CMOS—complementary metal oxide semiconductor; SiNW—silicon nanowire; VOCs—volatile organic compounds; AgNPs—silver nanoparticles; AuNPs—gold nanoparticles; ND—not determined; HER2—human epidermal growth factor receptor 2; PVP —poly(N-vinylpyrrolidone); PCL-PVP—poly(e-caprolactone)-b-poly(N-vinylpyrrolidone); MNFs—multifunctional nanofibers; FTO—fluorine-doped tin oxide; PEG—polyethylene glycol; SPC-ECL—surface plasmon coupling electrochemiluminiscence; WS$_2$ NW/TM—tungsten sulfide nanowire array on titanium mesh; FET—field effect transistor; PDA—polydopamine; SH-miRNA—short hairpin microRNAs.

### 13.2.2.3 Low concentration detection

Detecting target biomolecules at extremely low concentrations poses a significant challenge, particularly in complex biological samples where the target molecule may be present in trace amounts amidst a high background of other molecules.

### 13.2.3 Strategies to enhance sensitivity and specificity

Researchers are continually exploring innovative approaches to enhance the sensitivity and specificity of nanobiosensors [29, 30]. To tackle these obstacles successfully, it is essential to meticulously engineer the sensor's chemical barrier. This entails optimizing sensitivities to the desired reaction while minimizing interference from non-specific interactions (figure 13.2). Achieving optimal results in terms of selectivity and sensitivity hinges on striking a delicate balance in the arrangement and composition of the chemical layer [25].

### 13.2.3.1 Nanomaterials
Utilizing advanced nanomaterials with unique properties, such as quantum dots, metallic nanoparticles, or carbon nanotubes, can improve sensor performance by enhancing signal amplification and minimizing non-specific interactions.

### 13.2.3.2 Surface functionalization
Tailoring the surface chemistry of the sensor platform through functionalization with biomolecular recognition elements, such as antibodies, aptamers, or

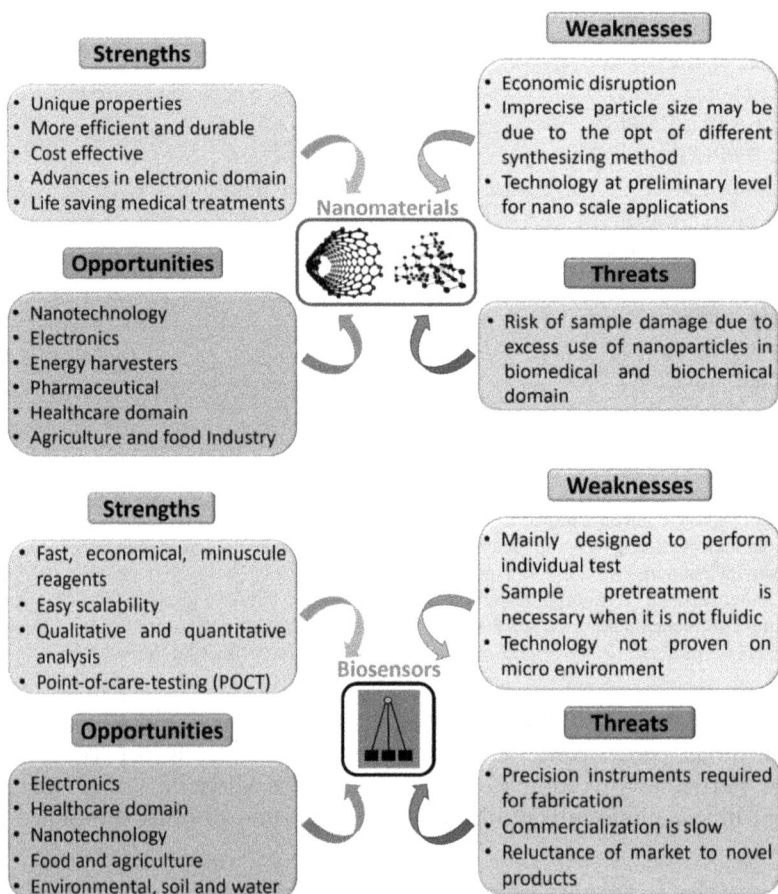

**Figure 13.2.** Diagram summarizing the advantages and disadvantages of nanomaterials in biosensor applications. (Adapted from [1]. CC BY 4.0.)

molecularly imprinted polymers, enhances specificity by selectively capturing the target molecule while minimizing non-specific binding.

### 13.2.3.3 Signal amplification

Employing signal amplification strategies, such as enzymatic reactions, nanoparticle-based amplification, or signal enhancement techniques, can boost the signal-to-noise ratio, improving sensitivity and enabling the detection of low-abundance biomolecules.

### 13.2.3.4 Multiplexing

Multiplexed detection platforms capable of simultaneously detecting multiple biomarkers enable comprehensive analysis of complex biological samples, enhancing diagnostic accuracy and specificity.

Achieving high sensitivity and specificity while minimizing non-specific binding and signal interference is essential for the successful development of nanobiosensors for diagnostic applications. Researchers are actively exploring innovative nanomaterials, surface functionalization techniques, and signal amplification strategies to overcome these challenges and enhance sensor performance. By improving the accuracy and reliability of nanobiosensors, we can advance early disease detection, personalized medicine, and improve patient outcomes in healthcare [31].

## 13.3 Stability and reproducibility

Ensuring the stability and reproducibility of nanobiosensors poses significant challenges. Factors such as nanomaterial degradation, surface fouling, and variations in fabrication processes can impact sensor performance and reliability over time. Nanomaterials, which are often the building blocks of nanobiosensors, can degrade due to environmental factors, chemical interactions, or biological processes. This degradation can compromise the structural integrity and functionality of the sensor, leading to inaccurate or unreliable results. Additionally, surface fouling, caused by the adsorption of biomolecules or contaminants onto the sensor surface, can interfere with target molecule detection and diminish sensor performance. Developing robust sensing platforms that exhibit long-term stability under physiological conditions is essential for real-world applications. Nanobiosensors intended for biomedical use must withstand the complex and dynamic environments found within biological systems, including temperature fluctuations, pH changes, and exposure to biological fluids. Designing sensor materials and surface coatings that are resistant to degradation and fouling is critical for maintaining sensor performance over extended periods [42, 43].

Moreover, achieving reproducibility across different batches of sensors is crucial for commercialization and widespread adoption. Variations in fabrication processes, material properties, and manufacturing conditions can lead to inconsistencies in sensor performance, making it challenging to produce sensors with consistent performance characteristics. Standardizing fabrication protocols, quality control measures, and validation procedures is essential for ensuring reproducibility and reliability across multiple sensor batches. Addressing the challenges of stability and reproducibility requires interdisciplinary collaboration and innovative engineering approaches. Researchers are exploring novel nanomaterials with enhanced stability properties, such as nanoparticles with protective coatings or biocompatible polymers with superior durability. Surface modification techniques, such as functionalization with self-assembled monolayers or polymer brushes, can mitigate surface fouling and enhance sensor stability [44–46]. Additionally, developing standardized fabrication protocols and quality control procedures can help improve reproducibility and ensure consistent sensor performance across different production batches. By addressing the challenges of stability and reproducibility, nanobiosensors can fulfill their potential as reliable tools for biomedical applications, including disease diagnosis, monitoring, and personalized medicine. Continued research and development efforts are essential for advancing the field of nanobiosensors and overcoming these technical hurdles to enable their widespread adoption in healthcare [47].

## 13.4 Biocompatibility and biodegradability

Nanobiosensors intended for biomedical applications must prioritize biocompatibility to minimize adverse effects on living organisms. Ensuring the compatibility of nanomaterials with biological systems, including cells, tissues, and bodily fluids, remains a paramount challenge. Biocompatibility is essential to prevent immune reactions, inflammation, or cytotoxicity, which can compromise the safety and efficacy of nanobiosensors in clinical settings. Moreover, the biodegradability of nanomaterials is crucial to prevent long-term accumulation and potential toxicity issues. Non-biodegradable nanoparticles may persist in biological systems, leading to bioaccumulation and adverse effects on cellular functions or organ systems [7, 9]. Therefore, designing nanobiosensors using biodegradable materials or engineering strategies for their safe disposal after use is a critical consideration in their development. Addressing the challenges of biocompatibility and biodegradability requires a thorough understanding of the interactions between nanomaterials and biological systems. Researchers employ various strategies to enhance biocompatibility, such as surface functionalization with biocompatible polymers or coatings to minimize adverse interactions with biological components. Additionally, optimizing the physicochemical properties of nanomaterials, such as size, shape, and surface charge, can mitigate cytotoxicity and improve biocompatibility [46].

Incorporating biodegradable materials into nanobiosensor design offers a sustainable approach to minimize environmental impact and reduce long-term health risks associated with non-biodegradable nanoparticles. Biodegradable polymers, such as polylactic acid (PLA) or poly(lactic-co-glycolic acid) (PLGA), are commonly used as matrix materials for nanobiosensors due to their biocompatibility and tunable degradation properties [48]. These materials degrade into non-toxic byproducts that can be metabolized or eliminated from the body, reducing the risk of bioaccumulation and long-term toxicity [49]. Furthermore, engineering strategies, such as stimuli-responsive materials or enzymatic degradation mechanisms, can enable controlled and targeted degradation of nanobiosensors in biological environments. These approaches facilitate the safe disposal of nano-materials after use, minimizing environmental impact and ensuring patient safety [7, 50]. In conclusion, addressing the challenges of biocompatibility and biodegrad-ability is essential for the successful development and clinical translation of nano-biosensors in biomedical applications. By prioritizing biocompatible materials and engineering strategies for controlled degradation, researchers can enhance the safety, efficacy, and sustainability of nanobiosensors, paving the way for their widespread adoption in healthcare. Continued research and innovation in this field are crucial for advancing nanobiosensor technology and realizing its full potential in improving patient care and outcomes.

## 13.5 Integration and miniaturization

Integration with existing diagnostic platforms and miniaturization of nanobiosen-sors are pivotal for enabling point-of-care applications and decentralized healthcare settings. The ability to seamlessly integrate nanobiosensors into compact, portable devices holds the promise of revolutionizing healthcare delivery by providing rapid, on-site diagnostics. However, achieving this integration without compromising performance poses significant technical challenges. Integrating com-plex sensing elements into compact, portable devices requires careful consideration of various factors, including sensor size, power consumption, and data processing capabilities. Nanobiosensors often incorporate advanced technologies and sophis-ticated sensing mechanisms, which must be adapted to fit within the constraints of miniaturized devices [1, 51, 52]. Furthermore, ensuring compatibility and interoper-ability with existing diagnostic platforms is essential for seamless integration into clinical workflows.

Miniaturization can impact sensor sensitivity, signal-to-noise ratio, and robust-ness, posing additional challenges in nanobiosensor development. Shrinking sensor components may lead to reduced sensitivity due to decreased surface area for target molecule interaction. Moreover, miniaturization can exacerbate signal interference from background noise or environmental factors, potentially compromising the accuracy and reliability of sensor measurements. Overcoming these challenges requires interdisciplinary collaboration and innovative engineering approaches. Researchers must leverage advances in nanotechnology, microfabrication techni-ques, and sensor design to develop compact, user-friendly nanobiosensor platforms. Integrating multiple sensing modalities, such as optical, electrical, and biochemical detection methods, can enhance sensor performance and versatility in diverse diagnostic applications.

Furthermore, optimizing signal processing algorithms and data analysis techni-ques is essential for extracting meaningful information from miniaturized nano-biosensors. Advanced signal processing methods, such as machine learning algorithms or digital signal processing techniques, can improve sensor sensitivity, specificity, and robustness in real-world environments. Interdisciplinary collabora-tion between engineers, material scientists, biologists, and clinicians is crucial for addressing the multifaceted challenges of integration and miniaturization in nanobiosensor development. By harnessing collective expertise and innovative thinking, researchers can overcome technical hurdles and pave the way for the widespread adoption of compact, user-friendly nanobiosensor platforms in point-of-care diagnostics and decentralized healthcare settings. Continued research and development efforts in this area are essential for realizing the full potential of nanobiosensors in improving patient care and outcomes [53–55]. Among the array of nanobiosensor technologies available, electrochemical biosensing tools offer distinct advantages. These include affordability, the capability for miniaturization, and scalability for mass production. Additionally, their suitability for deployment in healthcare facilities and home settings as POC systems enhances their appeal. Consequently, there is considerable interest and effort directed towards the development of highly specific and targeted electrochemical biosensors tailored for identifying cancer-specific antigens [25].

## 13.6 Regulatory and ethical considerations

Navigating regulatory pathways and ensuring compliance with ethical standards are critical challenges in the development of nanobiosensors for clinical use. Regulatory agencies mandate comprehensive validation of sensor performance, safety assessments, and clinical trials to demonstrate efficacy and reliability. Additionally, addressing ethical concerns related to patient privacy, data security, and informed consent is paramount to ensure the responsible and ethical use of nanobiosensors in healthcare settings. Regulatory approval is a prerequisite for the translation of nanobiosensors from the laboratory to clinical practice. Regulatory agencies, such as the Food and Drug Administration (FDA) in the United States and the European Medicines Agency (EMA) in Europe, establish stringent requirements for medical devices' safety, efficacy, and quality. Nanobiosensor developers must navigate complex regulatory pathways, which often involve preclinical testing, clinical trials, and regulatory submissions to obtain market authorization. Comprehensive validation of nanobiosensor performance is essential to demonstrate its accuracy, reliability, and clinical utility. This includes evaluating sensitivity, specificity, precision, and accuracy through rigorous analytical testing and validation studies. Additionally, safety assessments are critical to identify and mitigate potential risks associated with nanomaterials, such as toxicity, immunogenicity, or unintended biological interactions [56–58].

Addressing ethical considerations is equally important in the development and deployment of nanobiosensors. Safeguarding patient privacy, data security, and confidentiality are fundamental principles in healthcare ethics. Nanobiosensors often involve the collection, processing, and analysis of sensitive biological data, raising concerns about data privacy and unauthorized access. Implementing robust data encryption, access controls, and secure data storage protocols can help mitigate these risks and protect patient confidentiality. Furthermore, ensuring informed consent from study participants is essential to uphold their autonomy and rights. Informed consent involves providing individuals with clear and comprehensive information about the purpose, risks, benefits, and alternatives of participating in nanobiosensor research or clinical studies. Respecting individuals' autonomy and ensuring their voluntary participation in research are foundational ethical principles that must be upheld throughout the development and deployment of nanobiosensors. Collaborating with regulatory authorities, stakeholders, and ethicists from the early stages of development can help streamline the regulatory approval process and address ethical considerations effectively [59, 60]. Engaging in transparent communication, stakeholder consultation, and interdisciplinary collaboration fosters a holistic approach to regulatory compliance and ethical oversight. By integrating regulatory and ethical considerations into the nanobiosensor development process, researchers can enhance transparency, accountability, and trust in healthcare innovation.

In conclusion, navigating regulatory and ethical considerations is essential for the successful development, validation, and deployment of nanobiosensors in clinical practice. By adhering to regulatory requirements, conducting robust safety and efficacy assessments, and upholding ethical principles, researchers can ensure the responsible and ethical use of nanobiosensors in improving patient care and outcomes. Continued collaboration and dialogue between researchers, regulators, ethicists, and stakeholders are essential to address the evolving challenges and complexities of nanobiosensor development in healthcare [27, 61].

## 13.7 Cost-effectiveness and scalability

Achieving cost-effectiveness and scalability is pivotal for the widespread adoption of nanobiosensors in diagnosis. Despite their transformative potential in healthcare, the steep costs associated with nanomaterials, fabrication techniques, and specialized equipment pose a significant hurdle to commercialization and accessibility. To unlock their full potential, it is imperative to devise cost-effective manufacturing processes and scalable production methods capable of driving down the overall cost of nanobiosensors.

A primary cost driver in nanobiosensor development stems from the expense linked to nanomaterials. Advanced materials such as quantum dots or metallic nanoparticles, integral to sensor fabrication, often come with a hefty price tag. Moreover, specialized fabrication techniques such as lithography or chemical vapor deposition necessitate costly equipment and skilled personnel, further inflating expenses. Researchers are actively exploring alternative nanomaterials and fabrication methods to mitigate these challenges, striving to identify materials offering comparable performance at a lower cost, such as carbon-based nanomaterials or polymers synthesized through cost-effective routes [41, 42, 62, 63]. Additionally, the development of scalable fabrication processes such as inkjet printing or roll-to-roll manufacturing holds promise in substantially reducing production costs and enhancing throughput.

Considering the economic implications and reimbursement policies in healthcare systems is indispensable for ensuring the affordability and sustainability of nanobiosensors. While nanobiosensors hold immense clinical promise, their widespread adoption hinges on cost-effectiveness in relation to existing diagnostic technologies.

Demonstrating their economic value through rigorous analyses and reimbursement studies can facilitate seamless integration into healthcare systems [43, 64].

Furthermore, ensuring scalability is paramount to meeting the escalating demand for diagnostic tests in healthcare settings. Collaborative efforts between academia, industry, and government agencies are pivotal for advancing cost-effective and scalable nanobiosensor technologies. By pooling expertise, resources, and fostering innovation, stakeholders can expedite the development and commercialization of nanobiosensors for diagnostic applications. Engaging with regulatory agencies and policymakers to streamline pathways and incentivize investment in nanobiosensor development further bolsters their integration into clinical practice.

In conclusion, achieving cost-effectiveness and scalability is indispensable for widespread nanobiosensor adoption in diagnosis. Through innovative manufacturing processes, exploration of alternative materials, and consideration of economic factors, researchers can enhance affordability and accessibility. Scalable production methods, coupled with collaborative efforts, ensure nanobiosensors meet the burgeoning demand for diagnostic tests, ultimately improving patient care and outcomes. Continued innovation and collaboration are crucial to surmount challenges and unlock the full potential of nanobiosensors in healthcare [1, 65, 66].

## 13.8 Conclusion and future perspectives

Cancer is universally acknowledged as one of the most dangerous illnesses, claiming millions of lives annually. Given its devastating impact on individuals, it has garnered significant attention from scholars and specialists alike. Efforts to uncover the latest and most efficient techniques for detecting, studying, and treating cancer have been underway among researchers. Discovering a dependable method for diagnosing cancer early is paramount. Nanoparticles play a vital role in contemporary strategies, given their extensive use in medicine. These particles can effectively diagnose and treat cancer. This approach involves examining various targets, including bioluminescent enzymes, fluorescent proteins, and a range of nanoparticles, to assess microRNA (miRNA) function. They can also be combined in various configurations for multimodal imaging and therapy.

Another benefit of utilizing nanoparticles in imaging technology is their ability to serve as precise and accurate agents for locating cancer, enabling prompt medication and treatment. Nanoparticles possess multifunctional properties, suggesting their potential for detecting tumor subtypes such as heterogeneous and epigynous markings in the near future. Nanomaterials exhibit unique properties that align well with our requirements. Recent advancements in early cancer diagnosis using diverse nanostructures as biosensors, with a wide range of applications, represent a groundbreaking development. While the four major biomarkers—CTCs, circulating tumor (ctDNA), exosomes, and circulating miRNA—are comparatively well-explored, efforts should ensure their consistency. Exploration and validation of fluid biopsy predictors such as cell-free miRNA and exosomes are necessary, topics which have not been thoroughly addressed. Ultimately, fluid biopsy could potentially become a standard medical practice for many cancer patients in the foreseeable future [25].

Nucleic acids, such as DNA and RNA, function as adaptable recognition components in electrochemical biosensors, exhibiting remarkable effectiveness in detecting various cancer biomarkers with high sensitivity and specificity. These biosensors present benefits such as cost efficiency, swift response time, simplicity of operation, and minimal sample preparation requirements. It includes specific instances targeting pivotal cancer biomarkers such as prostate-specific antigen, miRNA-21, and carcinoembryonic antigen. These sensors exhibit sensitivity and specificity in detecting biomarkers for both non-communicable and communicable diseases. The self-assembly, programmability, catalytic activity, and dynamic nature of DNA and RNA enable versatile sensing platforms. They have the capability to improve biosensor biocompatibility, stability, signal transduction, and amplification when integrated with nanomaterials. In summary, electrochemical biosensors based on nucleic acids hold considerable promise for improving cancer detection and treatment by enabling early and precise diagnosis.

In future research on electrochemical biosensors utilizing nucleic acids, a crucial area of focus lies in the creation of novel nucleic acid structures and patterns. This aim is to augment the biosensors' capabilities in recognizing and catalyzing reactions, while also facilitating the integration of diverse functions and sensing modes. Efforts should prioritize the exploration of innovative nucleic acid engineering techniques, such as DNA origami, alongside the development of aptamer libraries tailored to meet specific biosensing requirements. Furthermore, to enhance signal transduction, amplification, and modulation in biosensors, it is imperative to optimize the interface between nucleic acids and carbon nanotubes, as well as other nanomaterials. This optimization process should involve refining the selection and design of aptamer sequences to enhance stability and resilience across varied environmental conditions [67].

Despite the significant strides made in nanobiosensor technology, numerous obstacles impede their widespread adoption in diagnosis, spanning technical, regulatory, and ethical realms. To fully exploit the potential of nanobiosensors in healthcare, these challenges demand concerted efforts from researchers, engineers, clinicians, regulators, and stakeholders across diverse disciplines. Collaborative initiatives are indispensable for navigating regulatory frameworks, refining sensor performance, and upholding ethical standards throughout the lifecycle of nanobiosensors.

The emerging era of nanobiosensors offers an affordable, portable, user-friendly, and non-invasive solution with exceptional sensitivity and specificity, showing significant potential for the early detection of cancer diseases. Nevertheless, further advancement is necessary in biosensor devices, particularly in enabling multiplex analysis of samples, reducing sample volume requirements, and shortening processing time. The advent of POC biosensors holds promise in curtailing infection rates among cancer patients through prompt diagnosis and prognosis (figure 13.3). Collaboration among scientists and engineers from various relevant fields is essential to advance and bring to market this highly promising technology. Biosensors find

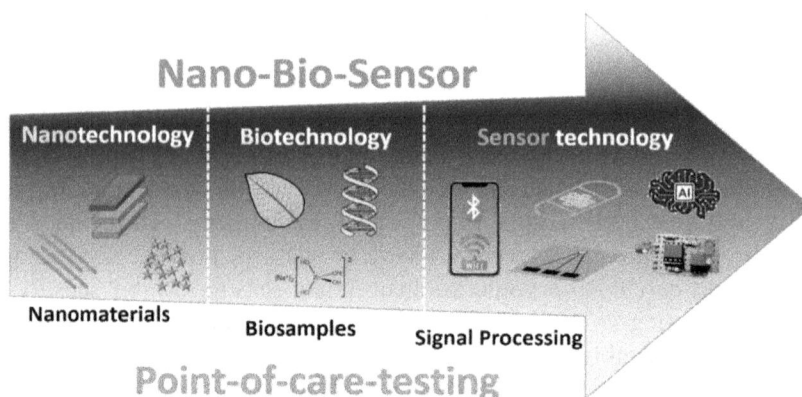

**Figure 13.3.** Advancing nanobiosensors: the future of point-of-care testing. (Adapted from [1]. CC BY 4.0.)

extensive application in biomedical research, healthcare, and pharmaceutical industries. They utilize molecular probes affixed to a solid surface to detect disease biomarkers. Encouragingly, recent progress in biotechnology, nanotechnology, and innovative immobilization methods has led to the emergence of nanobiosensors, offering enhanced efficacy in disease diagnosis [68].

Overcoming technical barriers, including bolstering sensitivity, ensuring stability, and seamlessly integrating with existing diagnostic platforms, is imperative for empowering nanobiosensors to deliver unparalleled capabilities in early disease detection, treatment monitoring, and personalized medicine. Additionally, ensuring compliance with regulatory standards and addressing ethical concerns are paramount for fostering trust among healthcare providers, regulators, and the public. Transparent communication, stakeholder engagement, and ethical adherence are fundamental for fostering confidence and fostering responsible innovation in healthcare technology.

Nanobiosensors possess the transformative potential to revolutionize healthcare delivery by enabling swift disease detection, personalized treatment, and enhanced patient outcomes. Their ability to furnish rapid, sensitive, and precise diagnostic information stands to revolutionize clinical practice and enhance healthcare access and equity. Continued innovation and collaboration are pivotal for unlocking the full potential of nanobiosensors in diagnosis and reshaping the healthcare landscape. By surmounting technical obstacles, ensuring regulatory compliance, and addressing ethical considerations, nanobiosensors can spearhead a new era of precision medicine, characterized by prompt diagnoses, tailored treatments, and optimized healthcare outcomes for all.

## Acknowledgments

Author MSS, PK and NS want to acknowledge IIT Delhi, IIT Kharagpur, DEI and DU for providing library facilities for the literature review.

# References

[1] Kulkarni M B, Ayachit N H and Aminabhavi T M 2022 Recent advancements in nanobiosensors: current trends, challenges, applications, and future scope *Biosensors* **12** 892

[2] Kulkarni M B, Ayachit N H, Aminabhavi T M and Pogue B W 2023 Recent advances in microfluidics-based paper analytical devices ($\mu$PADs) for biochemical sensors: from fabrication to detection techniques *Biochem. Eng. J.* **198** 109027

[3] Ukhurebor K E, Onyancha R B, Aigbe U O, Uk-Eghonghon G, Kerry R G, Kusuma H S, Darmokoesoemo H, Osibote O A and Balogun V A 2022 A methodical review on the applications and potentialities of using nanobiosensors for disease diagnosis *BioMed Res. Int.* **2022** 1682502

[4] Mikaeeli Kangarshahi B, Naghib S M and Rabiee N 2024 DNA/RNA-based electrochemical nanobiosensors for early detection of cancers *Crit. Rev. Cin. Lab. Sci.* **61** 1–23

[5] Iqbal M J *et al* 2022 Biosensing chips for cancer diagnosis and treatment: a new wave towards clinical innovation *Cancer Cell Int.* **22** 354

[6] Lan H, Jamil M, Ke G and Dong N 2023 The role of nanoparticles and nanomaterials in cancer diagnosis and treatment: a comprehensive review *Am. J. Cancer Res.* **13** 5751

[7] Khazaei M, Hosseini M S, Haghighi A M and Misaghi M 2023 Nanosensors and their applications in early diagnosis of cancer *Sens. Bio-Sens. Res.* **41** 100569

[8] Tobore T O 2019 On the need for the development of a cancer early detection, diagnostic, prognosis, and treatment response system *Future Sci. OA* **6** FSO439

[9] Swierczewska M, Liu G, Lee S and Chen X 2012 High-sensitivity nanosensors for biomarker detection *Chem. Soc. Rev.* **41** 2641–55

[10] Kamali H, Golmohammadzadeh S, Zare H, Nosrati R, Fereidouni M and Safarpour H 2022 The recent advancements in the early detection of cancer biomarkers by DNAzyme-assisted aptasensors *J. Nanobiotechnol.* **20** 438

[11] Kangarshahi B M and Naghib S M 2024 Nanogenosensors based on aptamers and peptides for bioelectrochemical cancer detection: an overview of recent advances in emerging materials and technologies *Discov. Appl. Sci.* **6** 1–26

[12] Yang T and Duncan T V 2021 Challenges and potential solutions for nanosensors intended for use with foods *Nat. Nanotechnol.* **16** 251–65

[13] Sadeghi M, Sadeghi S, Naghib S M and Garshasbi H R 2023 A comprehensive review on electrochemical nano biosensors for precise detection of blood-based oncomarkers in breast cancer *Biosensors* **13** 481

[14] Wasti S, Lee I H, Kim S, Lee J H and Kim H 2023 Ethical and legal challenges in nanomedical innovations: a scoping review *Front. Genet.* **14** 1163392

[15] 2009 *Nanotechnology and Society: Current and Emerging Ethical Issues* ed F Allhoff and P Lin (Dordrecht: Springer)

[16] Wagner V, Dullaart A, Bock A K and Zweck A 2006 The emerging nanomedicine landscape *Nat. Biotechnol.* **24** 1211–7

[17] Liu L, Wei Y, Jiao S, Zhu S and Liu X 2019 A novel label-free strategy for the ultrasensitive miRNA-182 detection based on $MoS_2/Ti_3C_2$ nanohybrids *Biosens. Bioelectron.* **137** 45–51

[18] Choudhary M, Singh A, Kaur S and Arora K 2014 Enhancing lung cancer diagnosis: electrochemical simultaneous bianalyte immunosensing using carbon nanotubes–chitosan nanocomposite *Appl. Biochem. Biotechnol.* **174** 1188–200

[19] Salahandish R, Ghaffarinejad A, Naghib S M, Majidzadeh-A K, Zargartalebi H and Sanati-Nezhad A 2009 Nano-biosensor for highly sensitive detection of HER2 positive breast cancer *Biosens. Bioelectron.* **117** 104–11

[20] Benvidi A, Tezerjani M D, Jahanbani S, Ardakani M M and Moshtaghioun S M 2016 Comparison of impedimetric detection of DNA hybridization on the various biosensors based on modified glassy carbon electrodes with PANHS and nanomaterials of RGO and MWCNTs *Talanta* **147** 621–7

[21] Chung S, Chandra P, Koo J P and Shim Y B 2018 Development of a bifunctional nanobiosensor for screening and detection of chemokine ligand in colorectal cancer cell line *Biosens. Bioelectron.* **100** 396–403

[22] Daneshpour M, Karimi B and Omidfar K 2018 Simultaneous detection of gastric cancer-involved miR-106a and let-7a through a dual-signal-marked electrochemical nanobiosensor *Biosens. Bioelectron.* **109** 197–205

[23] Ebrahimi A, Nikokar I, Zokaei M and Bozorgzadeh E 2018 Design, development and evaluation of microRNA-199a-5p detecting electrochemical nanobiosensor with diagnostic application in triple negative breast cancer *Talanta* **189** 592–8

[24] Bodkhe M, Chalke T, Kulkarni S and Goswami A 2024 A review on sustainable applications of nanobiosensors in various fields and future potential *BioNanoScience* **14** 1940–60

[25] Mustafa S K, Khan M, Sagheer M, Kumar D and Pandey S 2024 Advancements in biosensors for cancer detection: revolutionizing diagnostics *Med. Oncol.* **41** 1–15

[26] Moradi S, Khaledian S, Abdoli M, Shahlaei M and Kahrizi D 2018 Nano-biosensors in cellular and molecular biology *Cell. Mol. Biol.* **64** 85–90

[27] Chamorro-Garcia A and Merkoçi A 2016 Nanobiosensors in diagnostics *Nanobiomedicine* **3** 1849543516663574

[28] Ghorbani F, Abbaszadeh H, Mehdizadeh A, Ebrahimi-Warkiani M, Rashidi M R and Yousefi M 2019 Biosensors and nanobiosensors for rapid detection of autoimmune diseases: a review *Microchim. Acta* **186** 1–11

[29] Ukhurebor K E, Onyancha R B, Aigbe U O, Uk-Eghonghon G, Kerry R G, Kusuma H S, Darmokoesoemo H, Osibote O A and Balogun V A 2022 A methodical review on the applications and potentialities of using nanobiosensors for disease diagnosis *BioMed Res. Int.* **2022** 1682502

[30] Perdomo S A, Marmolejo-Tejada J M and Jaramillo-Botero A 2021 Bio-nanosensors: fundamentals and recent applications *J. Electrochem. Soc.* **168** 107506

[31] Thakur M, Wang B and Verma M L 2022 Development and applications of nanobiosensors for sustainable agricultural and food industries: recent developments, challenges and perspectives *Environ. Technol. Innov.* **26** 102371

[32] Gharra A *et al* 2020 Exhaled breath diagnostics of lung and gastric cancers in China using nanosensors *Cancer Commun.* **40** 273

[33] Nardi-Agmon I, Abud-Hawa M, Liran O, Gai-Mor N, Ilouze M, Onn A, Bar J, Shlomi D, Haick H and Peled N 2016 Exhaled breath analysis for monitoring response to treatment in advanced lung cancer *J. Thorac. Oncol.* **11** 827–37

[34] Hasanzadeh M, Babaie P, Jouyban-Gharamaleki V and Jouyban A 2018 The use of chitosan as a bioactive polysaccharide in non-invasive detection of malondialdehyde biomarker in human exhaled breath condensate: a new platform towards diagnosis of some lung disease *Int. J. Biol. Macromol.* **120** 2482–92

[35] Lu N, Gao A, Dai P, Song S, Fan C, Wang Y and Li T 2014 CMOS-compatible silicon nanowire field-effect transistors for ultrasensitive and label-free microRNAs sensing *Small* **10** 2022–8

[36] Zheng X, Tang H, Xie C, Zhang J, Wu W and Jiang X 2015 Tracking cancer metastasis *in vivo* by using an iridium-based hypoxia-activated optical oxygen nanosensor *Angew. Chem. Int. Ed.* **54** 8094–9

[37] Guo X, Liu S, Yang M, Du H and Qu F 2019 Dual signal amplification photoelectrochemical biosensor for highly sensitive human epidermal growth factor receptor-2 detection *Biosens. Bioelectron.* **139** 111312

[38] Liu S T, Liu X P, Chen J S, Mao C J and Jin B K 2020 Highly sensitive photoelectrochemical biosensor for microRNA159c detection based on a $Ti_3C_2$: CdS nanocomposite of breast cancer *Biosens. Bioelectron.* **165** 112416

[39] Zhang Q, Tian Y, Liang Z, Wang Z, Xu S and Ma Q 2021 DNA-mediated Au–Au dimer-based surface plasmon coupling electrochemiluminescence sensor for BRCA1 gene detection *Anal. Chem.* **93** 3308–14

[40] Cao W, Gao W, Liu Z, Hao W, Li X, Sun Y, Tong L and Tang B 2018 Visualizing miR-155 to monitor breast tumorigenesis and response to chemotherapeutic drugs by a self-assembled photoacoustic nanoprobe *Anal. Chem.* **90** 9125–31

[41] Tang Y, Dai Y, Huang X, Li L, Han B, Cao Y and Zhao J 2019 Self-assembling peptide-based multifunctional nanofibers for electrochemical identification of breast cancer stem-like cells *Anal. Chem.* **91** 7531–7

[42] Salahandish R, Zargartalebi H, Janmaleki M, Khetani S, Azarmanesh M, Ashani M M, Aburashed R, Vatani M, Ghaffarinejad A and Sanati-Nezhad A 2019 Reproducible and scalable generation of multilayer nanocomposite constructs for ultrasensitive nanobiosensing *Adv. Mater. Technol.* **4** 1900478

[43] Soy S, Sharma S R and Nigam V K 2022 Bio-fabrication of thermozyme-based nano-biosensors: their components and present scenario *J. Mater. Sci., Mater. Electron.* **33** 5523–33

[44] Semenova D, Gernaey K V, Morgan B and Silina Y E 2020 Towards one-step design of tailored enzymatic nanobiosensors *Analyst* **145** 1014–24

[45] Abdel-Karim R, Reda Y and Abdel-Fattah A 2020 Nanostructured materials-based nano-sensors *J. Electrochem. Soc.* **167** 037554

[46] Iftikhar F J, Shah A, Akhter M S, Kurbanoglu S and Ozkan S A 2019 Introduction to nanosensors *New Developments in Nanosensors for Pharmaceutical Analysis* (New York: Academic) pp 1–46

[47] Negahdary M, Sharma A, Anthopoulos T D and Angnes L 2023 Recent advances in electrochemical nanobiosensors for cardiac biomarkers *TrAC, Trends Anal. Chem.* **164** 117104

[48] Chavan Y R, Tambe S M, Jain D D, Khairnar S V and Amin P D 2022 Redefining the importance of polylactide-co-glycolide acid (PLGA) in drug delivery *Ann. Pharm. Fr.* **80** 603–16

[49] Miglani R, Parveen N, Kumar A, Ansari M A, Khanna S, Rawat G, Panda A K, Bisht S S, Upadhyay J and Ansari M N 2022 Degradation of xenobiotic pollutants: an environmentally sustainable approach *Metabolites* **12** 818

[50] Silva D F, Melo A L, Uchôa A F, Pereira G M, Alves A E, Vasconcellos M C, Xavier-Júnior F H and Passos M F 2023 Biomedical approach of nanotechnology and biological risks: a mini-review *Int. J. Mol. Sci.* **24** 16719

[51] Bhatia D, Paul S, Acharjee T and Ramachairy S S 2024 Biosensors and their widespread impact on human health *Sens. Int.* **5** 100257

[52] Behera P P, Kumar N, Kumari M, Kumar S, Mondal P K and Arun R K 2023 Integrated microfluidic devices for point-of-care detection of bio-analytes and disease *Sens. Diagn.* **2** 1437–59

[53] Prasad S 2014 Nanobiosensors: the future for diagnosis of disease? *Nanobiosens. Dis. Diagn.* **3** 1–10

[54] Mobarak M H, Mimona M A, Islam M A, Hossain N, Zohura F T, Imtiaz I and Rimon M I H 2023 Scope of machine learning in materials research—a review *Appl. Surf. Sci. Adv.* **18** 100523

[55] Chien Y R, Zhou M, Peng A, Zhu N and Torres-Sospedra J 2023 Signal processing and machine learning for smart sensing applications *Sensors* **23** 1445

[56] Dokholyan R S, Muhlbaier L H, Falletta J M, Jacobs J P, Shahian D, Haan C K and Peterson E D 2009 Regulatory and ethical considerations for linking clinical and administrative databases *Am. Heart J.* **157** 971–82

[57] Ferry B, Gervasoni D, Vogt C, Ferry B, Gervasoni D and Vogt C 2014 Regulatory and ethical considerations *Stereotaxic Neurosurgery in Laboratory Rodent: Handbook on Best Practices* (Berlin: Springer) pp 1–18

[58] Malik S, Muhammad K and Waheed Y 2023 Emerging applications of nanotechnology in healthcare and medicine *Molecules* **28** 6624

[59] Bhalla N, Pan Y, Yang Z and Payam A F 2020 Opportunities and challenges for biosensors and nanoscale analytical tools for pandemics: COVID-19 *ACS Nano* **14** 7783–807

[60] Goirand M, Austin E and Clay-Williams R 2023 Engaging stakeholders in a substantive and transparent way when implementing ethics in medical AI: a qualitative study *Stud. Health Technol. Inform.* **304** 101–2

[61] Mabillard V, Demartines N and Joliat G R 2022 How can reasoned transparency enhance co-creation in healthcare and remedy the pitfalls of digitization in doctor–patient relationships? *Int. J. Health Policy Manag.* **11** 1986

[62] Pramanik P K D, Solanki A, Debnath A, Nayyar A, El-Sappagh S and Kwak K S 2020 Advancing modern healthcare with nanotechnology, nanobiosensors, and internet of nano things: taxonomies, applications, architecture, and challenges *IEEE Access* **8** 65230–66

[63] Hossain N, Mobarak M H, Mimona M A, Islam M A, Hossain A, Zohur F T and Chowdhury M A 2023 Advances and significances of nanoparticles in semiconductor applications: a review *Res. Eng.* **19** 101347

[64] Hussain A, Abbas N and Ali A 2022 Inkjet printing: a viable technology for biosensor fabrication *Chemosensors* **10** 103

[65] Heidt B, Siqueira W F, Eersels K, Diliën H, van Grinsven B, Fujiwara R T and Cleij T J 2020 Point of care diagnostics in resource-limited settings: a review of the present and future of PoC in its most needed environment *Biosensors* **10** 133

[66] Fruncillo S, Su X, Liu H and Wong L S 2021 Lithographic processes for the scalable fabrication of micro-and nanostructures for biochips and biosensors *ACS Sens.* **6** 2002–24

[67] Mikaeeli Kangarshahi B, Naghib S M and Rabiee N 2024 DNA/RNA-based electrochemical nanobiosensors for early detection of cancers *Crit. Rev. Clin. Lab. Sci.* **61** 1–23

[68] Sharma A, James A, Kapoor D N, Kaurav H, Sharma A K and Nagraik R 2024 An insight into biosensing platforms used for the diagnosis of various lung diseases: a review *Biotechnol. Bioeng.* **121** 71–81

www.ingramcontent.com/pod-product-compliance
Lightning Source LLC
Chambersburg PA
CBHW082140210326
41599CB00031B/6047

* 9 7 8 0 7 5 0 3 6 2 3 5 1 *